350
Questions
for the
SITUATIONAL
JUDGEMENT
TEST

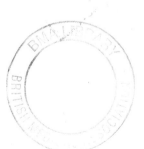

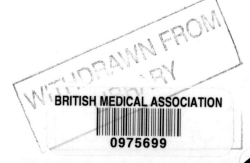

350
Questions
for the

SITUATIONAL
JUDGEMENT
TEST

Editor:
Harriet Walker, Core Surgical Trainee, Derriford Hospital, Plymouth, United Kingdom

Authors:
Sarah Craig, Core Medical Trainee, Leeds Teaching Hospitals NHS Trust, Leeds, United Kingdom

Giles Dixon, Resident Medical Officer, Palmerston North Hospital, Mid Central District Health Board, Palmerston North, New Zealand

Alice Pitt, Foundation Year 2 Doctor, Sheffield Teaching Hospitals NHS Foundation Trust, Sheffield, United Kingdom

Isobel Platt, General Practitioner Trainee, Sheffield Teaching Hospitals NHS Foundation Trust, Sheffield, United Kingdom

Catherine Sproson, Core Surgical Trainee, Sheffield Teaching Hospitals NHS Foundation Trust, Sheffield, United Kingdom

Andrew Viggars, Core Medical Trainee, Leeds Teaching Hospitals NHS Trust, Leeds, United Kingdom

Eileen Wedge, Foundation Year 2 Doctor in Emergency Medicine, Imperial College Healthcare NHS Trust, London, United Kingdom

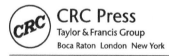

CRC Press
Taylor & Francis Group
Boca Raton   London   New York

CRC Press is an imprint of the
Taylor & Francis Group, an **informa** business

CRC Press
Taylor & Francis Group
6000 Broken Sound Parkway NW, Suite 300
Boca Raton, FL 33487-2742

Printed and bound by CPI UK on sustainably sourced paper
Version Date: 20151104

International Standard Book Number-13: 978-1-4987-5288-6 (Paperback)

This book contains information obtained from authentic and highly regarded sources. While all reasonable efforts have been made to publish reliable data and information, neither the author[s] nor the publisher can accept any legal responsibility or liability for any errors or omissions that may be made. The publishers wish to make clear that any views or opinions expressed in this book by individual editors, authors or contributors are personal to them and do not necessarily reflect the views/opinions of the publishers. The information or guidance contained in this book is intended for use by medical, scientific or health-care professionals and is provided strictly as a supplement to the medical or other professional's own judgement, their knowledge of the patient's medical history, relevant manufacturer's instructions and the appropriate best practice guidelines. Because of the rapid advances in medical science, any information or advice on dosages, procedures or diagnoses should be independently verified. The reader is strongly urged to consult the relevant national drug formulary and the drug companies' and device or material manufacturers' printed instructions, and their websites, before administering or utilizing any of the drugs, devices or materials mentioned in this book. This book does not indicate whether a particular treatment is appropriate or suitable for a particular individual. Ultimately it is the sole responsibility of the medical professional to make his or her own professional judgements, so as to advise and treat patients appropriately. The authors and publishers have also attempted to trace the copyright holders of all material reproduced in this publication and apologize to copyright holders if permission to publish in this form has not been obtained. If any copyright material has not been acknowledged please write and let us know so we may rectify in any future reprint.

Visit the Taylor & Francis Web site at
http://www.taylorandfrancis.com

and the CRC Press Web site at
http://www.crcpress.com

Contents

Preface   vii
Acknowledgements   ix
Editor and Authors   xi
An introduction to the situational judgement test   xiii

1. Commitment to professionalism   1
    Questions   1
    Answers   52
2. Coping with pressure   117
    Questions   117
    Answers   138
3. Effective communication   165
    Questions   165
    Answers   197
4. Patient focus   235
    Questions   235
    Answers   268
5. Working effectively as part of a team   309
    Questions   309
    Answers   334

Index   365

Preface

This book has been designed to give you a chance to familiarise yourself with the format of questions and the frame of mind required when thinking through clinical conundrums similar to those you will be likely to encounter in the actual exam. The questions have been written by FY1s and FY2s having just finished medical school and scoring highly on the SJT themselves and therefore will be based on real-life clinical encounters during the daily life of these junior doctors. The answers and rationales have been constructed using the recommendations from the General Medical Council (GMC) as to how you would be expected to behave in the clinical environment and have been extensively reviewed. It therefore accurately represents life as a junior doctor and highlights how you should be approaching these situations in your future clinical practice as well as helping you practice for your upcoming SJT exam. Each question has been coded according to the overriding professional domain that the picture portrays, although in actuality there is a great deal of overlap of all the professional attributes. It was felt that this would be beneficial to you as a student to help you to contemplate each area individually as you are familiarising yourself with the subject matter. We strongly recommend that you complete each question in a timed manner and then mark your answers after a period of time to help you to become used to answering them under exam conditions. Good luck, and remember to breathe!

Harriet Walker on behalf of the author team, 2015

Acknowledgements

We would like to thank our editorial advisors for their help and guidance:

- **Aarti Bansal,** GP and Academic Teaching Fellow, Academic Unit of Primary Medical Care, The University of Sheffield, Sheffield, UK
- **Kirsty Gillgrass,** Academic Research Training Fellow, Academic Unit of Primary Medical Care, Northern General Hospital, Sheffield, UK
- **Pirashanthie Vivekananda-Schmidt,** Curriculum Lead for Medical Ethics and Law and the Personal and Professional Development Programme for the MBChB Course, The University of Sheffield, Sheffield, UK

Editor and Authors

Editor

Harriet Walker
Core Surgical Trainee
Derriford Hospital
Plymouth, United Kingdom

Authors

Sarah Craig
Core Medical Trainee
Leeds Teaching Hospitals NHS Trust
Leeds, United Kingdom

Giles Dixon
Resident Medical Officer
Palmerston North Hospital
Mid Central District Health Board
Palmerston North, New Zealand

Alice Pitt
Foundation Year 2 Doctor
Sheffield Teaching Hospitals
    NHS Foundation Trust
Sheffield, United Kingdom

Isobel Platt
General Practitioner Trainee
Sheffield Teaching Hospitals NHS
    Foundation Trust
Sheffield, United Kingdom

Catherine Sproson
Core Surgical Trainee
Sheffield Teaching Hospitals NHS
    Foundation Trust
Sheffield, United Kingdom

Andrew Viggars
Core Medical Trainee
Leeds Teaching Hospitals NHS Trust
Leeds, United Kingdom

Harriet Walker
Core Surgical Trainee
Derriford Hospital
Plymouth, United Kingdom

Eileen Wedge
Foundation Year 2 Doctor in
    Emergency Medicine
Imperial College Healthcare
    NHS Trust
London, United Kingdom

Authorship by Question/Answer

Sarah Craig	1.22, 1.23, 1.28, 1.29, 1.30, 1.31, 1.37, 1.52, 1.53, 1.61, 1.62, 1.74, 1.80, 1.81, 1.96, 1.97, 1.110, 2.16, 2.17, 2.27, 2.28, 2.29, 2.35, 2.36, 2.43, 2.44, 3.1, 3.2, 3.6, 3.11, 3.19, 3.45, 3.46, 3.59, 3.60, 4.1, 4.7, 4.8, 4.28, 4.36, 4.37, 4.69, 4.80, 5.9, 5.10, 5.43, 5.54, 5.55
Giles Dixon	1.7, 1.8, 1.9, 1.21, 1.34, 1.55, 1.56, 1.65, 1.66, 1.67, 1.77, 1.78, 1.79, 1.89, 1.90, 1.91, 1.105, 1.106, 2.4,

2.5, 2.10, 2.14, 2.23, 2.31, 3.4, 3.8, 3.15, 3.16, 3.25, 3.26, 3.39, 3.40, 3.57, 3.58, 4.5, 4.17, 4.52, 4.70, 4.71, 5.3, 5.4, 5.13, 5.14, 5.15, 5.25, 5.32, 5.49, 5.50

Alice Pitt

1.16, 1.17, 1.18, 1.19, 1.20, 1.36, 1.47, 1.48, 1.49, 1.50, 1.57, 1.70, 1.71, 1.72, 1.73, 1.82, 1.83, 1.84, 1.85, 1.98, 1.99, 1.100, 1.112, 1.113, 2.3, 2.15, 2.45, 3.9, 3.29, 3.30, 3.44, 3.53, 3.54, 3.61, 3.62, 3.67, 3.68, 4.2, 4.25, 4.26, 4.27, 4.32, 4.61, 4.62, 4.67, 5.8, 5.20, 5.21, 5.23, 5.26, 5.45, 5.56

Isobel Platt

1.6, 1.27, 1.40, 1.51, 1.63, 1.64, 1.92, 1.93, 1.107, 1.108, 2.1, 2.2, 2.6, 2.11, 2.21, 2.32, 2.33, 2.34, 2.39, 2.40, 3.7, 3.10, 3.13, 3.14, 3.22, 3.23, 3.24, 3.37, 3.38, 3.66, 4.6, 4.13, 4.14, 4.15, 4.16, 4.50, 4.51, 4.64, 4.77, 5.1, 5.2, 5.12, 5.27, 5.33, 5.34, 5.35, 5.36, 5.37, 5.38, 5.51

Catherine Sproson

1.1, 1.2, 1.3, 1.4, 1.5, 1.32, 1.33, 1.38, 1.39, 1.54, 1.94, 1.95, 1.109, 1.111, 2.7, 2.18, 2.19, 2.26, 2.41, 2.42, 3.3, 3.12, 3.17, 3.18, 3.20, 3.21, 3.33, 3.34, 3.35, 3.36, 3.52, 4.9, 4.10, 4.11, 4.12, 4.31, 4.38, 4.39, 4.63, 5.11, 5.22, 5.39, 5.40, 5.41, 5.42, 5.52, 5.53

Andrew Viggars

1.13, 1.14, 1.15, 1.24, 1.44, 1.45, 1.46, 1.58, 1.59, 1.60, 1.68, 1.69, 1.75, 1.86, 1.101, 1.102, 2.8, 2.9, 2.24, 2.30, 2.37, 3.5, 3.47, 3.48, 3.49, 3.55, 3.56, 3.63, 4.3, 4.20, 4.21, 4.22, 4.23, 4.24, 4.29, 4.30, 4.34, 4.56, 4.57, 4.58, 4.59, 4.68, 4.72, 4.73, 5.7, 5.19, 5.24, 5.46, 5.47

Harriet Walker

4.35

Eileen Wedge

1.10, 1.11, 1.12, 1.25, 1.26, 1.35, 1.41, 1.42, 1.43, 1.76, 1.87, 1.88, 2.4, 2.5, 2.10, 2.14, 2.23, 2.25, 2.31, 3.27, 3.28, 3.31, 3.42, 3.43, 3.50, 3.51, 3.64, 3.65, 4.4, 4.18, 4.19, 4.53, 4.54, 4.55, 4.65, 4.66, 4.74, 4.75, 4.78, 5.5, 5.6, 5.16, 5.17, 5.18, 5.28, 5.30, 5.31, 5.44, 5.48

An Introduction to the Situational Judgement Test

The situational judgement test (SJT) has been used by the UK Foundation Programme Office (UKFPO) for recruitment into the foundation programme since the 2013 round of applications. Combined with an educational performance measure (EPM) score, this provides a mark by which candidates are compared against each other for consideration of individual preferences for foundation year allocation. It was designed to replace the traditional 'white-space questions' which were heavily criticised for being influenced by an applicant's creative writing skills and therefore being potentially biased. The test itself consists of 70 questions (10 of which are pilot questions for the following year and therefore do not contribute to the final score) in which the candidate is required to make a judgement about the correct way to behave in a particular scenario that they may reasonably encounter as a junior doctor. In this sense, it is designed to test professional attributes, interpersonal and communication skills as opposed to clinical knowledge in order to ensure that a final year medical student would be able to adequately answer the question. This is additionally beneficial since these attributes are notoriously difficult to assess in a written exam despite the fact that they are vital skills required of a doctor.

There are two different formats of questions that are used in the SJT: one in which the student ranks a series of statements based on the desirability of the action and the other being a multiple choice '3 of the best of 8'. Both of these formats serve slightly different purposes with multiple choice questions being favoured when there is more than one correct answer and ranking questions being appropriate when comparing multiple options based on suitability. The situations described are designed to present a moral or ethical dilemma for which the candidate needs to judge what would be the most effective behaviour from the options listed to achieve the required outcome. There are five professional domains that have been identified as being fundamental to life as a proficient junior doctor: commitment to professionalism, coping with pressure, effective communication, patient focus and working effectively as part of a team. The key documents published by the General Medical Council (GMC) that the classification of these domains is based on are *Good Medical Practice* (2013) and *Tomorrow's Doctors* (2009).

The main advantage of using the SJT, as opposed to an interview or the previously utilised white-space questions, is that a national exam can be standardised, which therefore allows for a fair and direct comparison of candidates. Thus, the UKFPO can perceive more easily who has an understanding of how they should be behaving in their future role as junior clinicians. It also allows for quicker turnaround of the marks since the moderation process is less arduous and time-consuming. In a highly varied and complex field such as medicine in which employees will encounter different challenges on a daily basis, the use of a situational-based test also has the advantage of giving the candidates an insight into likely scenarios they will face in their daily job. This means that the test is indirectly setting out a job specification that the applicants can use as a framework for their future clinical practice. SJTs are also used as part of the recruitment process for specialty training in general practice and public health and may well be included in others in the future, so this can be viewed as a good 'practice run' for future career applications.

The major disadvantage of the exam is that there is no easy way to revise for it apart from familiarising yourself with the professional domains as outlined by the GMC and the structure of the examination in order to ensure that the questions can be analysed efficiently and answered successfully. Due to the fact that the hypothetical situations posed by the questions are subject to a great deal of interpretation, there may also not be an absolutely correct (or incorrect) answer; however, it is designed to ensure that the candidates consider the problem in a logical manner based on how they envisage that they are expected to behave as set out in the guidelines.

The exam that you will sit will have been written based on advice from clinicians from FY1 level through to consultancy, who will draw upon their clinical experience to create a number of realistic scenarios, similar to the practice questions that you will find in this book. Each question then goes through a thorough review process to ensure that both the envisaged clinical situation and subsequent answer are as accurate as possible. The exam itself lasts 2 hours and 20 minutes, which when broken down by the number of questions (70) gives you 2 minutes per question. This is quite a tall order and does make for a pressured (and exhausting) exam, so it is important that you practice answering questions with this in mind. It is also important to make sure that you remember that all the information that you require will be present in the scenario; therefore, you should not make assumptions about what might or might not be happening in the clinical picture. Reading the key documents mentioned earlier is a good way to identify how best to answer the questions as this will give you an idea of how you are expected to behave. Remember to answer according to how you 'should' behave and not necessarily how you 'would' behave (as these two may or may not be mutually exclusive). The multiple choice questions are marked out of 12 (4 points per correct answer), so you should ensure that you select 3 options; however, if you select 4, then you will score 0 points in that question. The ranking questions are marked according to a more intricate framework – there are 20 possible marks (4 per option) based on where you have put the particular option compared to the mark scheme, that is in the exact same place, similar or in a completely different location. Again, you cannot be awarded marks for omitted answers to ensure that you do rank all of the options.

Chapter 1

COMMITMENT TO PROFESSIONALISM

QUESTIONS

1.1 Relationships

You are working as an FY1 on an orthopaedic ward. One of your patients has been on the ward for two weeks and will be going home in the next couple of days. One evening the patient asks to speak to you. They tell you that they have become really fond of you while you have been caring for them and would like to take you on a date once they are discharged.

Rank in order the following actions in response to this situation (1 = Most appropriate; 5 = Least appropriate).

A   Explain that, while you are flattered by the offer, it is inappropriate for doctors and patients to pursue relationships.

B   Explain that you cannot arrange a date while they are in hospital but swap numbers and promise to arrange a date once they are discharged.

C   Say nothing but avoid the patient from now on.

D   Swap numbers and arrange a date for the following week.

E   Tell the patient that you do not want to go on a date.

1.2 Police caution

It is the end of your first month working as an FY1, and you go out to celebrate with a few drinks. When you are walking home, you see a garden gnome in a neighbour's garden, and you drunkenly decide it would be a good idea to take it home as a souvenir of the night. As you are continuing on your way home, carrying the gnome, a police officer stops you. They have seen you steal the gnome and decide to issue you with a caution. When you wake up the next day, you are mortified to realise that you now have a police caution.

Choose the **THREE most appropriate** actions to take in this situation.

A   Contact a lawyer for advice.

B   Contact your medical defence union for advice.

C   Go to the police station to try and persuade the police to withdraw the caution.

D   Notify the General Medical Council (GMC) of your caution immediately.

E   Reflect about the incident in your e-portfolio.

F   Tell no one and try to forget about the incident since you are so embarrassed.

G   Tell the trust's foundation programme lead immediately.

H   Wait until you are next asked to fill out a criminal records bureau (CRB) form and declare the caution then.

1.3 Gifts

You have been caring for an elderly lady for a number of weeks. She is getting better but will need to stay in hospital for a few more days. Her husband asks to see you. He thanks you for looking after his wife and insists that he would like to give you a large bouquet of flowers and a bottle of champagne.

Rank in order the following actions in response to this situation (1 = Most appropriate; 5 = Least appropriate).

A Accept the gift and tell him that you are so grateful that from now on you will take extra special care of his wife.
B Accept the gift but resolve to put the flowers in the patient waiting room and give the champagne to charity so as to not feel as if you have benefitted.
C Decline the gift and explain that you don't like champagne.
D Explain that a gift is not necessary but thank him and accept the gift.
E Thank the patient but decline the gift and explain that staff are unable to accept gifts from patients or their family.

1.4 Facebook

You have only been working as an FY1 for a few days. One of your new FY1 colleagues comments to you that they have seen your profile on a social media website. They mention that many of your recent photographs picture you appearing extremely drunk, including some in which you are dancing on a table. They suggest that you remove the pictures as they feel that it is inappropriate for a doctor to be seen behaving in this way.

Rank in order the following actions in response to this situation (1 = Most appropriate; 5 = Least appropriate).

A Delete your social media profile completely and resolve not to use social media.
B Ignore your colleague's advice but delete all your colleagues from your friends list to prevent a similar situation in the future.
C Leave all of your photographs on your profile but ensure that only your friends, rather than the public, can view your profile.
D Remove all compromising photographs from your profile and ensure that only your friends, rather than the public, can view your profile.
E Tell the colleague to mind their own business and ignore their advice.

1.5 Documenting

It is your first on-call night shift, and you are asked to see a patient who has become unwell. They are hypotensive, tachycardic and pyrexial. You examine the patient but are not sure why they are unwell or how you might manage them. You therefore write a plan in the notes to discuss with a senior. After 30 minutes, you eventually find a registrar. He tells you that the patient probably has an infection and that you should have already done a number of things, including taking blood cultures and starting antibiotics. When you get back to the patient, they are even more unwell and you are now worried that you should have done these things sooner.

Choose the **THREE most appropriate** actions to take in this situation.

A   Add your discussion with the registrar and the plan that he gave you into the original entry in the notes.
B   Ask your registrar to review the patient himself.
C   Cross out the original entry in the notes so that it can no longer be read and write a new entry with your management plan as suggested by the registrar.
D   Go back to your original entry in the notes and add in the management plan given to you by your registrar, as if you had made the plan yourself at the time.
E   Immediately do the things that your registrar told you to do, including taking blood cultures and starting antibiotics.
F   Reflect on the incident in your e-portfolio.
G   Rip the page from the notes and write a new entry with your management plan being that given by the registrar.
H   Write a new entry in the notes detailing your discussion with the registrar and the management plan that he gave.

1.6 Friend's test results

You are an FY1 doctor. Your housemate tells you that she has had blood samples taken at her GP surgery because she has been feeling tired all the time. She is worried about the results and asks you to look at them at work and let her know what they are.

Choose the THREE most appropriate actions to take in this situation.

A   Advise her to get the results from her own doctor.
B   Agree but ask her not to tell anyone.
C   Ask another of your colleagues to look at the results so that it can't be traced back to you.
D   Give her a patient information leaflet about feeling tired all the time.
E   Refuse to look at the results.
F   Talk to her about why she might be concerned.
G   Tell her that the results are likely to be normal.
H   Tell her that you're not her doctor so you don't have a duty of care to her.

1.7 Lying about results

You are working as an FY2 doctor in a GP surgery and are about to see a patient who has type 2 diabetes. She is attending for her annual review and would like to know the results of her blood tests which were done last week. The blood tests were processed by the local hospital and the results sent to the

GP practice in a letter. Before the patient consultation, you realise that you have lost the letter and therefore don't have the results.

Choose the **THREE most appropriate** actions to take in this situation.

A   Apologise to the patient for losing her results.
B   Ask the practice nurse to retake the blood tests, booking your patient in for a repeat appointment in a week's time.
C   Cancel the appointment, request another copy of the results and send a letter to the patient informing her of the results when you receive them.
D   Inform the patient that the hospital hasn't processed the results yet and then phone the hospital asking for a copy of the letter.
E   Phone the hospital and ask them to read the results of the tests to you over the phone if possible.
F   Reassure your patient that the blood test results are fine and attempt to find the letter after the consultation to double-check.
G   Tell the patient that the results have been 'lost in the system' and she must have another blood test.
H   Tell the patient that you need to book her in for another appointment with another GP in a week's time.

1.8 Lying about experience

You are working as an FY1 in the medical assessment unit. You have been clerking a patient with suspected meningitis. The patient requires a lumbar puncture to help diagnose his condition. You inform the medical registrar of this, and he agrees to supervise you while you perform the procedure. You have seen many lumbar punctures in the past few weeks and have received practical teaching about the procedure on models. You have never carried out a lumbar puncture on a real patient before. You consent your patient, warn him of the risks of the procedure and get your equipment together. As you are about to start, your patient leans round and says, 'You have done this before, haven't you?'

Rank in order the following actions in response to this situation (1 = Most appropriate; 5 = Least appropriate).

A   Ask the medical registrar to complete the procedure.
B   Ask the medical registrar to talk to the patient and explain the situation.
C   Explain to the patient that you have received training and seen the procedure done many times and that you will be supervised throughout.
D   Tell the patient that you have done lumbar punctures before, without mentioning it was on a model.
E   Tell the patient you have done many lumbar punctures on several patients.

1.9 Honesty on death certificates

You are an FY1 doctor completing a death certificate for a patient whose case is well known to you. The patient recently had a gastrointestinal bleed and passed away shortly after. The family of the patient wants his body released as soon as possible so that they can have a funeral. The family have no concerns over their relative's death. As you are completing the death certificate you realise that you have not identified a cause for his bleed. The patient was otherwise quite healthy and was only 64 years old. You are unaware of any co-morbidities.

Choose the **THREE most appropriate** actions to take in this situation.

A   Ask your senior house officer to complete the certificate.
B   Complete the death certificate, giving the cause of death as 'gastrointestinal bleed' with no further information.
C   Complete the death certificate, giving the cause of death as 'gastrointestinal bleed' with peptic ulcer as a factor that led to the bleed.
D   Consult the patients' medical notes to look for potential causes that could explain his gastrointestinal bleed.
E   Inform the family that the patient's body won't be released for a few weeks.
F   Seek advice from the local pathologist and coroner over completing the death certificate.
G   Seek advice from the secretarial staff who help to organise the death certificates.
H   Seek advice from your registrar or consultant about completing the death certificate.

1.10 Insurance fraud

You are an FY1 in a district general hospital. One of your colleagues is using their new laptop computer in the mess and tells you that they acquired it by claiming to their insurance company that their old laptop was stolen, when actually it wasn't. They talk jovially about how you have to claim on insurance occasionally, otherwise it's a waste of money.

Rank in order the following actions in response to this situation (1 = Most appropriate; 5 = Least appropriate).

A   Change the subject and take no further action.
B   Explain that, now they have told you this, you have no choice but to report them to the police.
C   Explain that, now they have told you this, you have no choice but to report them to the General Medical Council (GMC).
D   Inform the FY1's educational supervisor.
E   Warn the FY1 that they should keep this to themselves.

1.11 Handover task forgotten

You are an FY1 working on a medical ward cover over a weekend. On Saturday morning, the night FY1 hands over that a patient needs a blood test to measure the antibiotic level. This is urgent since they didn't get the chance to do it before handover. Unfortunately, you become distracted by an urgent call to a patient with acute chest pain and forget to do the blood test. In the evening, the registrar does a ward round and reviews the patient who needed the blood test. The patient asks whether the level of antibiotics was high the day before and if this is why they haven't had their dose. Away from the patient, the registrar is frustrated and says to you that they had asked the night FY1 to get this sorted out at the Friday evening handover.

Choose the **THREE most appropriate** actions to take in this situation.

A   Apologise to the patient.
B   Document in the notes why the blood test was delayed.
C   Do the blood test now.
D   Explain to the patient that the night doctor was very busy and forgot.
E   Explain to the patient that they weren't due for the blood test until now.
F   Explain to the registrar that it was handed over appropriately but you forgot.
G   Say nothing to the registrar about who is responsible for the blood test not being performed.
H   Tell the registrar that you weren't aware of the issue.

1.12 Forgot to document

You are the FY1 working on an acute medical unit. You are clerking in a patient who is presented with suspected meningitis. You check thoroughly for a rash and conclude that there is no rash present. However, you forget to write this down in the clerking notes. Later that day the patient deteriorates and your senior house officer (SHO) notices a petechial rash. Antibiotics are initiated for septicaemia, and your team starts to organise a transfer to the intensive care unit (ICU).

Choose the **THREE most appropriate** actions to take in this situation.

A   Add a current entry explaining that no rash was present on your earlier examination.
B   Add to your earlier entry that there was no rash present.
C   Arrange to meet with your clinical supervisor to discuss the event.
D   Ask your SHO not to mention the rash in their documentation.
E   Call your medical defence organisation for advice.
F   Don't make any addition to the notes.
G   Explain to your team that you had checked for a rash earlier.
H   Write a reflection for your e-portfolio about the situation.

1.13 Mr or Dr

You are working with a senior house officer (SHO) who has recently passed the first part of the surgical membership exam. Since then, they have started introducing themselves to patients and on the phone as 'Mr Wilson' rather than 'Dr Wilson', implying that they are a fully qualified surgeon rather than a surgical trainee.

Rank in order the following actions in response to this situation (1 = Most appropriate; 5 = Least appropriate).

A After the SHO sees a patient, enter the room and tell them that they have not been seen by a surgeon.
B Explain to the consultant what is happening.
C Ignore the matter; by working for a surgical firm, the SHO is giving a surgical opinion.
D Inform the Royal College of Surgeons about what is happening.
E Tell the SHO that it is not in their best interests to let people think that they are more qualified than they are.

1.14 Medical students

You are supervising a medical student and take them with you to see a patient. On introducing themselves to the patient, you notice that they only say their name and do not mention that they are a medical student. When you have finished, the patient thanks your student, saying 'thank you, doctor', and the medical student does not correct them.

Rank in order the following actions in response to this situation (1 = Most appropriate; 5 = Least appropriate).

A Ask the student to return to the patient and explain that they are not a qualified doctor.
B Discuss with the student how they need to fully inform the patient about who they are.
C Go back yourself and explain that you are the doctor overseeing the medical student and will be organising their tests.
D Leave the matter; you are supervising the medical student fully anyway.
E Stop the medical student from seeing any further patients.

1.15 Colleagues accepting gifts

You are working on a care of the elderly ward, and one day, you overhear the senior house officer (SHO) telling a patient how they have pulled some strings with the radiologist to make their computed tomography (CT) scan a priority. Later you see the SHO accept some money from the patient's husband 'for all he has done for them'.

Choose the **THREE most appropriate** actions to take in this situation.

A Advise the SHO to refuse gifts from patients in the future to prevent him from looking like he is doing things for the wrong reason.
B Discuss the matter with your education supervisor.
C Discuss the SHO with the nursing staff.
D Recommend to the SHO that he donates the money to charity.
E Report the SHO to the General Medical Council (GMC).

F   Tell the patient that she has had the normal standard of care and that doctors should not be accepting bonuses from patients.
G   Tell your consultant that your SHO is accepting money from patients.
H   Try and use the same technique on your patients.

1.16 Open disclosure of mistake

You are the FY1 doctor working on a busy medical admissions unit (MAU). One of your patients, a 75-year-old woman, has been admitted with suspected community-acquired pneumonia (CAP), and you have prescribed a penicillin antibiotic in line with local protocols. When revisiting her inpatient drug prescriptions later in the day, you realise that she has a penicillin allergy and has already been given one dose of the drug. The patient is sitting up in bed, drinking her cup of tea and reading *Reader's Digest* and is not obviously in any distress clinically.

Choose the **THREE most appropriate** actions to take in this situation.

A   Comprehensively assess the patient for any adverse signs using an ABCDE approach.
B   Draw a line through the original antibiotic you prescribed and prescribe an alternative suitable for patients with a penicillin allergy.
C   Enter this experience into your e-portfolio and use it as an opportunity for reflection.
D   Explain to the patient your mistake, apologise and reassure her that it will not happen again.
E   Find the nurse who administered the antibiotic and ask why the allergy status of the patient was not checked before giving the drug.
F   Speak to the specialist registrar (SpR) on the ward about what to do.
G   Write up a change in allergy status and continue the penicillin.
H   Write up a new drug prescription chart for the patient and throw away the old one without telling anyone what has happened.

1.17 Lying about hangover

It is the morning after the payday social, and you have just received a text message from your FY1 colleague asking you to tell your consultant that they will not be at work today as they have the flu. Your housemate mentioned over breakfast that they had seen this person very drunk at the social last night. Due to your colleague's absence, one of the senior house officers (SHOs) in your team will have to miss some of their scheduled teaching to help you out on the ward.

Rank in order the following actions in response to this situation (1 = Most appropriate; 5 = Least appropriate).

A   Do not respond to the message and, when asked by the consultant, deny any knowledge of where your colleague is.
B   Ring your colleague to clarify why they are absent from work today before your consultant arrives on the ward.

C Ring your colleague to tell them that they have to come into work because you are understaffed and that their reason for being absent is not good enough.
D Speak to the SHO on your ward and explain your situation.
E Tell the consultant that your colleague is very hungover and will not be in to work today.

1.18 Drugs

You need to make an important phone call regarding a patient on the ward, so you decide to use the telephone in the doctor's office, where it is quieter. As you open the door, you accidentally knock an FY1 colleague's bag on the floor and what appears to be a small bag of marijuana falls out.

Rank in order the following actions in response to this situation (1 = Most appropriate; 5 = Least appropriate).

A Get advice from a senior nurse on the ward about what to do.
B Go back to the ward and confront your colleague about what you have found.
C Immediately contact your educational supervisor about what you have found.
D Pocket the bag of marijuana for yourself and don't mention it to anyone.
E Talk with your colleague in privacy, and ask them to explain, encouraging them to talk to their educational supervisor.

1.19 Consenting

Your consultant is attending an emergency in theatre with the registrar, and you are the only doctor available for the ward. A senior nurse approaches you asking you to obtain consent from Mr Jones, who is already running late to be prepped for a laparoscopic cholecystectomy. This is a procedure that you have observed many times as a medical student and FY1.

Choose the **THREE most appropriate** actions to take in this situation.

A Approach the patient with all the relevant paperwork, apologise for the delay and gain consent for the operation.
B Call your consultant in theatre and tell him that he needs to attend the ward to obtain consent from Mr Jones for his operation.
C Explain to the nurse that you have not been trained in carrying out the procedure nor have you been given training to gain consent; therefore, it would be inappropriate to do as she asks.
D Explain to the patient the reason for the delay in going to theatre but that a doctor will be with him as soon as possible to complete the paperwork.
E Get advice from another doctor who is qualified to perform the operation and explain the situation, asking whether they would mind coming to the ward to gain consent from Mr Jones.
F Give Mr Jones a patient information leaflet, ask him to sign the form and explain that you will collect it when you get the chance.

G   Inform theatre that they should cancel Mr Jones's operation as he has not
    yet formally given written consent.
H   Tell the nurse that you are just too busy with more urgent patients and that
    Mr Jones will have to wait.

1.20 Alcohol on breath

You are the FY1 for hepatobiliary surgery and have just arrived on the ward
for the morning's handover. You take a seat next to the specialist registrar (SpR), who is complaining that they have not had enough sleep last night.
As they are talking to you, you think you can smell alcohol on their breath.

Rank in order the following actions in response to this situation (1 = Most
appropriate; 5 = Least appropriate).

A   Ask to have a quiet word with the SpR in question after the handover and
    explain that you are concerned.
B   Confront the SpR in the room before the handover starts and explain that
    you think it is very unprofessional for them to come in to work in that state.
C   Do nothing about it; you are probably mistaken and the colleague in ques-
    tion is more senior, so it is likely no one will believe you.
D   Go to your educational supervisor for advice about whom you should voice
    your suspicions to.
E   Speak to your consultant, who is also present at the handover, and voice
    your concerns in private.

1.21 Stopping at an accident

You are an FY1 doctor driving home from a shift in the emergency department.
While you are driving on a small country road, you see a car that has had an
accident and hit a tree. There are two people inside who are obviously in pain
and have sustained injuries. There are no other cars passing, and no one has
stopped to offer assistance.

Rank in order the following actions in response to this situation (1 = Most
appropriate; 5 = Least appropriate).

A   Assess whether it is safe to stop your car and provide assistance.
B   Continue driving as getting involved in the situation could be dangerous
    alone.
C   Stop your car and offer assistance.
D   Telephone 999 and inform them about the accident before continuing on
    your journey.
E   Telephone 999 and then approach the car to offer assistance.

1.22 Angry partner

You are an FY1 caring for a 24-year-old woman who has been admitted with a
broken arm after falling down the stairs. She asks you not to let her boyfriend

know that she is in hospital because he will be angry with her for being clumsy. Later that afternoon, one of the nurses approaches you and tells you that there is an angry man on the phone claiming to be your patient's boyfriend and demanding to know what her current medical plan is. He is threatening to come to the ward immediately and 'trash the place' if you do not give him the information he wants.

Rank in order the following actions in response to this situation (1 = Most appropriate; 5 = Least appropriate).

A   Call the police.

B   Hang up the phone and call security.

C   Pass the phone over to your patient so that she can speak with the man and diffuse the situation.

D   Speak to the man, apologise and calmly tell him that you are not allowed to give out any information over the telephone without your patient's permission.

E   Ask the patient if it is alright for you to tell her boyfriend that she is well so that he doesn't worry.

1.23 Unskilled procedure

You are the FY1 on call for neurosurgery. A nurse asks you to review a patient and to deliver the intra-ventricular antibiotics that have been prescribed to them. You have never seen or done this before, but the nurse tells you that it is easy – you simply inject the antibiotic solution into the line that has already been sited intra-ventricularly. You attempt to call your registrar for advice, but he is stuck in theatre with an emergency and say he will be several hours. The patient in question is very unwell, and you don't wish the antibiotics to be delayed any further.

Rank in order the following actions in response to this situation (1 = Most appropriate; 5 = Least appropriate).

A   Call the on-call consultant for advice.

B   Ask the on-call general surgical registrar for advice.

C   Search the internet for information about how to deliver these antibiotics and do it yourself.

D   Write a message on the evening handover board instructing the FY1 on nights to speak with your registrar regarding the antibiotics once he is out of theatre.

E   Perform the procedure under the nurse's guidance since she said she has seen this procedure done several times before.

1.24 Death certification

You are working with an FY2 in gastroenterology, and you are both in the bereavement office of the hospital filling out forms for two patients who have recently died under the care of your team. As you are entering the details of your patient, you hear the FY2 on the phone to the coroner's office regarding the other patient. You notice that he is missing out some of the details of the case and does not mention a recent endoscopy and biopsy performed on the patient.

Choose the **THREE most appropriate** actions to take in this situation.

A   Ask the FY2 to explain the case to you and discuss the importance of the biopsy in the report.

B   Call the coroner yourself and give your version of the story.

C   Call the medical examiner and ask them to review the case.

D   Discuss the matter with your consultant to get their understanding of the case.

E   Ignore the matter.

F   Mention to the bereavement office staff what your heard and seek their advice.

G   Take the phone off the FY2 in the middle of his conversation and tell the office that he is lying.

H   Tell the FY2 after he has finished the phone call that what he has done is inappropriate.

1.25 Dishonest form for patient

You are an FY1 working on a medical ward. One of your patients is being discharged after an admission with gastroenteritis, probably acquired from a takeaway restaurant. They ask you to sign a form to support their application to the local council for rehousing. They have cited health grounds as the reason they need rehousing and have written that they were admitted to hospital with an infection acquired as a result of living in a damp house.

Rank in order the following actions in response to this situation (1 = Most appropriate; 5 = Least appropriate).

A   Confirm with the patient that they are really living in housing that is damp and in poor condition, then sign the form.

B   Refuse to sign the form, and call the local council to get anonymous advice about how to report the patient to them.

C   Explain that you cannot sign the form because the information they have asked you to verify is not true.

D   Call the police and report the patient for fraud.

E   Explain to the patient that you cannot sign the form because you are too junior, and they would need to ask a more senior member of your team to do so.

1.26 Inappropriate drunken stories

You are an FY1 and you are out at a party, chatting in a group with another doctor and several lay people. One of the doctors is quite drunk and starts to talk about work. They are saying that they see patients coming in to the emergency department with some 'hilarious' presentations. They say 'this one patient…'.

Rank in order the following actions in response to this situation (1 = Most appropriate; 5 = Least appropriate).

A See what the doctor goes on to say.
B Tell the other doctor to stop because they are being inappropriate.
C Interrupt and try to change the subject.
D Interrupt apologetically and ask if you can speak to them privately for a minute.
E Report them to the General Medical Council (GMC) the next day.

1.27 Hours monitoring

You are an FY1 working for a general surgical firm. Your hospital is currently carrying out monitoring of doctors' working hours. As your firm is busy, you are working overtime during the monitoring. Your consultant asks to see you and tells you that if you reveal the extra hours you are working, then you would be putting the department into trouble. She asks you not to put down these hours.

Rank in order the following actions in response to this situation (1 = Most appropriate; 5 = Least appropriate).

A Put down the true hours (including the overtime) that you have been working without telling your consultant.
B Say that you can't be dishonest and put down the true hours.
C Put down the false hours (not including the overtime).
D Seek advice from senior colleagues.
E Seek advice from the British Medical Association (BMA).

1.28 False audit

You are working on an audit on consenting for hernia repair surgery. You are working with your consultant, and it is becoming clear to you that the department is not performing well regarding informing patients of the risks. You are only involved in data collection, and your consultant is doing the statistics. When he presents the audit at your departmental meeting, it shows that the department has done extremely well and gained a financial bonus from the trust. You cannot understand how this has happened as it was very clear to you during the data collection that the department was failing.

Rank in order the following actions in response to this situation (1 = Most appropriate; 5 = Least appropriate).

A Analyse the data yourself to check if your consultant's conclusions are right.
B Ask the advice of a senior doctor you trust about how to take this further.
C Ask to see your consultant after the meeting to ask how the department had done so well when you thought it was failing.
D Assume you must have been mistaken in your conclusions and congratulate the department.
E Send an email to the trust, containing your data, asking them to look into this audit in more detail.

1.29 Flu jab

It is autumn in your first rotation as an FY1. You attend a teaching session and are reminded that you should get a flu vaccination from occupational health or a number of drop-in clinics. You feel that you do not need the flu vaccine for your own protection as you are fit and well and have heard that it can make you feel unwell.

Rank in order the following actions in response to this situation (1 = Most appropriate; 5 = Least appropriate).

A Do not have the flu jab and keep it quiet from your colleagues.
B Have the flu jab as soon as is convenient: it is important to protect your patients.
C Opt to have the flu jab before the weekend so that, if you feel unwell, you can recover at home.
D Tell everyone that you have already had the flu jab but actually never have it.
E Write a letter to the chief executive officer of your hospital informing them of your right to opt out.

1.30 Out of practice

You decided to take a year out of medicine between medical school and FY1. When you return to the wards, you feel out of practice in many of the skills and procedures you are required to carry out on a daily basis, such as venepuncture, arterial blood gasses and catheterisation.

Rank in order the following actions in response to this situation (1 = Most appropriate; 5 = Least appropriate).

A Ask your colleagues to teach you and watch you do a few of each procedure before you do them alone.
B Attempt the procedures anyway; you used to know how to do it.
C Avoid these procedures and ask your colleagues to perform them instead.
D Discuss retraining opportunities with your educational supervisor.
E Revise the skills in the medical education department using your old medical school notes to re-familiarise yourself.

1.31 Shooting

You are working a surgical take shift and clerk a patient with a gunshot wound to his thigh. The patient has been assessed by your registrar and is cardiovascularly stable with no bone injuries. You are completing the clerking when he asks you not to inform the police of the injury. He says the injury was an accident, self-inflicted, and he doesn't want to bother the police with something so trivial.

Rank in order the following actions in response to this situation (1 = Most appropriate; 5 = Least appropriate).

A   Discuss this issue of confidentiality with the hospital Caldicott Guardian.
B   Discuss with your registrar how to continue.
C   Explain to your patient that the police must be informed in the case of such an injury regardless of how it happened.
D   Explore the patient's concerns regarding police involvement.
E   Inform the police without the patient's consent.

1.32 Good Samaritan

You have been working as an FY1 for two months, and you decide to take a well-earned holiday. You are halfway through your flight, and you have had a small glass of wine. You then hear an announcement asking if any doctors on the plane could come forward and assist a passenger with breathing difficulties.

Rank in order the following actions in response to this situation (1 = Most appropriate; 5 = Least appropriate).

A   Decide to keep quiet and enjoy the rest of your flight.
B   Go forward and help the patient.
C   Inform the passenger and the crew that you have had a small glass of wine but offer your assistance.
D   Offer your advice to the crew but do not go and see the passenger.
E   Wait and see if someone else goes forward to help.

1.33 Death certificate

You have just finished an on-call night shift when you receive a bleep from the bereavement office asking you to complete a death certificate for one of your patients. You knew the patient well and had verified his death during your previous night shift. Your shift has now finished, and you will not be in work for the next two days.

Choose the **THREE most appropriate** actions to take in this situation.

A   Bleep another member of your team who knew the patient and ask them to complete the certificate.
B   Call the ward sister and ask her to find a member of the team to complete the death certificate.
C   Complete the death certificate during your next shift.
D   Decline to complete the death certificate.
E   Give the bereavement office the bleep number of a fellow FY1 who also knew the patient.
F   Go home to sleep before coming back to the hospital to complete the death certificate.
G   Hand over to the next on-call FY1 who has not met the patient.
H   Tell the bereavement office that your shift has now finished and advise them to try and contact another doctor who made an entry in the notes prior to your last entry.

1.34 Near-miss event

You are an FY1 working on a stroke ward caring for a patient who has recently had a haemorrhagic stroke. As a result of the stroke, your patient requires feeding through a nasogastric (NG) tube. When you arrive at work, one of the nurses informs you that the patient has not been fed through his NG tube because it was in the wrong place. You remember checking the chest x-ray and documenting that you thought it was safe to feed. On further investigation, you discover that the radiology registrar telephoned the ward after you left work telling them to remove the tube.

Rank in order the following actions in response to this situation (1 = Most appropriate; 5 = Least appropriate).

A   Ask a senior to review every NG tube placement chest x-ray in the future.
B   Complete an e-learning program on NG tube placement so that you don't make this mistake again.
C   Ensure the tube has been removed from the patient and check that he has not come to any harm.
D   Ignore the situation as no harm came to the patient.
E   Inform your clinical supervisor of the 'near miss' and ask him for advice.

1.35 Advising friend

You are coming to the end of your FY1 year and are feeling much more confident about your abilities. You meet a non-medical friend for lunch on one of your days off, and they tell you that they are worried about a mole on their shoulder that seems to have changed in appearance. They ask you to take a quick look at it and advise them on what to do. They show you the lesion, and you feel that it looks very normal with no worrying features.

Rank in order the following actions in response to this situation (1 = Most appropriate; 5 = Least appropriate).

A   Offer to take a picture of the mole and show it to a more senior doctor at work.
B   Reassure your friend that the mole looks absolutely fine.
C   Reassure your friend that the mole looks fine, but suggest that they show it to you again in a few weeks so that you can check for any change in appearance.
D   Say that the mole doesn't look too worrying to you but that you would recommend they showed it to their GP anyway.
E   Tell your friend that you really cannot give them advice, and they should go and see their GP promptly.

1.36 Consenting

You are the FY1 in gastroenterology. Halfway through the morning ward round, your consultant is called away to see an acutely unwell patient. As he leaves, he asks you to consent the next patient for an OGD (oesophago-gastro-duode-noscopy), which is happening later that day. You have never done this before and have only seen the procedure being performed once as an undergraduate.

Rank in order the following actions in response to this situation (1 = Most appropriate; 5 = Least appropriate).

A Access the intranet for local guidelines on consenting patients for OGDs and familiarise yourself with these before proceeding to consent the patient.
B Call your specialist registrar (SpR) who has performed the procedure before and ask them to consent the patient.
C Chat to the nurses while waiting for your consultant to return as you have never consented for an OGD and should therefore let him do this.
D Explain what you can remember about an OGD with the help of your *Oxford Handbook of Clinical Medicine*, telling the patient that you will find out later about the risks and benefits, then proceed to consent them.
E Print out an information sheet from the internet for the patient to read.

1.37 Removing chest drain

You are an FY1 working on a general surgery ward, and one of your patients has a chest drain in situ. On the ward round, your team are happy for the chest drain to be removed. There are no nurses able to remove the chest drain on your ward, and you and your FY1 colleague haven't seen or done one. Your FY1 colleague is very confident and says that they will remove the chest drain. They want to learn through experience and doubt that it can be very difficult.

Rank in order the following actions in response to this situation (1 = Most appropriate; 5 = Least appropriate).

A Agree to assist them so that you can learn as well.
B Ask the nurses to keep your FY1 colleague away from the patient because they are dangerous.
C Ask your FY1 colleague not to tell you any more about their plans to remove the drain as you don't want to be implicated if something goes wrong.
D Ask your registrar to come back from theatre between cases to supervise your colleague.
E Discuss with a respiratory doctor the details of chest drain removal and whether they would recommend you removing it unsupervised.

1.38 Poor teaching

Once a week you are required to attend FY1 teaching. You are managing to find the time to go every week but you are disappointed by the quality of the teaching. You have discussed this with your colleagues; they agree that the topics are repetitive, and the speakers seem ill-prepared. You do not feel that you are learning as much as you should from the sessions.

Choose the **THREE most appropriate** actions to take in this situation.

A   Accept that the sessions are a waste of time and continue to attend.
B   Discuss your concerns with your educational supervisor.
C   Encourage your colleagues to discuss the quality of teaching with their educational supervisors.
D   Fill in an anonymous feedback form detailing your concerns.
E   Stop going to the sessions and ask to sit in on an out-patient clinic instead.
F   Stop going to the sessions and use the time to do your own reading.
G   Suggest to the teaching coordinator some topics that you and your colleagues would like to be included in the sessions.
H   Volunteer to lead one of the sessions.

1.39 Mentoring

You are an FY1 working on a general medical ward. A medical student has just started her general medical placement and is attached to your ward. She has told you that she needs some experience of intravenous cannulation. You have a patient who needs a cannula, and the medical student is keen to do it. She tells you that she has only performed cannulation on a dummy arm.

Rank in order the following actions in response to this situation (1 = Most appropriate; 5 = Least appropriate).

A   Ask the student to demonstrate her cannulation technique on a dummy arm.
B   Ask the student to observe you while you cannulate the patient.
C   Ask the student to perform the cannulation.
D   Go and put the cannula in yourself.
E   Observe the student while she cannulates the patient.

1.40 Procedure confidence

As an FY2 in a GP surgery, you see a 24-year-old female who tells you that she is experiencing post-coital bleeding and dyspareunia (pain during sexual intercourse). As part of your assessment of this patient you need to perform a speculum examination; however, you haven't done this examination since medical school and do not feel confident of doing this without assistance.

Rank in order the following actions in response to this situation (1 = Most appropriate; 5 = Least appropriate).

A   Advise the patient to return to the surgery in two months if she is still experiencing difficulties.
B   Ask another GP to observe and assist you while you perform the examination.
C   Book an appointment for the patient with another GP in the practice.
D   Observe another GP examining your patient.
E   Perform a speculum examination anyway.

1.41 Time pressures and teaching

You are the FY1 on a general surgical team. A medical student has been attached to the team and has asked you to help them improve their cannulation skills. They have practised on a plastic model but have not carried out the skill on a patient yet and do not feel confident. You have a long list of jobs to do today, including three cannulas, several discharge summaries and clerking in a new patient.

Choose the **THREE most appropriate** actions to take in this situation.

A   Ask the FY2 to supervise the student when they have time.
B   Ask the patient to consent to cannulation by the student but do not specify their level of experience.
C   Ask the student to carry out the cannulation so that you can complete your other jobs, but tell them to come and find you if they have any problems.
D   Ask the student to clerk in the waiting patient while you complete the discharge summaries, then you can do the cannulas together.
E   Get the student to observe you inserting the cannulas today and say that they can carry out the procedure themselves another day.
F   Inform the patient that cannulation is a new skill for the student and ask for their consent.
G   Send the student to clinical skills to practise more on plastic models.
H   Supervise the student throughout the procedure.

1.42 Prescribing limits

You are the FY1 on the medical admissions unit and are clerking in a patient with community-acquired pneumonia. They have a past medical history of kidney transplantation and, as a result, take an immunosuppressant drug to prevent rejection of the transplant. You need to ensure their drug chart is completed with the necessary medicines prescribed for this admission.

Rank in order the following actions in response to this situation (1 = Most appropriate; 5 = Least appropriate).

A   Do not prescribe anything but alert your registrar that there is a complex patient who requires their input.
B   Call the patient's transplant team for advice.
C   Prescribe antibiotics according to trust protocol for the pneumonia and the regular immunosuppressant, copying the details from the patient's repeat prescription paperwork.
D   Prescribe antibiotics according to trust protocol for the pneumonia, but do not prescribe the immunosuppressant and alert your registrar that they need to complete this prescription.
E   Prescribe antibiotics according to trust protocol for the pneumonia, but do not prescribe the immunosuppressant because the patient has an acute infection.

1.43 Choosing training

You are an FY1 in paediatrics, the specialty you are intending eventually to train in. Your next rotation, which starts next month, is in cardiology. This will include being part of the arrest team that is called to all adult cardiac arrests in the hospital. You have received basic life support training in medical school but have not yet attended any postgraduate courses on resuscitation. You are considering your current training priorities.

Rank in order the following actions in response to this situation (1 = Most appropriate; 5 = Least appropriate).

A Don't use your days off for training, just get some rest. Study leave is available in FY2, so training can wait until then.
B Use a day off during the next month to attend a course on paediatric life support.
C Use a day off to attend a revision course for the Royal College of Paediatrics and Child Health part one exam.
D Use two days off during the next month to attend a course on adult advanced life support (ALS).
E Wait until the next rotation, then arrange time off to attend an ALS course.

1.44 Surgical error

You are working on the general surgical ward, looking after a patient who is two days post-op after a laparoscopic cholecystectomy. Ever since the operation they have been in pain, and on your examination this morning, they exhibited signs of peritonitis with tenderness and guarding in the right upper quadrant. You are worried that this may be a complication of the surgery and look back at the operation notes. There is no mention of any complications; however, you notice that the primary surgeon was a junior registrar. You ask this registrar for advice, and they decide to take the patient back to theatre as, during the operation, they suspected that they may have damaged the common bile duct but didn't want to admit this to the consultant or patient at the time. They ask you not to tell anyone about this.

Choose the **THREE most appropriate** actions to take in this situation.

A Agree to do as the registrar asks as they are more senior than you and you do not wish to challenge them.
B Ask the registrar to discuss the matter with the consultant and explain the need to return the patient to theatre.
C Ask the registrar to explain the problem to the patient as they have a right to know about the potential complication from their previous surgery.
D Discuss this at your next educational supervision meeting to find out how you could have handled the situation differently.

E Discuss this with the consultant, explaining the reason for returning the patient to theatre as this will need to be taken up at a morbidity and mortality meeting.
F Discuss this with the registrar's educational supervisor as perhaps they are performing theatre procedures too advanced for them.
G Explain to the patient that they need to go back to theatre due to an unforeseen complication with the surgery, not mentioning the mistake by the registrar.
H Go and see the patient before the operation and explain to them that the need to go back to theatre was due to a mistake made by the registrar.

1.45 Performing new tasks

You are a surgical FY1 and your consultant has offered you the chance to come to theatre for the day. As you are scrubbed up for the third case of the day, the consultant asks if you would like to close so that they can go and see and consent the rest of the patients on the list. You have not performed this procedure on a patient before, but you have been trained by simulation.

Choose the **THREE most appropriate** actions to take in this situation.

A Ask the consultant if you can observe this time but say you would like to perform suturing on a later case when the consultant has more time to observe you.
B Decide not to say anything and perform the suturing.
C Decide not to say anything with the consultant there and ask the scrub nurse to observe your technique to ensure you do it properly.
D Decline the opportunity this time.
E Do not admit to feeling unsure of your competence and instead ask the consultant if you can come and watch the consenting process to learn that skill instead.
F Explain that you are unsure about your competence to the consultant and allow them to make the decision about what happens next.
G Perform the suturing yourself, but ask the consultant to come back and check the sutures later.
H Tell the consultant that you do not feel confident in performing the procedure without supervision, and ask if they will stay to observe you this time.

1.46 Career progression

You are having a conversation with your FY2 about future training paths. He tells you that, as he wishes to enter into a career in psychiatry next year, he is no longer attending any medical training days as they don't seem worth it.

Rank in order the following actions in response to this situation (1 = Most appropriate; 5 = Least appropriate).

A Raise this issue with his educational supervisor.
B Recommend that, instead of attending the medical training days, he could attend extra psychiatry training instead.

C Suggest that, even though in psychiatry he will not see the management of medical conditions as often, he still needs to remain up to date in the mean time.

D Suggest that, if he does not attend the required amount of training, he is unlikely to meet the requirements to complete FY2.

E Tell your FY2 that this is not an appropriate way of thinking.

1.47 Tourniquet

You have just returned to the ward after teaching, when the sister approaches you and asks you whether you took a particular patient's blood that morning. She says that one of the nurses has just found a tourniquet still on the patient's arm and that his hand and wrist has turned blue. You remember that it was indeed you who had bled this patient.

Choose the **THREE most appropriate** actions to take in this situation.

A Apologise to the patient and let him know that you are taking steps to ensure that it doesn't happen again.

B Ask your FY1 colleague on the ward for advice about what you should do.

C Check the arms of the other patients on the ward that you bled to make sure you didn't leave a tourniquet on anyone else's arm.

D Deny that it was you that took the blood and quickly return to your jobs.

E Don't let the nurse know that it was you who had taken the blood but go and apologise to the patient when you have a spare minute.

F File an incident report stating exactly what happened and who was involved.

G Own up to the fact that it was you that had bled the patient.

H Ring up your educational supervisor and let him know what has happened.

1.48 Ordering incorrect test

You are the FY1 on a busy respiratory ward. Yesterday, on the ward round, your consultant asked you to order a computed tomography (CT) scan of the thorax for one of your patients who has been complaining of haemoptysis and weight loss. He also has an abnormal chest x-ray. While chasing the results, you realise that you have requested a CT scan of the abdomen by mistake, which has unfortunately been carried out.

Rank in order the following actions in response to this situation (1 = Most appropriate; 5 = Least appropriate).

A Ask your consultant to return to the ward so that you can explain your mistake.

B Fill in another CT request form and don't tell anyone about your mistake.

C Inform the patient and apologise for your mistake.

D Request another CT, ensuring that you fill out the card correctly this time.

E Ring your consultant to explain your mistake.

1.49 NG tube

It is the end of the morning ward round, and your last patient is reported by the nursing staff to be having difficulty swallowing. Your consultant tells you to pass a nasogastric (NG) tube as he is late for his morning clinic. You have seen one being done before, but you have never performed the procedure yourself. The nurses are not qualified to perform this clinical procedure.

Rank in order the following actions in response to this situation (1 = Most appropriate; 5 = Least appropriate).

A Bleep your senior house officer (SHO) so that they can come and supervise you while you pass the NG tube.
B Inform your consultant that you are happy to pass the NG tube but need supervision as you have never done it before on a patient.
C Ring up your registrar who is on the next ward, and ask them to come and pass the NG tube.
D Take a nurse with you, pass the NG tube yourself and get a chest x-ray to confirm the position.
E Wait until lunchtime when your consultant's clinic has finished, and ask him to come up and pass the NG tube.

1.50 Audit

Following efficiency savings in your hospital, you have noticed that the work-load of the elective surgical ward upon which you work has reduced. You are finding that you have finished most of the jobs by midday and are getting bored in the afternoons.

Rank in order the following actions in response to this situation (1 = Most appropriate; 5 = Least appropriate).

A Contact your clinical supervisor about your situation and ask for their advice.
B Contact your consultant to ask whether you could conduct an audit for the department.
C Go and find your friend, another FY1 in the hospital, and help out with their jobs.
D Go to the doctors' mess and watch the news.
E Tell your team you are going to the theatres to see if any of the surgeons operating will let you assist them.

1.51 Unfamiliar with equipment

You are an FY1 on a general medical on-call shift. You are called to attend a cardiac arrest, and the person leading the arrest asks you to prepare and administer adrenaline (a drug used in cardiac arrests). You find that you are unfamiliar with the equipment and that you are unable to do this. Another of your colleagues takes over and administers the drug correctly.

Rank in order the following actions in response to this situation (1 = Most appropriate; 5 = Least appropriate).

A Ask a colleague to demonstrate how to prepare the drug in a non-emergency setting.
B Fill in an incident form about the situation.
C Contact your foundation programme director to arrange appropriate training for this skill.
D Make sure that you are doing airway management at the next cardiac arrest you attend, where you feel more confident.
E Revise the basic life support (BLS) guidelines.

1.52 Confused patient pre-theatre

You are taking blood from a patient who is due to go to theatre later this afternoon. While conversing with her, you discover that she is quite confused, and when asking her about the operation, she becomes distressed and tells you that she refuses to undergo the surgery and that she just wants to be left alone.

Choose the **THREE most appropriate** actions to take in this situation.

A Ask the nursing staff for more information regarding the patient's confused state.
B Ask your registrar to re-consent the patient for theatre using the principles of best interest as she now lacks the capacity to make the decision herself.
C Discuss the patient's confusion and capacity with your registrar.
D Get an emergency psychiatric review of the patient.
E Ignore the patient's new onset confusion.
F Inform the operating theatre that the surgery should be cancelled.
G Perform a mini-mental state examination and investigate the patient's new confusion.
H Return to the patient in a couple of hours to see if the confusion has resolved.

1.53 Coercion end of life

You are working in respiratory medicine, and one of your patients has terminal lung cancer. He has been admitted with a chest infection and has become very weak. His end-of-life wishes have been known for some time: he has always said that he has a fear of dying of thirst and requested that, if he becomes too weak to swallow, he would like to be intravenously (IV) hydrated if appropriate. This has been the case all along; however, after a visit from one of his sons (whom you have not met before), he tells you that he has changed his mind and would like his IV fluids stopped to allow a natural death.

Rank in order the following actions in response to this situation (1 = Most appropriate; 5 = Least appropriate).

A Ask to speak to the patient's son regarding his father's sudden change of mind.

B Call your medico-legal insurer asking for advice regarding this patient, who you think may have been coerced by his family.

C Discuss these new views thoroughly with the patient to ensure that you understand what he means completely.

D Speak to the palliative care team about the patient's end-of-life care.

E Speak to your registrar about the patient's sudden change of mind.

1.54 Needlestick

You are taking routine bloods from a patient on your ward when you accidentally give yourself a needlestick injury. You have had a lot of involvement with this patient and have no reason to suspect that the patient has a communicable disease.

Rank in order the following actions in response to this situation (1 = Most appropriate; 5 = Least appropriate).

A Ask another member of staff to get consent from the patient for HIV and hepatitis testing.

B Decide to forget about it since you think it is unlikely that the patient has any sort of communicable disease.

C Go back later and consent the patient for HIV and hepatitis testing.

D Inform your ward manager immediately so that the appropriate procedures for a needlestick injury can be followed.

E Send the blood that you have already taken from the patient for HIV and hepatitis testing without gaining consent from the patient.

1.55 Consenting

You are the FY1 doctor working with an ENT (ear, nose and throat) firm in a busy teaching hospital. You receive a phone call from a theatre nurse who tells you that your registrar forgot to consent the next patient who is going to theatre. You know that he is performing the operations on the list today, and your consultant is observing. She says he is currently scrubbed, and she doesn't want to delay the start of the next operation. You have never consented for this procedure before and have only seen it once in theatre.

Rank in order the following actions in response to this situation (1 = Most appropriate; 5 = Least appropriate).

A Ask a consultant from a different team, who also performs this procedure, to consent the patient.

B Ask the consultant who is in theatre with the registrar to consent the patient.

C Ask the theatre nurse to inform the registrar that the next patient hasn't been consented and tell him that he must complete it himself.

D Consent the patient, describing what you can remember of the procedure.

E Research how to consent the patient on the hospital intranet and consent him yourself.

1.56 Consent for student

You are an FY1 doctor on a neurology ward treating patients who have suffered strokes. A number of medical students have been attached to your team and are keen to practise examining patients in preparation for their final exams. Your consultant suggests that this is a good opportunity for you to practise your teaching skills. After finishing your ward jobs you decide to offer some teaching. You have identified a patient who would be appropriate for the students to examine and obtain consent from. As the final group of students come to the bedside, the patient complains of being tired and dizzy and would like to go to sleep. The students seem disappointed as their colleagues have all received teaching.

Rank in order the following actions in response to this situation (1 = Most appropriate; 5 = Least appropriate).

A Apologise to the students for the inconvenience before continuing with your other jobs.
B Ask the students to complete the examination quickly while trying not to exert the patient.
C Ask your registrar to review the patient while you teach the students with another patient.
D Assess the patient to make sure they are well and leave the bedside offering alternative teaching to the students.
E Leave the bedside and apologise to the students, arranging for them to see another patient.

1.57 Dementia and consent

You are the FY1 working on a general surgery ward. One of your patients, a 65-year-old man with a history of gallstones and Pick's disease (frontotemporal dementia), has been admitted with right upper quadrant pain, vomiting and a positive Murphy's sign. Your consultant thinks that a laparoscopic cholecystectomy is the most suitable method of management in view of his recurrent admissions.

Choose the **THREE most appropriate** actions to take in this situation.

A Ask the family and carers to come into hospital so that you can have a discussion with them about surgical management options.
B Ask the sister on the ward to come with you to consent the patient for surgery.
C Ask your registrar to ring up the family and carers so that they can come in for a discussion about appropriate management.
D Assess the patient's capacity to make the decision about whether he wants surgery or not.
E Explain to the patient, his carers and relatives what the surgery would involve, including the risks and benefits.
F Put the patient on the list for surgery the following day.

G Speak to the patient about the procedure and prepare a consent form for your consultant, so he can consent the patient after his clinic.
H Tell the carers/relatives that the patient is going to be having surgery as this is what is in his best interests.

1.58 Disclosure after death

You are working on a care of the elderly ward and have recently been caring for a woman, Mrs Green, who passed away the previous night. While you are sitting at the nurses' station, you answer the phone. It is Mrs Green's lawyer, who has been informed by Mrs Green's husband that she passed away, and he wants you to confirm this so that he can start the process of releasing her will.

Rank in order the following actions in response to this situation (1 = Most appropriate; 5 = Least appropriate).

A Ask him for a number that you can call him back at to discuss the matter further.
B Confirm that Mrs Green has died but do not disclose any medical details about her.
C Give the phone to the nurse in charge so that she can sort the matter out.
D State that you can neither confirm nor deny her death or that she has been treated in the hospital as this would be breaching her confidentiality.
E Tell the lawyer that she died last night but as you have not signed the death certificate, he will not be able to release the will until it is formally confirmed.

1.59 Drug problems

You are the FY1 working in psychiatry. At the weekly meeting, the consultant starts discussing a patient who has recently relapsed and restarted taking heroin. You realise that the patient in question is the husband of someone you lived with during your first years of university. She had never mentioned that her partner had a drug problem, and you know that they have a young baby at home.

Choose the **THREE most appropriate** actions to take in this situation.

A Discuss with your consultant after the meeting what you know about the patient and your concerns about the child's welfare.
B Find a contact number for the patient and ring him so that you can tell him your concerns about his child.
C Following the meeting, discuss with the consultant that you know the patient and therefore would rather not attend meetings in which they are discussing his case.
D Leave the room so that you do not hear any more information about the patient.

E   Organise a meeting with your friend and the patient and bring up his drug problem so that you can discuss it together.

F   Ring the patient's GP and inform him of the relapse so that he can follow up on the family.

G   Tell your friend about the patient's drug addiction as they are at risk since this is a potential child protection problem.

H   Use the fact that you know the patient's history and social circumstances to help the multidisciplinary team (MDT) in their management of the patient as you are concerned about the baby.

1.60 Friends with problems

You are doing a taster day in a GP surgery. The GP you are shadowing is doing some telephone consultations. She brings up one of the patients on the screen, and you note that they have a history of depression. You subsequently realise that she is talking to someone that you know from your local running club. He has never mentioned anything about this to you.

Rank in order the following actions in response to this situation (1 = Most appropriate; 5 = Least appropriate).

A   In future, check the name of the patient before each consultation to avoid similar situations.

B   Leave the room during the consultation so that you don't hear any more of the conversation.

C   Look through the rest of his medical records later so that you can get an idea of the severity of his depression.

D   Next time you see your friend, ask him if everything is ok and let him know you are available if he wants to talk.

E   Speak to the GP following this and discuss the best way to proceed.

1.61 DVLA

One of the patients on your ward was admitted with status epilepticus. He previously had well-controlled epilepsy but is now having frequent seizures. He is a self-employed taxi driver, and when you advise him to inform the Driver and Vehicle Licensing Agency (DVLA) about his seizures, he tells you that he can't because they would stop him from driving. He needs to continue working as a taxi driver to support his family. He refuses to take time off from work or to inform the DVLA.

Rank in order the following actions in response to this situation (1 = Most appropriate; 5 = Least appropriate).

A   Call the police.

B   Ask for consent to talk to his wife, then ask her to convince him not to drive.

C   Sit down with the patient to fully explain to him the dangers of driving with poorly controlled epilepsy.

D   Call the DVLA yourself and inform them of the situation.
E   Speak to your trust's Caldicott Guardian regarding breaking the patient's confidentiality.

1.62 Fish and chips

You are working on a gastroenterology ward and are caring for a patient with a flare-up of ulcerative colitis. His name is Mr Green, and he owns a fish and chips shop. As part of your routine work, you send a stool sample for culture that grows the organism *Campylobacter jejuni*. The microbiology report recommends that you report this to the public health official at your hospital. However, when you inform Mr Green of his notifiable infection, he begs you not to report it as he is worried that he will lose his business.

Rank in order the following actions in response to this situation (1= Most appropriate; 5= Least appropriate).

A   Notify the public health team of this infection behind Mr Green's back.
B   Write an anonymous letter to the local newspaper informing them of a potential disease outbreak from the fish and chips shop.
C   Discuss Mr Green's concerns with him and explain that the disclosure of information will be limited to medical professionals.
D   Advise Mr Green to close his business for a while to avoid the potential spread of infection.
E   Ask one of the public health doctors to see Mr Green to explain the investigations that will need to go ahead.

1.63 Lost patient list

You are working on a care of the elderly ward. You realise that you have lost your patient list which has confidential information on it. A nurse approaches you and tells you that she has found a patient reading it after it was left on the patient's table.

Rank in order the following actions in response to this situation (1 = Most appropriate; 5 = Least appropriate).

A   Alter your list, removing patients' names from it.
B   Apologise to the patient, explaining the importance of confidentiality.
C   Complete an incident form.
D   Inform your consultant.
E   Tell the nurse not to tell anyone else what you have done.

1.64 Driving against medical advice

You work in a GP surgery and see a 21-year-old female who was attended after experiencing an unprovoked generalised seizure. She had been discharged from the emergency department with counselling about her obligation not to drive and advised to inform the Driver and Vehicle Licensing Agency (DVLA).

She wished to discuss her seizure further with you. The following week, you see this patient in the community driving her car.

Rank in order the following actions in response to this situation (1 = Most appropriate; 5 = Least appropriate).

A   Call the police.
B   Contact the patient to rediscuss the importance of the situation with her.
C   Do nothing as you can only offer advice.
D   Inform the DVLA.
E   Run after the car to confront the patient directly.

1.65 Transferring computer files

You are the FY1 doctor in the respiratory department and are asked to put together a presentation, including a number of chest radiographs of patients with tuberculosis. You compile a list of patients whom you wish to discuss during the presentation and obtain consent from them to use their images, provided they are made anonymous. As you are compiling your presentation, you wish to transfer the file to the computer in the lecture theatre. You are unsure of the best way to do this.

Rank in order the following actions in response to this situation (1 = Most appropriate; 5 = Least appropriate).

A   Ask the information technology (IT) department for advice over how to transfer the images.
B   Leave the images out of the presentation and replace them with text.
C   Rewrite the presentation on the lecture theatre computer reacquiring the images.
D   Send the images over the dedicated trust network to the lecture theatre.
E   Use your personal memory stick to transfer the images to the lecture theatre.

1.66 Food poisoning

You are an FY1 doctor working in the emergency department and are treating a young man with suspected gastroenteritis. You are about to discharge the patient to the community, where he will be treated with oral rehydration therapy and rest, when he informs you he is going to work. He tells you he works as a takeaway chef and is planning on working that night. He tells you that he is at risk of being fired if he doesn't work as his manager will not understand the situation. He asks you not to tell anyone he has a 'tummy bug', and he wishes to leave.

Rank in order the following actions in response to this situation (1 = Most appropriate; 5 = Least appropriate).

A   After further discussion with the patient, agree that he will stay away from work for five days and self-certify his illness to his manager.
B   Allow the patient to leave but give him some extra antibiotics.

C Discuss the situation further with your patient and offer to contact his manager to help explain that he will have to take five days off work because of his illness.
D Inform the patient that you are unable to maintain confidentiality and inform the local public health authorities.
E Refer the case to the medical team for admission.

1.67 Domestic violence and children

While working as an FY1 doctor in the emergency department you assess a woman who has several cuts and bruises on her body. She confesses to you that her partner and the father of her young children hit her last night when he was drunk. She says he has never done this before and is a 'loving father'. However, she doesn't want to inform anyone else and would like to be treated without involving the authorities. Her children are currently at home with their father.

Rank in order the following actions in response to this situation (1 = Most appropriate; 5 = Least appropriate).

A Ask your senior colleague for advice on what to do.
B Inform her that you cannot agree to confidentiality and phone the police to arrest the husband immediately.
C Inform her that you cannot agree to confidentiality since her children are potentially at risk.
D Treat her injuries and discharge her after trying to persuade her to inform the police.
E Treat her injuries, discharge her and then telephone social services and inform them of the situation.

1.68 Coffee house discussion

You and the rest of your team decide to take a trip to a café outside the hospital to have a team coffee break. You are having a general discussion about the ward when one of the team says something about the care of one specific patient, referring to their full name. You don't think anyone around the table noticed, and you are pretty certain that no one in the rest of the café heard either.

Rank in order the following actions in response to this situation (1 = Most appropriate; 5 = Least appropriate).

A Change the subject immediately to avoid any other breaches in confidentiality.
B Go straight to the ward on your return to the hospital and let the patient know that someone broke their confidentiality in a public place.
C Say nothing as no one seems to have heard and therefore it doesn't matter.
D Stop the conversation and say that the doctor has broken confidentiality.
E Wait until you get back to the hospital and are in private and then bring the fact that he potentially broke confidentiality to the doctor's attention.

1.69 Case note security

You are due to have a meeting with your consultant for a case-based discussion (CBD). When you get to their office, you knock and enter as you normally do with your consultant. You discover that the consultant isn't there, but the patient's notes that you are due to discuss are open on the desk.

Choose the **THREE most appropriate** actions to take in this situation.

A   Close the door and wait for your consultant outside.
B   Discuss the case and try and bring confidentiality around note-keeping into the conversation to remind the consultant about confidentiality.
C   Do nothing as the notes are in a different part of the hospital to where the patient was as an in-patient, so it is unlikely that anyone other than staff would come across the notes.
D   Remind your consultant that the patient's information is confidential and therefore if the notes are in an unattended office, the office door should be locked.
E   Remove the notes from the office to prove a point about keeping notes in the office.
F   Say nothing initially, but then once you have left, ask the data protection officer for the trust to send out a blanket email about case note security.
G   Say nothing; the consultant has likely just nipped out of the office and will only have been gone a couple of minutes.
H   Wait in the office with the notes so that they are no longer unattended.

1.70 Food poisoning

You are the FY1 working in a busy emergency department. An ambulance has just arrived with a couple referred in by their GP with severe diarrhoea, vomiting and rigors for the past 24 hours. Two days ago the couple visited a new, local Argentinian restaurant in town. Since the restaurant opened, you have seen many similar cases.

Rank in order the following actions in response to this situation (1 = Most appropriate; 5 = Least appropriate).

A   Assess the patients using an ABCDE approach and treat them appropriately.
B   Inform your local authority officers as per Health Protection Authority regulations.
C   Let your colleagues know about your concerns so that they can be vigilant for any further cases.
D   Speak to the consultant on call during that shift and voice your concerns.
E   Visit the restaurant yourself on your evening off and see if you get ill too.

1.71 Discussing patients

You have just finished a busy day on the medical admissions unit (MAU) and have been invited by another FY1 on the ward for a drink at your local pub.

You join him a bit late, and as you are arriving, you notice that your colleague has his handover sheet from today's shift out on the table and is relaying a story to some friends about one of your current patients.

Rank in order the following actions in response to this situation (1 = Most appropriate; 5 = Least appropriate).

A Chip in with your own hilarious story about another patient that you saw that day.
B Interrupt the conversation as soon as you can and explain to the group that this information is confidential and that it should not be discussed in public.
C Laugh along with the rest of the group about the story and don't mention anything to your colleague as you find the story funny too.
D Politely ask your colleague to stop talking about the patient and have a word with them in private about discussing confidential information.
E Report your colleague to his educational supervisor.

1.72 Disclosing to a third party

You are the FY1 working on the urology admissions unit and have just seen a male patient whom you know to be your brother's best friend. He is to be admitted pending treatment for testicular torsion. As you finish your shift that evening you bump into your brother. He asks you to tell him what's wrong with his friend, who won't tell him as he doesn't want anyone to worry.

Choose the **THREE most appropriate** actions to take in this situation.

A Approach the patient alone and explain that your brother is here and asking you what is wrong.
B Ask the patient what he would like you to say to your brother.
C Call security and ask them to remove your brother from the premises.
D Direct your brother to the ward sister on duty, who will explain what's been going on.
E Explain to your brother that you can't reveal patient details without their express consent regardless of who the people involved are.
F Invite your brother to go to the local pub with you and you will explain everything.
G Take your brother to his friend and explain things in front of the patient and your brother so that the patient can hear what you say.
H Tell your brother where his friend's bed is and let them sort things out for themselves.

1.73 Diabetes and driving

You are working on a general medical ward and have just clerked in a patient from the medical admissions unit (MAU) who has recently been diagnosed with type 2 diabetes mellitus, treated with insulin. She has been admitted with, what your team believes to be, an episode of hypoglycaemia. During the history she mentions that she has had some similar funny turns in the past, often early in the morning when she is driving to work. She says that she hasn't informed the DVLA (Driver and Vehicle Licensing Agency) as she needs the car to get to her place of work, which is 20 miles away.

Rank in order the following actions in response to this situation (1 = Most appropriate; 5 = Least appropriate).

A   Advise the patient that she should inform the DVLA at the earliest opportunity and that you have a professional obligation to do so if she doesn't.
B   Inform the DVLA straight away without the patient's knowledge.
C   Provide the patient with some written information about diabetes and driving.
D   Reassure the patient that her condition does not automatically mean she will lose her licence.
E   Speak to your consultant about how you should handle the situation.

1.74 Media

You are working on an acute medical ward and answer the ward phone. It is a journalist from the local newspaper asking if you would be willing to discuss your opinion on staffing levels in acute medicine. They have done some research that suggests the hospital may be understaffed out of hours.

Choose the **THREE most appropriate** actions to take in this situation.

A   Ask the journalist not to call the ward as it distracts clinical staff. Advise them to speak to hospital management.
B   Discuss your feelings with them but ask to remain anonymous.
C   Give a glowing report of the excellent staffing levels, even though you know very little about it.
D   Hang up the phone on the journalist.
E   Offer the journalist a private interview outside of work.
F   Pass the phone over to the nursing staff so that they can give their opinion.
G   Recommend that they speak to your foundation programme director about junior staffing if they wish to know more.
H   Take the contact details from the journalist and speak to a senior about how to respond and then call them back.

1.75 Interpersonal relationships

You are due to go for a mid-point meeting with your consultant, and on arriving at his office, you notice the door is already ajar, so you decide to knock and enter. On pushing open the door, you notice the consultant and your senior house officer (SHO) in a compromising position behind the desk.

Rank in order the following actions in response to this situation (1 = Most appropriate; 5 = Least appropriate).

A   Arrange for your SHO to see a counsellor for rape counselling.
B   Discuss how to proceed with this matter with the nursing staff on your ward.

C Discuss how to proceed with this matter with your fellow FY1 colleagues.
D Discuss how to proceed with this matter with your foundation programme director.
E Ignore what you saw; it is not your business what two consenting adults do together.

1.76 Raising concerns

You are an FY1 working in a large teaching hospital. Your senior house officer (SHO) tells you about a problem he had a few days ago with getting an interventional procedure organised in the radiology department. The consultant on call had told him that it would not be possible to do the procedure that day because he had a private list in the afternoon. The procedure was very urgent. You have heard from other FY1s that it can be difficult to get procedures done when this consultant is on call.

Rank in order the following actions in response to this situation (1 = Most appropriate; 5 = Least appropriate).

A Discuss the difficulty with your clinical supervisor.
B Email the radiologist and tell them that they need to stop doing private lists when on call.
C Contact the General Medical Council (GMC) to raise concerns about the radiologist.
D Encourage the SHO to discuss the situation with the consultant responsible for the patient.
E Do nothing.

1.77 Acting on hearsay

You are working as an FY1 doctor in a big teaching hospital where there are a large number of medical students. A number of students approach you with full blood culture bottles in their hands asking to be 'signed off' for having completed a practical exercise on taking blood cultures. You have not seen them complete the procedure and therefore politely decline to sign them off. As they are walking away, you overhear them saying that your colleague has agreed to do this for them for a wide range of clinical skills without actually seeing them complete the tasks.

Rank in order the following actions in response to this situation (1 = Most appropriate; 5 = Least appropriate).

A Inform your colleague of what you have heard and ask them whether this is true.
B Inform the medical school dean that your colleague should not be allowed to sign further forms.
C Chase after the students and ask them which tasks your colleague has signed them off for and ask them to repeat the skills while you watch.

D   Inform your clinical supervisor of what you have heard, allowing them to make the decision of whether to refer this on to the appropriate persons.
E   Ignore the situation; you cannot challenge your colleague based on this as it is nothing more than a rumour at this point.

1.78 Inappropriate requests

You are working as an FY1 doctor in a GP surgery. One of your friends, a fellow doctor who has been a senior colleague of yours in the past, is registered as a patient at the practice. You are nearing the end of an on-call shift at the practice when your friend telephones asking for a prescription. He asks for some antibiotics for his wife, who has a productive cough and some strong painkillers for himself as he has hurt his ankle playing football.

Rank in order the following actions in response to this situation (1 = Most appropriate; 5 = Least appropriate).

A   Offer your colleague and his wife appointments with another GP the following day so they can be assessed and treated appropriately.
B   Offer the antibiotics for his wife but not the painkillers as you are worried he may have an opiate addiction.
C   Inform your friend that his request is inappropriate and potentially dangerous and that you will have to inform the General Medical Council (GMC).
D   Take a history from your friend over the phone, relaying this to your GP trainer, who can telephone him back later.
E   Prescribe some ibuprofen and paracetamol for your friend and tell him to take his wife to the local emergency department.

1.79 Newspaper cutting of colleague

You are an FY1 doctor on annual leave, and you are reading your local newspaper. You read an article about an assault in the city centre earlier that year, and you are shocked to see that your FY1 colleague was involved and has been charged with assault. You are unsure whether anyone else at the hospital is aware of this incident as your colleague hasn't mentioned it.

Rank in order the following actions in response to this situation (1 = Most appropriate; 5 = Least appropriate).

A   Approach your colleague privately asking him about the incident.
B   Ignore the issue as your colleague has always been pleasant and friendly in your experience.
C   Inform the General Medical Council (GMC) immediately of the situation.
D   Take the article into work and confront your colleague during the next ward round.
E   Wait and see if he is found guilty of the offence before raising the issue.

1.80 Phony thank you's

It is coming to the end of your FY1 year, and you are updating your CV. You realise that you have very little feedback from patients about your care to incorporate, and many of your colleagues are in the same position. One of your colleagues suggests that you all write fake thank you letters from patients for each other so you can boost your CVs.

Rank in order the following actions in response to this situation (1 = Most appropriate; 5 = Least appropriate).

A Report your colleague to the General Medical Council (GMC) for attempting to lie on their CV.
B Decline to be involved in writing the letters.
C Speak to your educational supervisor about how to boost your CV honestly.
D Write and receive some fake thank you letters.
E Advise your colleagues against doing this as the GMC may take serious action if they were aware of this.

1.81 Sexism

You are working in general medicine with a female FY1 colleague. You have always been pleased with the way your consultant treats you, and you think he is supportive and encouraging; however, you notice that he does not behave in the same way with your female colleague. He has attempted to joke with you in the past about her poor career prospects because she will have children in the future and often remarks to her that medicine is 'not a woman's job'.

Rank in order the following actions in response to this situation (1 = Most appropriate; 5 = Least appropriate).

A Speak with your consultant privately to discuss his sexist behaviour.
B Speak with another consultant in the team about your consultant's behaviour.
C Encourage your colleague to raise this issue with the British Medical Association (BMA).
D Advise your colleague to avoid the consultant and keep a low profile until the end of the rotation.
E Discuss your consultant's behaviour with your educational supervisor, including whether and how to report this issue.

1.82 Breast exam

You are clerking in a patient who is complaining of lower back pain and intermittent paraesthesia in both her legs, when she also discloses the fact that she has noticed a lump in her left breast, which has been there for quite a few months. You think it is necessary to perform a breast examination in addition to arranging an MRI of her spine.

Rank in order the following actions in response to this situation (1 = Most appropriate; 5 = Least appropriate).

A Ask the patient to remove the clothing on her top half so that you can examine her breasts.
B Find a suitable chaperone for a breast examination.
C Don't examine the breasts during the clerking and leave it for your senior house officer (SHO) to do the following day.
D Document the examination, the lack of chaperone present and your findings.
E Gain consent to perform a breast examination, explaining the procedure and the reasons why you think it is necessary.

1.83 Doctor harassing nurse

You have finished the jobs on your ward and are about to go and get some lunch. As you pass the corridor to the doctors' office you notice one of your FY1 colleagues with his arm around a nurse, whispering in her ear. She doesn't look comfortable with the situation, and when she sees you, she immediately runs back to the ward.

Choose the **THREE most appropriate** actions to take in this situation.

A Ask your educational supervisor in confidence for advice.
B Find an appropriate time later in the day to ask the nurse whether she would like to talk in private.
C Follow the nurse back to the ward and demand that she tell you what is going on between her and the other FY1.
D Ignore the situation and walk on to get lunch.
E Politely ask your FY1 colleague what is going on and give him a chance to explain his actions.
F Report your FY1 colleague to his educational supervisor.
G Tell the rest of your colleagues what you saw, at the ward party that evening, and ask what you should do.
H Tell your FY1 colleague that his behaviour is inappropriate and that you are going to report him.

1.84 Embarrassing colleague photos

You have just returned to work after annual leave and are catching up with your FY1 colleague. She is boasting about the fact that on New Year's Eve she got so drunk at a party that she ended up running along her street naked with some friends. She then proceeds to show you the photos on her online social media profile.

Rank in order the following actions in response to this situation (1 = Most appropriate; 5 = Least appropriate).

A Refuse to comment and leave the room, feeling quite sick.
B Make the other staff on the ward aware of the photos.

C Suggest that she takes the photos off her online profile as she doesn't know which colleagues or potential patients might be able to see them.
D Recommend that your colleague reads the guidance on the use of social media among doctors from the General Medical Council (GMC).
E Seek advice from your senior house officer (SHO) about whether you should say anything about her behaviour.

1.85 Patient–doctor relationship

You are working on a respiratory firm, and you have noticed that one of the female patients on your ward has been asking a lot about your male FY1 colleague. He has spent a lot of time treating her, but you are a little concerned that this patient may have developed a romantic attachment to him.

Rank in order the following actions in response to this situation (1 = Most appropriate; 5 = Least appropriate).

A Tell your colleague that he should ask the patient out for a date when she is discharged as you suspect that she likes him.
B Voice your concerns to your colleague in private and suggest that he talks to the patient.
C Tell the patient that it would be unprofessional of your colleague to pursue a relationship with a patient.
D Ask your colleague if he feels any attraction towards this particular patient.
E Tell your senior house officer (SHO) that the patient likes your colleague and ask for advice about what to do.

1.86 Gynaecology complaints

You are an FY1 working in gynaecology. You go to see one of the post-operative patients who needs some bloods checking. She had her procedure done under regional anaesthetic and mentions that during the procedure she heard the consultant make a comment to the registrar about her personal hygiene which upset her.

Choose the **THREE most appropriate** actions to take in this situation.

A Ask one of the nursing staff to talk to the patient.
B Contact the consultant and let them know what the patient heard.
C Discuss with the patient what was said and how she feels.
D Leave the matter; you weren't there, so you cannot comment.
E Mention the matter to the registrar when you next see them.
F Raise this matter at the next team mortality and morbidity (M&M) meeting.
G Recommend that if she was upset, she should make a formal complaint.
H Tell the patient that she must be mistaken as this would not happen.

1.87 Alcohol and misdemeanours

You are an FY1 working in a district general hospital. At several social events one of your FY1 colleagues has become very intoxicated, which has led to some inappropriate behaviour in public. They recently urinated in a side-street and narrowly avoided being caught by the police. You are not aware of any instances where they have been intoxicated or hungover at work.

Choose the **THREE most appropriate** actions to take in this situation.

A   Contact the General Medical Council (GMC).
B   Discuss your concerns with the other FY1s.
C   Explain to your colleague that they need to be careful about how they behave, even outside work.
D   Inform their educational supervisor of your concerns.
E   Inform the programme director of your concerns.
F   Keep track of how much the FY1 drinks at the next social event.
G   Take the FY1 somewhere quiet and private to discuss the matter.
H   Tell them that their recent behaviour is unacceptable.

1.88 Sexist consultant

You are the FY1 on a surgical ward. One of your consultants has a tendency to make comments about female members of staff, including remarks about their appearance. These comments sometimes include statements about the size of their bottoms or breasts. He frequently remarks that women aren't capable of achieving as much as men.

Rank in order the following actions in response to this situation (1 = Most appropriate; 5 = Least appropriate).

A   Speak to your educational supervisor about your concerns.
B   Ignore the comments.
C   Ask one of the other consultants on the ward to speak to the consultant about his behaviour.
D   Next time he makes a comment on the ward, respond by telling him that it is inappropriate.
E   Contact the General Medical Council (GMC) about his behaviour.

1.89 Inappropriate comments in mortuary

You are working as an FY1 doctor in a busy teaching hospital, and you are attending the mortuary to see one of your patients who has sadly passed away. As you are identifying the body, you overhear a conversation between a fellow FY1 doctor and a member of the mortuary staff. You can't hear the whole conversation, but you do hear the doctor referring to the patient as 'really fat' and 'too big for the freezer'.

Choose the **THREE most appropriate** actions to take in this situation.

A   Ask the mortuary staff member afterwards if he had any concerns about the situation and discuss this with the doctor involved.
B   Ask your senior colleagues for advice without mentioning your colleague's name.

C   Complete an incident form on the situation.
D   Discuss your concerns with the FY1 suggesting that his comments were inappropriate.
E   Ignore the comments as they have not caused harm to anyone.
F   Raise the situation at the weekly FY1 teaching programme asking your colleague to explain why he made his comments.
G   Report the situation to the consultant in charge of the foundation programme in the hospital.
H   Write a letter to the patients' family explaining the situation and apologise for any offence caused.

1.90 Recommending illegal substances

You are working as an FY2 doctor in a GP surgery and are seeing a patient with motor neurone disease. She tells you that as part of her disease she has been experiencing severe pain in her legs. After discussing the situation further, she tells you that she has read information online suggesting that cannabis could help with her pain. She wants to know your advice on taking cannabis for medicinal purposes.

Rank in order the following actions in response to this situation (1 = Most appropriate; 5 = Least appropriate).

A   Ask the patient to book a further consultation with yourself and seek advice from your educational supervisor in the meantime.
B   Inform your patient that cannabis is illegal and refuse to discuss the situation further.
C   Outline the risks and benefits of cannabis, tell her that you have heard of other patients who have benefitted from cannabis and suggest that she could try it for her pain.
D   Suggest that the patient shouldn't try cannabis and offer alternative advice and medications for her pain.
E   Tell the patient you will book her into a pain control clinic and that she should wait until then for further advice.

1.91 Smart phone pictures

You are working as an FY2 doctor in an emergency department, and you are seeing a patient who has been involved in a road traffic accident. He has a large laceration to the outside of his leg which needs to be seen by a plastic surgeon. The plastic surgery department is located within another hospital in the same city, and the patient will need to be transferred. You telephone the plastic surgery registrar on call at the hospital who accepts your referral. She then asks you to take a photo of the injury using your smart phone and send it as a message to them so that they can begin to plan the operation. You have seen other doctors doing this, but you are unsure whether this is the correct practice. The nurses inform you that they are going to dress the wound and ask you to make a decision.

Rank in order the following actions in response to this situation (1 = Most appropriate; 5 = Least appropriate).

A Ask the hospital photographer to take photographs urgently so that they can be transferred with the patient.
B Ask the nurse not to dress the wound, leaving it open, so the plastic surgeon can see the wound on arrival.
C Refuse to take the image and ask the nurses to dress the wound ready for transfer.
D Take the photo and send it to the registrar via your smart phone asking them to delete the image immediately after they have seen it.
E Take a photo using your smart phone and email it on the secure server to the surgeon, then delete the photo from your phone.

1.92 Gift

You are an FY1 working on a care of the elderly ward. A patient of yours is discharged following a long hospital stay. The patient's family is extremely happy and grateful for the care that they have received. They give you a card expressing their thanks and a £20 note enclosed as a gift.

Rank in order the following actions in response to this situation (1 = Most appropriate; 5 = Least appropriate).

A Ask them to donate money to your chosen charity instead.
B Accept the card but not the gift.
C Thank them and accept the gift.
D Accept neither the card nor the gift.
E Ask the family to take you out for a meal instead.

1.93 Termination of pregnancy

While working as an FY2 in a GP surgery, a female patient attends your clinic and says that she would like to end her pregnancy. For both religious and personal reasons, you object to termination of pregnancy (TOP).

Choose the **THREE most appropriate** actions to take in this situation.

A Advise her to take alternative options, such as adoption.
B Arrange for her to see another GP at the practice who does not object to TOP.
C Ask her to take another week to consider her options.
D Discuss her reasons why she would like a TOP.
E Explain that TOP goes against your personal beliefs.
F Give her a patient information leaflet about TOP.
G Refuse to refer her to a TOP service.
H Sign the abortion certificate and make the referral to TOP services.

1.94 Aggressive patient

You are leaving work one evening when you see someone dressed in a hospital gown behaving strangely in the car park. He is hitting cars, talking to himself and being aggressive to passers-by. You see him try to punch someone who approaches him.

Choose the **THREE most appropriate** actions to take in this situation.

A Approach the patient and attempt to calm him down.
B Ask those nearby to help you restrain the patient.
C Call 999 and ask for police assistance.
D Call the hospital security team.
E Call the psychiatric team to come and review the patient.
F Continue walking to your car since your shift has now finished.
G Stop others attempting to approach the patient.
H Tell the patient to stop damaging the cars.

1.95 Racist comments

You walk into the doctors' office and overhear two registrars making racist comments about a consultant who works in your department. They turn to you and ask for your opinion.

Rank in order the following actions in response to this situation (1 = Most appropriate; 5 = Least appropriate).

A Ask your educational supervisor for advice.
B Explain to the registrars that you find their comments inappropriate.
C Inform the consultant about the comments that have been made.
D Offer no opinion and change the topic of conversation.
E Print out some General Medical Council (GMC) information regarding equality and diversity and pin it up in the doctors' office for future reference.

1.96 Child protection

You are caring for a 15-year-old patient who has been admitted with a suspected fractured elbow. You notice that over the past two years he has also had admissions for a broken wrist, broken ribs, lacerations, burns and minor head injuries. He confides in you that he is being bullied in school, and the bullies are responsible for his injuries. He does not wish you to tell his parents because they will remove him from the school, and he is just about to sit for his exams and wants to do well enough to go to college.

Rank in order the following actions in response to this situation (1 = Most appropriate; 5 = Least appropriate).

A Don't tell the parents: he is old enough to understand the risks of returning to school with violent bullies and can make this decision himself.

B   Encourage him to raise this issue with his parents and offer to be there during the conversation for moral support.
C   Raise the issue with your designated doctor for child protection.
D   Call the police: these are serious cases of assault and need to be reported.
E   Call social services to discuss the issue with them and request some input from them regarding his school.

1.97 Relationships

Your rotation as an FY1 on a urology ward is drawing to a close. One of your patients has been admitted on the ward for the entirety of your job and has required a lot of treatment, including catheterisation and intimate examinations by yourself. You and the patient have bonded well; they are of similar age as yourself, and you have enjoyed friendly and easy conversation with them on the ward. When you inform them of your departure, they thank you for all your help, pass you their phone number and ask you to call them when you are free for a date as you are now no longer their doctor.

Choose the **THREE most appropriate** actions to take in this situation.

A   Accept the phone number but write in the notes that you have destroyed it and have no intentions of pursuing a personal relationship.
B   Accept the phone number graciously but never call the patient and avoid any situation that you might run into them.
C   Accept the phone number since you were hoping to write up their case for publication and you think they are more likely to agree if you accept their number.
D   Accept the phone number to save the patient's feelings but inform your registrar of the situation and your intentions never to call.
E   Accept the phone number with the intention of calling; it is difficult to meet potential partners with your shift pattern after all.
F   Reject the phone number, explaining that it is unprofessional and could get you into a lot of trouble with the General Medical Council (GMC).
G   Reject the phone number, explaining that you have enjoyed the professional bond with the patient but that, for the protection of both them and you, you cannot accept.
H   Reject the phone number, explaining that your relationship was always professional and that they must have been confused during their illness to think otherwise.

1.98 Colleague missing teaching

You are an FY1 attending a mandatory training day in another hospital. You notice that your FY1 colleague who works on the same ward as you is not present despite being timetabled to be there. Between sessions, you overhear some people saying that he went out drinking last night and had called them to say that he was too hungover to attend training today.

Rank in order the following actions in response to this situation (1 = Most appropriate; 5 = Least appropriate).

A Tell the programme director for the day that your colleague is not here because he is too hungover.
B Seek advice from your friend, another FY1 at the training day.
C Ring up your colleague for an explanation as to why he isn't at the training.
D Tell everyone at the training that he is skiving that day because he can't handle his drink.
E Ring your colleague and say that he should try and come in for the afternoon lectures.

1.99 Prescribing error

You are in the middle of a week on call on a busy ear, nose and throat (ENT) ward and have just arrived on the ward to prepare the patient list for the ward round. Your specialist registrar (SpR) approaches you and asks whether you clerked in a woman yesterday with a sore throat. He says that she was prescribed amoxicillin and has since come out in a florid rash. You remember that you did see this patient just before you left last night, but you are sure that she didn't have any allergies.

Rank in order the following actions in response to this situation (1 = Most appropriate; 5 = Least appropriate).

A Apologise to the patient for your mistake and reassure them that it won't happen again.
B Tell the nurses not to continue the course of amoxicillin.
C Deny knowledge of this patient to your SpR but cross out the amoxicillin on the drug chart.
D Admit the mistake and ensure that the antibiotic is crossed off the drug chart.
E Inform your consultant that you made an error.

1.100 Receiving a gift

You are the FY1 on an endocrine ward and have been looking after a patient who has undergone surgery for papillary thyroid cancer. She is due to be going home today, but before she leaves she hands you an envelope with a cheque and says 'thank you for bending over backwards to make sure I received the best care possible'.

Rank in order the following actions in response to this situation (1 = Most appropriate; 5 = Least appropriate).

A Accept the gift gracefully and share it among the team looking after her.
B Ask the patient to donate it to the hospital charity.
C Accept the money and offer to take the patient out for a meal with the money.

D Decline the money saying that you appreciate the gesture, but you are not able to accept it.
E Accept the money and let your educational supervisor know about the gift.

1.101 Colleague's appearance

You work with an FY2 who consistently arrives at work wearing stained clothes which don't seem to have been ironed for some time. The nursing staff have been commenting on his appearance.

Choose the **THREE most appropriate** actions to take in this situation.

A Ask the sister on the ward to say something to him.
B Ask your fellow FY1s if they have noticed anything.
C Discuss the matter further with the nursing staff.
D Leave the matter; how he chooses to dress is up to him.
E Let the consultant know the nursing staff's opinions.
F Make sure that the FY2 is well and not struggling in any way.
G Suggest to the nursing staff that, if this is something they have noticed, they should let the FY2 know.
H Tell the FY2 that the way he dresses does not seem appropriate for a doctor.

1.102 Keeping promises

You are busy on call one evening and have a long list of jobs to complete. You see a patient and decide that she requires a blood test to help clarify her clinical picture. The patient is very anxious about the results of the test and asks you if you will let her know the results of the test as soon as they are back, which you promise to do. However, on walking home you realise that you handed over that task to your colleague taking over after your shift, and you are not aware of the result yourself.

Rank in order the following actions in response to this situation (1 = Most appropriate; 5 = Least appropriate).

A Call the nighttime FY1 and ask them to communicate the results to the patient.
B Go and see the patient with her results first thing in the morning. Apologise for not informing her of the results earlier and explain to her what they mean.
C Go and see the patient with the results the following day and say that they have only just come back that morning.
D Turn back, check the results and let the patient know.
E You have handed over the job, therefore it is no longer your responsibility.

1.103 Hungover

You are the FY1 working on an acute medical ward. You are out having a few drinks with friends on a Friday night when you receive a text from a colleague reminding you that you are covering their on-call shift the next day. You had agreed to this several weeks before as your colleague is going to a wedding. You have already had a bit too much alcohol and are worried that you will be significantly hungover the next morning.

Rank in order the following actions in response to this situation (1 = Most appropriate; 5 = Least appropriate).

A Stay out with your friends and call in sick in the morning.
B Go home immediately, have a glass of water, go to bed and go to work the next day.
C Explain to your colleague that you forgot and can no longer work in the morning, apologising profusely.
D Go home, have a glass of water, go to bed and call in sick the next day if you don't feel capable of working.
E Contact the rest of your fellow FY1s asking if anyone could work tomorrow at late notice, and if nobody can then inform your colleague that they will have to work, apologising profusely.

1.104 Train late

You are an FY1 on a medical ward, who is expected to be at work on Monday morning. You have been away for the weekend visiting family. You decided to take an early train back on Monday morning because it was your father's birthday on Sunday and you wanted to stay for dinner. Unfortunately, the train breaks down halfway through your journey. It is unclear how long the delay is going to be. There are other FY1s who will also be working on the team today.

Rank in order the following actions in response to this situation (1 = Most appropriate; 5 = Least appropriate).

A Apologise when you arrive at the hospital and explain why you are late.
B Call the hospital and ask to be put through to the registrar on call for your team, and tell them that you are sick and cannot come to work today.
C Call the hospital and ask to be put through to the registrar on call for your team, and explain the situation to them.
D Email your clinical supervisor explaining the situation.
E Call one of your FY1 colleagues and explain the situation, asking them to relay the information at the morning handover meeting.

1.105 E-learning certificate plagiarism

You are working on your first rotation as an FY1 doctor in a busy teaching hospital. As part of your induction programme, you are required to complete a set of e-learning modules covering various topics ranging from anticoagulation to the use of insulin. You have completed all the modules and uploaded your certificates to your e-portfolio. The night before the deadline a close friend of yours, who is also an FY1 colleague in the same hospital, telephones you saying that he can't complete a module covering equality and diversity because his laptop has broken. He asks if he can have a copy of your certificate, which he will edit and upload to his e-portfolio. He promises that he will complete the module in the next week and re-upload his genuine certificate.

Choose the **THREE most appropriate** actions to take in this situation.

A Allow him to have a copy of your certificate as this will not affect patient safety and ask to see his genuine certificate when he has completed the module.
B Contact a senior colleague to ask him what you should do.
C Ignore his request and inform your friend's educational supervisor of his attempted plagiarism.
D Reprimand your colleague for not completing the module earlier and refuse to help him.
E Suggest that he attends work early in the morning to complete the module before his ward round starts.
F Suggest that he can leave the module as you didn't learn anything useful from it.
G Suggest that he comes over to use your laptop to complete the module.
H Suggest that he contacts the foundation programme director asking for an extension to the deadline.

1.106 Illegible colleague signature

You are working as an FY1 doctor in a district general hospital and are completing your gastroenterology rotation. While finishing your ward rounds with the senior house officer (SHO), you notice that they have not been documenting their name after their entries in the medical notes. Instead, the SHO has been entering a short, illegible signature which cannot be identified easily.

Rank in order the following actions in response to this situation (1 = Most appropriate; 5 = Least appropriate).

A Contact human resources and ask them if they can produce a rubber stamp that your colleague could use to document his details in the notes.
B Offer to carry out all the writing on the ward rounds.
C Suggest to your colleague that he completes his entries with his full name and GMC number clearly legible as well as his signature.
D Suggest to your colleague that he acquires a rubber stamp with his details so he can clearly document his details in the notes.
E Write your colleague's details in the notes after his name so that he can be clearly identified.

1.107 Diarrhoea and vomiting

You are an FY1 doing a rotation in general surgery. It is the evening before a weekend on call, and you start to develop diarrhoea and vomiting.

Rank in order the following actions in response to this situation (1 = Most appropriate; 5 = Least appropriate).

A   Go into work but don't carry out any tasks involving patient contact.
B   Call into work the next morning to say you won't be able to go in to work.
C   Take some medication to prevent diarrhoea, such as loperamide, and go in to work, making sure that you have excellent hand hygiene.
D   Call into work in the evening, informing them that you will not be able to go to work the next day.
E   Inform the Health Protection Agency (HPA).

1.108 Prescribing for a friend

You are an FY2, and your housemate asks you to prescribe an antibiotic for her urinary tract infection (UTI). She has had these a few times before and usually requires a short course of antibiotics to clear it up. It is Friday evening, and the local out-of-hours centre is about to close.

Choose the **THREE most appropriate** actions to take in this situation.

A   Advise her to drink plenty of fluids and cranberry juice.
B   Gain a more thorough history of her presenting complaint.
C   Give her the antibiotic prescription and inform her GP on Monday.
D   Prescribe the antibiotic.
E   Refuse to prescribe the antibiotic.
F   Take a sample of her urine to the hospital laboratories.
G   Take her to the emergency department.
H   Tell her to make an appointment to see her GP on Monday.

1.109 Dress code

You have been working in a medical team for three months. You have noticed that your fellow FY1 has started wearing jeans to work. You do not feel that she looks as smart as the rest of the team.

Rank in order the following actions in response to this situation (1 = Most appropriate; 5 = Least appropriate).

A   Ask the other junior members of your team what they think about your colleague's clothes.
B   Do nothing since she is entitled to wear what she likes to work.
C   Start wearing jeans too since they are more comfortable than your smart trousers.
D   Suggest to your colleague privately that she would look smarter in something other than jeans.
E   Tell your consultant that you do not think that your colleague looks as smart as the rest of the team.

1.110 Other commitments

You are an FY1 dedicated to a career in academic medicine. You have spent the last year working on a research project that has yielded promising results. You and your supervisor wish to submit the work to a specialist conference for presentation. The deadline for submissions is sooner than you thought, and you only have one day to complete the data analysis and abstract, which you estimate will take eight hours to complete. Unfortunately, you are working a 13-hour shift both today and tomorrow as part of your on-call rota.

Choose the **THREE most appropriate** actions to take in this situation.

A Ask your supervisor to complete the data analysis and just do the abstract yourself.
B Call in sick for tomorrow's shift so that you have time to do the work.
C Don't submit to the conference; your job takes precedence.
D Go into work but turn off your bleep and sit in the doctors' office to complete your work.
E Make up the rest of the data for your study and submit on time.
F Speak to your registrar about having a few hours off in the morning to complete your work so you can work and sleep.
G Try and swap shifts last minute with another FY1 on the same on-call rota.
H Work through the night in between your long shifts to get the work completed.

1.111 Domestic violence

You are working as an FY1 in orthopaedics. You clerk in a 19-year-old woman with a broken arm. She tells you that it was an accidental injury, but from the bruising on her face and arms, you suspect that she may have been attacked. When you ask her about it, she admits that her boyfriend hit her and has done so on numerous occasions. She asks you not to tell the police because he has promised never to do it again.

Rank in order the following actions in response to this situation (1 = Most appropriate; 5 = Least appropriate).

A Contact the police without informing the patient that you are doing so.
B Encourage the patient to let you contact the police.
C Explain to the patient that you are concerned about her welfare and therefore intend to contact the police without her consent.
D Give the patient a leaflet about a charity that supports victims of domestic violence.
E Tell the patient that you will not contact the police without her consent.

1.112 Patient discrimination

You have just arrived on the ward and are preparing the patient list ready for the consultant's ward round. One of the staff nurses approaches you and wants to talk about the other FY1 on your ward. She overheard him yesterday making derogatory comments about one of your patients to another colleague. She says he was saying that the patient could 'wait for his analgesia to be prescribed as he doesn't belong in this country and can wait for his turn to get treatment'.

Rank in order the following actions in response to this situation (1 = Most appropriate; 5 = Least appropriate).

A Tell the nurse that she should speak directly to the FY1 in question.
B Report the incident to the FY1's educational supervisor.
C Speak to your senior house officer (SHO) about the nurse's concerns and ask for their advice.
D Speak directly to the FY1 in question about the nurse's concerns.
E Ask the patient whether he had any concerns over the treatment he received yesterday.

1.113 Criticising collegues on hearsay

You are working on the medical admissions unit (MAU) and are at the nurses' station chasing bloods whilst your FY1 colleague is clerking a patient. The patient is complaining that the doctor in accident and emergency (A&E) took a long time to come and see her and then kept disappearing to answer his phone whilst in the middle of the consultation. Your colleague apologises for the patient's wait and then remarks that the A&E doctor 'has a reputation for being slapdash' and that he agrees it is 'very unprofessional, and in my view, he should be suspended'.

Choose the **THREE most appropriate** actions to take in this situation.

A Ask to speak to your colleague when he has finished the consultation.
B Ask your colleague to go back to the patient and apologise for what he has said about the doctor in A&E.
C Don't do anything about the comments but keep an ear out for any similar remarks he makes about colleagues.
D Explain to your colleague that it is not professional to disseminate adverse information about a colleague, especially to patients, even if it may be true.
E Interrupt the consultation to have a word with the FY1 in private.
F Report the FY1 to the sister in charge.
G Speak to your educational supervisor.
H Tell the doctor in A&E that the FY1 is spreading rumours about him.

ANSWERS

1.1 Relationships

A E C B D

Patients need trust in their doctors and must be able to act honestly and openly without feeling that the doctor may see them as a potential partner. It is therefore unacceptable to pursue a relationship with a current patient, as in option D. Relationships with former patients are often inappropriate, but this depends on a number of factors including the length of time elapsed since attending the patient. In the case of option B, only a short time will have elapsed between the patient's discharge and the start of your potential relationship. More importantly, however, you would already be engaging in a relationship while they remain in hospital since there is the promise of arranging a date. While option C may seem a less awkward way of dealing with the situation and avoids a relationship, you must not allow the patient's advances to affect your doctor–patient relationship. If you were to feel that a patient's advance had affected the doctor–patient relationship, then you should bring the professional relationship to a definite end rather than simply avoiding the patient. Option E again avoids a relationship but would risk offending your the patient, therefore compromising the doctor–patient relationship. Diplomatically declining the offer (A) is the best option since it is most likely to preserve a good professional relationship.

Recommended reading

General Medical Council (2013), Explanatory guidance, in *Ending Your Professional Relationship with a Patient*.

General Medical Council (2013), Explanatory guidance, in *Maintaining a Professional Boundary Between You and Your Patient*.

General Medical Council (2013), *Good Medical Practice*, paragraphs 53, 62.

Medical Protection Society (2012), *MPS Guide to Ethics: A Map for the Moral Maze*, chapter 5, Morality and decency.

1.2 Police caution

B D G

There is a legal and professional obligation to declare all criminal investigations, cautions or convictions to both the GMC and your employer without delay (options D and G). In this case, it is unlikely that there will be any serious consequences for stealing a garden gnome; however, failing to disclose this information may have dire consequences, even the loss of your professional registration. Since there are potentially serious consequences to this situation, it would be prudent to seek further advice. A lawyer may be able to give advice (A), but a medical defence union (B) is a specialist organisation and would therefore be a better first step. If you do try and overturn the caution (C), your first action should still be to declare the caution and seek advice since it has already been issued to you and is unlikely to be rescinded. Ignoring the issue (F) and delaying further action (H) are both inappropriate since you need to act without delay. While it is important to reflect on the incident (E), this is not your immediate priority.

Recommended reading

General Medical Council (2013), *Good Medical Practice*, paragraphs 68, 75.
General Medical Council (2013), *Guidance on Convictions, Cautions and Determinations.*

1.3 Gifts

D B E C A

The issue of doctors accepting gifts from patients is a difficult one and often dependent on the nature of the gift. Intimate gifts such as lingerie are clearly inappropriate, cash gifts are generally viewed as unacceptable and expensive gifts should either be declined or registered with your employer. Expense is dependent on the patient's means although gifts worth in excess of £100 should usually be declined or declared. Whatever the circumstances, the receipt of a gift should not be seen to affect a patient's treatment. Option A is therefore the least appropriate response. Declining gifts can also be problematic as it may cause offence. The most appropriate response is therefore option D since it is clear that the gift does not affect the care of the patient but it shows gratitude. While option B avoids causing offence, the gifts were not offered with the intention that you should give them away. Option E may be appropriate although it has the potential to cause unnecessary disappointment or offence. In the case of option C, it would be rude to decline the gift based on your dislike of champagne.

Recommended reading

General Medical Council (2013), *Good Medical Practice*, paragraph 80.
Medical Protection Society (2011), *GP Registrar: How to be Good*, pages 6–7.

1.4 Facebook

D C A B E

Doctors are entitled to a personal life; however, they must maintain a level of professionalism. The currently accepted standards are ill defined, but the public needs to have confidence in both the individual and the profession. Doctors should consider that content uploaded onto social media may influence public confidence. In this scenario, it would be prudent to remove potentially damaging images from social media websites, and doctors are encouraged to review their privacy settings regularly. Option D is therefore the best response. Altering your privacy settings without removing the images (C) leaves the potential for your images to be viewed by people who may be adversely influenced, given that social media websites cannot guarantee complete privacy.

While refraining from the use of social media (A) would remove all risk to professional image, you should be allowed to take advantage of its benefits should you wish to. This is therefore a valid but less favourable solution. Options B and E may damage working relationships with your colleagues, and neither addresses the issue of professionalism.

Recommended reading

British Medical Association (2011), *Using Social Media: Practical and Ethical Guidance for Doctors and Medical Students.*

General Medical Council (2013), *Good Medical Practice*, paragraph 65.

Medical Protection Society (2012), *MPS Guide to Ethics: A Map for the Moral Maze*, chapter 12, Personal conduct.

1.5 Documenting

B E H

In this situation, regardless of your worries about whether you have potentially made a mistake or not, it is important to correct this as soon as possible. It is therefore appropriate to carry out the recommended investigations and treatment without delay (E). It would be prudent to ask the registrar to review the patient with you (B) since you were initially unsure of how to manage the patient and they have now deteriorated further. Documenting events in the notes is a crucial part of being a doctor, especially since the medical notes constitute a legal document. It is therefore important to clearly and accurately document what has happened in this situation (H). You should never destroy any part of a patient's notes (G) or obscure entries within the notes (C). Similarly, you should never alter a previous entry (options A and D). Option D is actually deceptive. Option A, while preferable to option D since you would be acknowledging that the management plan was formulated by your registrar and adding in a true account of your discussion with him, is still factually misleading as it will appear that this discussion took place at an earlier time. It would be useful to reflect on this case (F), but this is not something of immediate importance.

Recommended reading

General Medical Council (2013), *Good Medical Practice*, paragraphs 19–21.

Medical Protection Society (2012), *MPS Guide to Ethics: A Map for the Moral Maze*, Chapter 6, Honesty.

1.6 Friend's test results

A E F

As a doctor you will find that friends and family will regularly confide in you about their medical problems and ask you for information. In this scenario, you should tell your friend that you cannot access her results for her (E), advise her to get the results from the doctor who requested the tests (A) and talk to her about her concerns (F). The General Medical Council (GMC) warns against treating family and close friends for many reasons, including emotional involvement and thus a lack of objectivity; patients receiving care outside a practice setting may not receive the same standard of care, and doctors may not feel able to ask sensitive questions or conduct intimate examinations on friends or relatives.

You should not access the results (B) or get a colleague to access them for you (C). Both of these options would be unprofessional as you should never access the results of patients not directly under your care. By accessing your friend's results, you are actively getting involved in your friend's management. Asking someone else to access them for you would be dishonest and may get them in trouble as well. Giving her a patient information leaflet (D) may be appropriate, but in the first instance, you should talk to her about her concerns. Telling her that the results are likely to be normal (G) would be inappropriate as you have not ordered the test and you may not be completely aware of your friend's medical history. Telling her that you don't have a duty of care to her as you are not her doctor (H) is unnecessarily harsh; instead, it would be better to say that she should discuss it with the doctor who ordered the tests.

Recommended reading
General Medical Council (August 2011), *The Development of Good Medical Practice*, Treating family members.
Medical Protection Society (2012), *MPS Guide to Ethics: A Map for the Moral Maze*, chapter 6, Honesty.

1.7 Lying about results

A B E
An underlying principle in our healthcare system is the need for honesty and transparency. In this situation, if you respond with anything but honesty, it is likely that there will be negative repercussions. Blood results are now very rarely confirmed by letter; however, many other inter-professional communications within medicine are still done in paper form. In this scenario, you have made an honest mistake. The most appropriate course of action is to apologise to the patient (A) and make every effort to resolve the situation. This could be achieved by phoning the hospital for the results (E) or asking the practice nurse to retake the blood tests (B). Both of these options retain honesty while protecting patient safety. Although option D could be seen as a 'white lie' that is unlikely to harm the patient, dishonesty in any guise should be discouraged. Cancelling the appointment and sending a letter (C) may provide the patient with the results; however, a diabetic review requires a range of other questions and examinations such as checking for peripheral neuropathy. Transferring the issue to another GP (H) would be just delaying the issue and is likely to affect your professional relationship with your colleague. Perhaps the most dangerous option here is to reassure your patient without knowing the results (F); you may find it difficult to take a step back if the results are not what you expected. The excuse of 'lost in the system' is counterproductive in all scenarios, and in this case, it would also be a lie and is therefore inappropriate (G).

Recommended reading

General Medical Council (2013), *Good Medical Practice*, Duties of a doctor.
General Medical Council (2013), *Good Medical Practice*, paragraphs 1, 63.

1.8 Lying about experience

C   B   A   D   E

It is the nature of learning a new skill that there will always be a first time to complete a procedure. As a foundation doctor you are allowed to perform procedures such as lumbar punctures, pleural drains and ascitic drains, as well as the core procedures required by the foundation programme curriculum, as long as you have had the relevant teaching and training and have appropriate supervision. When completing any procedure, you may often be asked by the patient whether or not you have performed it before. It is always essential to be honest with your patient and the General Medical Council makes it very clear that every doctor should maintain integrity and honesty with their patients and colleagues. Option C would allow you to be honest with the patient, while also offering them reassurance of the fact that you will be supervised during the procedure and maintaining the learning opportunity for yourself. The patient may also be reassured after an explanation from a more senior and experienced doctor, so asking the medical registrar to explain the situation could also be helpful (B). Asking the registrar to carry out the procedure (A) will ensure that an experienced doctor is performing the task; however, this would remove the opportunity for your own learning and development. Option E ranks last because lying to your patient is completely unacceptable, and this response would display a disregard for patient autonomy. Option D involves an omission of the truth, which, although preferable to lying outright to the patient, is still misleading and therefore also inappropriate.

Recommended reading

General Medical Council (2008), Explanatory guidance, in *Consent: Patients and Doctors Making Decisions Together*, paragraphs 3, 10, 12.

1.9 Honesty on death certificates

D   F   H

Completing death certificates is a common task for FY1 doctors and a potentially difficult one. The death certificate is a legal document, and you must comply with the specific rules and regulations on how they should be completed. For the majority of certificates, the cause of death and the events leading to the death are obvious and can be completed without discussion with the coroner. However, in this scenario, you have no identifiable cause for the gastrointestinal bleed in a patient who was otherwise healthy. The most appropriate course of action would be to actively seek advice from professionals experienced in the area. This could be your registrar or consultant (H) or a pathologist or coroner (F). There may also be other aspects in the patient's history that you are unaware of which could explain his gastrointestinal bleed (D).

Completing the cause of death as gastrointestinal bleed without giving causes or risk factors that led to the bleed (B) may not be accepted by the coroner. This would lead to unnecessary delay for the patient's family. Completing the death certificate dishonestly by declaring he had a peptic ulcer without investigating this (C) would be wholly inappropriate. Asking your colleague to complete the certificate without attempting to seek advice first (A) would be passing off the problem onto somebody else, whereas this is something you should try to resolve first, and you may be able to learn from this scenario in the future. Giving non-specific information to the family (E) would be incredibly damaging during times of great distress around a death. While the secretarial staff may offer solutions to practical problems, this is a medical issue that needs to be sorted with professional help, so asking them here is not appropriate (G).

Recommended reading
Office for National Statistics (2010), *Guidance for Doctors Completing Medical Certificates of Cause of Death in England and Wales*, section 5, How to complete the cause of death section.

1.10 Insurance fraud

B   C   D   A   E

Insurance fraud is a criminal offence and once you are aware of it you have an obligation to report it to the police (B) because you are bound by the professional values of being a doctor. Informing the GMC (C) is not the best option since they are not the most appropriate body to investigate this situation from a criminal perspective. The GMC will need to be involved, particularly if the doctor is convicted, but the role of the police is more important at this stage. Telling the FY1's educational supervisor (D) is a somewhat passive way of taking action, when it is you who has heard the information. The worst options involve not taking any action to report the doctor. Morally, the worst response is to warn the doctor about the need to keep this a secret (E) as you are then admitting that you recognise the illegality of what they have done and are making yourself complicit in covering up this action. Although you are somewhat complicit as soon as you are aware, option A does not actively support the criminal activity and is therefore preferable to option E.

Recommended reading
Medical Protection Society (2012), *MPS Guide to Ethics*, chapter 6, Honesty, section: Indirect threats; chapter 12, Personal conduct, section: Morality.

1.11 Handover task forgotten

A   C   F

You must be honest with the registrar and accept responsibility for the delay (F) and include an explanation of why you were distracted so that the registrar fully understands the situation. It would be dishonest and unfair to your night colleague to either actively deny that they had handed over the job (H) or passively allow the registrar to continue with this assumption (G). You must also be honest and open with the patient rather than blaming your colleague (D), which unfairly undermines the patient's trust in them. It would also be dishonest to try to convince the patient that there had been no delay (E), which could damage their trust in you. Whenever a mistake has been made, the most important thing to do is to put it right in a timely manner (C). Although there would be nothing wrong with documenting the events in the notes (B), and this would be thorough and open of you, there are three more important priorities. Documenting will not help to correct the mistake in the way option C does, will not change the registrar's criticism of your undeserving colleague as F does and will not set the patient's mind at rest, as in option A. You should always apologise to patients for mistakes that could negatively impact their care.

Recommended reading

General Medical Council (2013), *Good Medical Practice*, paragraphs 25, 55.
Medical Protection Society (2012), *MPS Guide to Ethics: A Map for the Moral Maze*, chapter 6, Honesty, section: Open disclosure.

1.12 Forgot to document

A   G   H

First, you should talk to your team and let them know that when you examined the patient earlier you had checked for a rash (G), since this is an important piece of information and will reassure the team that it was not missed. It is vital that all medical records are contemporaneous, so you should not go back and alter your earlier entry in any way (B). This would be a dishonest thing to do, even though what you are adding is truthful. It is a good idea to document that you had checked for a rash and found none, which should be done in the current place in the notes with the current time, and you can write that it is a retrospective comment about your earlier examination (A). This is advisable in case questions are raised later, and it is better than not recording anything (F). The SHO should not be required to be dishonest in order to cover your back (D), and they are likely to be unimpressed by your lack of professionalism if you ask this of them. It is very unlikely that they would agree to omit this information from the notes because it would bring their own conduct into question if investigated. You haven't done anything unethical or made any major error in this scenario, you have simply forgotten to document a negative finding that later turned out to be pertinent information. For the same reasons, you do not need to seek legal advice (E) or formal support from your supervisor (C). However, it would be beneficial for your learning and development to reflect on the experience and how you will learn from it (H), to ensure your examination documentation is thorough in the future.

Recommended reading

General Medical Council (2013), *Good Medical Practice*, paragraph 19.
Medical Protection Society (2012), *MPS Guide to Ethics: A Map for the Moral Maze*, chapter 6, Honesty, section: Records.

1.13 Mr or Dr

E B D C A

As a doctor, you should not make it appear as if you hold higher qualifications than you do. If someone is doing this, then they need to be made aware that it is inappropriate for both their patients and colleagues to think that they are talking to someone more qualified than they are. The best action therefore is to explain this to the SHO (E) and also to make your consultant aware of the situation (B). Of the remaining options, talking to the relevant Royal College (D) is the best as the rest involve either undermining the SHO in front of patients (A) or leaving the SHO to practise dangerously (C).

Recommended reading

General Medical Council (2013), *Good Medical Practice*, paragraph 66.
Medical Protection Society (2012), *MPS Guide to Ethics: A Map for the Moral Maze*, chapter 6, Honesty.

1.14 Medical students

A B C E D

Despite not being part of a registered body, medical students still have to follow the same rules as doctors. There is specific guidance for medical students from the General Medical Council (GMC) about personal conduct; therefore, the most appropriate thing to do is to ask the medical student to go back and fully inform the patient (A). The medical student needs reminding that they have a role in patient care and protecting patients, a big part of which involves being truthful with the patient (B). The third best option here is to discuss the matter with the patient yourself (C), although it would be better for the student to do this themselves. The two worst options are E and D: to leave the patient thinking that they have been seen by a doctor when they have not is completely inappropriate (D), making option E a better response than D, in which you do nothing.

Recommended reading

General Medical Council (2009), *Medical Students: Professional Values and Fitness to Practice*, paragraphs 23, 24, 26 and 28.

1.15 Colleagues accepting gifts

A B G

Accepting gifts from patients is an ethical grey area, and different people have differing opinions. However, it is agreed that you should not accept gifts in the form of money. Certainly, in this scenario, it sounds as though the SHO is coercing patients a little, by making it sound as if he is doing more than he actually is to influence patient care. Option A is correct because you should talk to the SHO in question and try and advise him otherwise. Talking to your supervisor (B) is also sensible as getting advice from someone with more experience is helpful. Telling the consultant who is in charge of the patient's care (G) is also important. Discussing it with the nurses is tantamount to gossiping and is therefore best avoided (C). Giving the money to charity is, of course, a good moral option (D), but it does not address the root of the problem. Immediately reporting the SHO to the GMC prior to talking to them (E) is also not recommended. Talking directly to the patient will leave them distrustful of the health service and will also make them feel bad about trying to give a gift (F). Obviously, trying similar methods to receive gifts from your patients is not appropriate (H).

Recommended reading

General Medical Council (2013), *Good Medical Practice*, paragraphs 77–80.
Medical Protection Society (2012), *MPS Guide to Ethics: A Map for the Moral Maze*, chapter 6, Honesty.

1.16 Open disclosure of mistake

A B D

This scenario assesses professionalism, particularly with regard to open and honest disclosure of mistakes. Despite the fact that your patient is sitting up in bed reading, option A should be one of your immediate actions as it should be when assessing any patient. There may be clues as to her clinical state that are only evident on closer physical examination. Option B is also a priority to prevent the antibiotic being given again, which could further compromise patient safety. Although the patient may not have come to any harm as a result of your mistake, it is important to be honest with patients in these situations and to reassure them that it will not happen again (D). This helps to build rapport and foster a respectful doctor–patient relationship. While recording this event in your e-portfolio is a conscientious decision, it is not an action that should be of top priority at this time. Similarly, it is important to document what appears to be a change in allergy status (G) but only when you can be sure there is no delayed reaction. This information should then be communicated to the patient's GP. Seeking advice from a senior (F) would not be incorrect; however, as an FY1 doctor, you should be competent at performing an initial assessment prior to seeking senior assistance. For example if your patient had had an adverse reaction and you required assistance in stabilising them, your SHO would be a suitable help. Option E does not immediately address the problem nor does it foster positive professional working relationships. Disposing of the evidence (H) is dishonest, legally indefensible and does not involve assessing the patient's present clinical state.

Recommended reading

General Medical Council (2013), *Good Medical Practice*, paragraphs 16, 23, 25, 55.
Medical Protection Society (2012), *MPS Guide to Ethics: A Map for the Moral Maze*, chapter 6, Honesty.

1.17 Lying about hangover

B D C A E

This scenario requires you to act professionally as part of a team as well as to maintain patient safety and work in the best interests of the patients. Option B is the most appropriate initial response as it is important to maintain respect for your colleagues and you do not know for certain that they are not suffering from the flu. Seeking advice from another, slightly more senior colleague (D) is often good practice if you are unsure how to act, and it is more appropriate than option C, which is too confrontational. While it is important for an FY1 to act without delay if you believe a colleague's practice is putting patients at risk, it is not your responsibility to reprimand colleagues for what you consider poor professional behaviour. Option E is the least appropriate as, at present, you have no firm evidence that your colleague is absent due to a hangover and it does not help to maintain good professional relationships. Option A is also unsuitable as you are not actively helping to provide the best care for your patients; however, it is marginally preferable to option E since, by denying knowledge of the situation, you are not actively making unsubstantiated claims regarding a colleague.

Recommended reading

General Medical Council (2013), *Good Medical Practice*, paragraphs 25, 35–37, 43, 59.

Medical Protection Society (2012), *MPS Guide to Ethics: A Map for the Moral Maze*, chapter 11, Relating to colleagues, chapter 12: Personal conduct.

1.18 Drugs

E C A B D

The General Medical Council's *Duties of a Doctor* states that in situations where you suspect that your conduct or that of a colleague may be compromising patient safety, you have a duty to act without delay. In this situation, possession of illegal substances is wrong regardless of the person's profession, and you have a duty to be honest, trustworthy and act with integrity. Option D is therefore the least suitable response. There is a professional duty to raise concerns, but you should speak directly to the colleague in question in private first to give them a chance to explain themselves and to help maintain a good professional working relationship. Option E is therefore the most suitable response in preference to C, while B would be inappropriate. Option C would be suitable further down the line if the colleague in question did not take any further action themselves. Asking a senior nurse for advice (A) may be appropriate; however, they do not have a direct supervisory role and are therefore a less suitable person to approach than your educational supervisor.

Recommended reading

General Medical Council (2009), *The New Doctor*, paragraphs 63, 101–102.

General Medical Council (2013), *Good Medical Practice*, paragraphs 35–37, 43.

Medical Protection Society (2012), *MPS Guide to Ethics: A Map for the Moral Maze*, chapter 11, Relating to colleagues, page 86.

1.19 Consenting

C D E

Informed consent is always required before any procedure, and to be quali-fied to gain consent, you need to have had training, either in carrying out the procedure or in gaining consent for it. As an FY1, option C would therefore be appropriate but option A would not. If you are unsure, getting advice from another senior colleague would be sensible, and if someone else were avail-able who was trained in the procedure, they could gain consent (E). You must always make the care of your patient your first concern, so communication of the circumstances to Mr Jones (D) is also courteous. Option H is inappropri-ate as it is neither polite nor conducive to maintaining positive professional relationships. Although it is unfortunate that Mr Jones has been waiting, his situation is not life-threatening and therefore attending to his problem has to be prioritised below that of the patient currently being operated on by the consultant (B). You must give patients information in the way they want and can understand; however, while a patient information leaflet can be an effec-tive way of relaying clinical information, the patient needs a conversation with a doctor about the procedure and its risks and benefits prior to giving consent, so option F is therefore inappropriate. Option G may be suitable, but it is a bit drastic in this situation.

Recommended reading

General Medical Council (2013), *Good Medical Practice*, paragraphs 2, 17, 32, 35–37, 46–48, 56.

1.20 Alcohol on breath

A E D B C

As a doctor you have a duty to respond promptly and appropriately if you think that patient safety is being compromised. It is possible that your SpR is still under the effects of alcohol or at least not in a fit state to be making decisions and looking after patients. Even though the drinking did not occur in the hospital, your personal conduct outside the hospital is relevant to your job if it is impacting your ability to work. Option A is the best response as you have a duty to maintain good working relationships and you have no evidence that what you suspect is true. It gives your colleague the chance to explain, which is courteous, and still immediately addresses a potentially serious situation. Discussing it with a more senior colleague (options E and D) could also be appropriate if you are unsure of what to do, and your consultant (E) would be slightly more preferable as there are immediate issues over patient safety. However, it is best practice to talk to the colleague in question first. Confronting the SpR in the meeting (B) would be unprofessional, and you do not have proof yet of your suspicions. However, your duty ultimately lies with your patients and to do nothing could potentially lead to harm; therefore, option C is the least appropriate response.

Recommended reading

General Medical Council (2009), *Tomorrow's Doctors*, paragraph 133.
General Medical Council (2013), *Good Medical Practice*, Duties of a doctor.
General Medical Council (2013), *Good Medical Practice*, paragraph 25c.
Medical Protection Society (2012), *MPS Guide to Ethics: A Map for the Moral Maze*, chapter 12: Personal conduct, page 91.

1.21 Stopping at an accident

A   C   E   D   B

As qualified medical professionals, doctors are likely to come across situations outside of work where they could usefully provide assistance to individuals who have had accidents or are suffering from a medical condition. While UK law states that there is no legal obligation for doctors to stop at accidents, the General Medical Council (GMC) does offer guidance. *Good Medical Practice* states: 'You must offer help if emergencies arise in clinical settings or in the community, taking account of your own safety, your competence and the availability of other options for care.' In this scenario, you have come across two members of the public requiring urgent medical care. The best option involves confirming your own safety first (A), but you should proceed to offer assistance to the people in the car (C). Option E may be a sensible decision; however, assessing the situation to acquire further details may help the operator to assess the urgency of the situation, so E is only the third most appropriate response. Although you are not legally obliged to stop, GMC guidelines suggest that not offering assistance (B) would be inappropriate. Alerting the emergency services but continuing on your way (D) ensures that the people involved in the accident will receive care but not offering assistance yourself would be incorrect if it was safe to do so. Any assistance you do offer should take account of your degree of training and other professionals available at the scene.

Recommended reading

General Medical Council (2013), *Good Medical Practice*, paragraph 26.

1.22 Angry partner

D   E   C   B   A

The best response (D) is the one that attempts to diffuse the situation by apologising and calmly describing that you are unable to give the man any information as this would involve breaking confidentiality. The next best option (E) is to revisit your patient and tell her that her boyfriend is on the phone, clarify whether she would be happy for you to explain that she is well so that he doesn't worry or whether she really wants you to say nothing at all. Option C, although unfair on your patient as it would put pressure on her to engage in a conversation that she would probably rather not have, would be the next best choice since it attempts to address the situation directly. The question implies that there may be some domestic abuse occurring, and your patient may wish to shelter in the hospital and not be faced with her violent partner.

The next best option would be to hang up the phone and call security (B), but this would be likely to anger the man who is threatening violence against the hospital. You have a responsibility to all of your patients on the ward, and you need to do all you can to calm the situation down rather than risk escalating it into a potentially dangerous situation. The least appropriate option would be to call the police (A) as it would be difficult to explain the situation to them without breaking the confidentiality of your patient.

Recommended reading

General Medical Council (2013), *Good Medical Practice*, Confidentiality, paragraph 53.

General Medical Council (2013), *Good Medical Practice*, confidentiality: reporting concerns about patients to the DVLA or DVA.

1.23 Unskilled procedure

A B D E C

This question assesses your integrity about knowing when you should not perform a procedure that you have not been trained to implement. Unless the situation involves life and death and doing nothing would undoubtedly be catastrophic for the patient, you should not perform procedures that you have not been satisfactorily trained in because you could potentially cause serious harm. In this example, in fact it is vital to draw off the same volume of cerebrospinal fluid (CSF) as the antibiotics so as not to cause raised intra-cerebral pressure. If you had performed the procedure without knowing this, the patient could have come to serious harm and be much worse off than they would be if there was a delay in their treatment. Asking an experienced clinician such as a consultant if they can come to assist you with the task, or at least tell you how to perform the task in detail, would be the safest and best option in this case (A). Option B is the next best option; some general surgeons will have experience from their earlier training in neurosurgery and might be able to assist or advise. Option D to leave the job until the expert is able to give advice and supervise, is the next best response as it is better than performing the job yourself with potentially inadequate advice from the internet or nursing staff. Of the two final options, option E is better than option C as a nurse may well have seen this procedure several times and know exactly how you are supposed to do it, whereas information on the internet may be much less reliable.

Recommended reading

General Medical Council (2013), *Good Medical Practice*, Duties of a doctor.

1.24 Death certification

A D F

Doctors have a legal obligation to tell the whole truth to protect the patients even though they have passed away. The best thing to do, therefore, is to discuss the matter with the FY2 himself (A), or with someone more senior and more experienced than you. In this situation, that would be the consultant in charge of the case (D). The other people to talk to would be those most used to this sort of event: the bereavement office staff may be of help here (F). Calling the coroner yourself (B) would be overstepping your role and competence as an FY1 and should not be your first move. Ignoring the matter is not acceptable for obvious reasons (E) nor is taking the phone from the FY2 (G). Simply telling the FY2 that he is inappropriate would only antagonise your colleague and is therefore not a good course of action (H).

Recommended reading

General Medical Council (2013), *Good Medical Practice*, End of life care: Certification, post-mortems and referral to a coroner or procurator fiscal, paragraphs 85–87.

Office for National Statistics (2010), *Guidance for Doctors Completing Medical Certificates of Cause of Death in England and Wales*, http://www.gro.gov. uk/images/medcert_July_2010.pdf.

1.25 Dishonest form for patient

C   E   B   A   D

You should never sign a document if you know that it contains information that is not truthful and accurate (A). However, you cannot report the patient to the police (D) as they have not done anything criminal, so disclosing would breach their confidentiality. The only circumstance in which you could talk to an external agency would be to get anonymous advice (B), although this is unlikely to be particularly helpful as your approach must be dictated by your professional obligations. It would be best to speak to the patient directly (C) as you may even find that they are not being intentionally deceitful and actually believe that their housing issues are the cause of their illness. Even if they are aware that they are not being entirely honest, a simple explanation and refusal from you may be enough for them to realise that the document needs to be honest. Option E defers the situation to a senior member of your team, which is not strictly necessary, but isn't unethical either. It therefore ranks higher than discussing with an external agency or signing the form (options B and A).

Recommended reading

General Medical Council (2013), *Good Medical Practice*, paragraph 71.
Medical Protection Society (2012), *MPS Guide to Ethics: A Map for the Moral Maze*, chapter: Honesty, section: Misleading statements.

1.26 Inappropriate drunken stories

D   B   C   E   A

It seems as though the doctor is about to tell a story that makes fun of patients, which will undermine the medical profession in the eyes of those present. It would not be acceptable behaviour even if the stories are anonymous as it still breaches the trust of those patients. You should therefore interject (options B, C and D) rather than let the doctor go on (options A and E). Reporting your colleague to the GMC (E) is better than simply allowing the situation to continue (A) because it demonstrates concern, although it makes no attempt to try and intervene at the time. If you can stop your colleague politely, this will be best as it avoids confrontation (D). Option B will embarrass the other doctor and may seem overdramatic to the rest of the group; however, it is a better response than option C because it lets the doctor know that they are being inappropriate. By simply changing the subject (C), they have not been warned about their behaviour, so they are more likely to try to return to the topic later on.

Recommended reading
General Medical Council (2013), *Good Medical Practice*, paragraph 65.
Medical Protection Society (2012), *MPS Guide to Ethics: A Map for the Moral Maze*, chapter 12: Personal conduct, sections: Expectations of statutory bodies, Alcohol.

1.27 Hours monitoring

B D E A C
As a young doctor, it is hard to question or challenge practice that seems to be taken for granted, especially by your senior colleagues. You must remember that you have your professionalism and integrity to uphold. The most appropriate option is to tell the consultant that you cannot be dishonest and put down your true working hours (B). You may feel unable to do this, so the next most appropriate option would be option D: to seek advice from senior colleagues about how to handle the situation. Seeking advice from your professional advocacy organisation such as the BMA (E) may be required, but it would be best to talk to colleagues within your department first to voice your concerns. Putting down the true hours without telling the consultant (A) may be appropriate, but your consultant is likely to find out later, and this will not stop the consultant from putting pressure on your other colleagues in the same way in the future. Claiming you have worked the false number of hours (C) is the most inappropriate option. Not only is this unprofessional and dishonest, it will not help the department in the long term since it is likely that you and your colleagues are being overworked and need more support with staffing levels.

Recommended reading
Medical Protection Society (2012), *MPS Guide to Ethics: A Map for the Moral Maze*, chapters 6 and 11.

1.28 False audit

C B A E D
The assumption in this question is that the consultant has been dishonest and altered the results of the audit to gain financial reward from the trust. This has patient safety implications since, instead of learning how to do better,

the department thinks that it is already excellent. The best response here is option C. You did not do the data analysis and could have made a mistake in your assumptions that the department was failing. Option B is the next best response: dishonesty for financial gain is a serious allegation and a senior doctor would be able to offer advice about how to investigate this potential case and which channels to use to escalate the issue if need be. Reanalysing the results yourself (A) would offer you a way of testing whether your conclusions are actually correct, taking into account that different statistical methods can yield slightly different results. You would then be in a stronger position to raise the alarm if you find your suspicions to be correct. Sharing your concerns with the trust (E) is the next best answer; as part of whistleblowers' protection rights, you should be able to send named emails without fear of repercussions, and it would be easier for them to investigate using your data if you did this. Option D ranks last as turning a blind eye to this shows a lack of integrity and morality.

Recommended reading

General Medical Council (2013), *Good Medical Practice*, paragraphs 65–80.
NHS Employers, Raising concerns at work, http://www.
   nhsemployers.org/your-workforce/retain-and-improve/
   raising-concerns-at-work-whistleblowing.

1.29 Flu jab

B   C   E   A   D

It is one of the General Medical Council's (GMC) recommendations that 'you should protect your patients, your colleagues and yourself by being immunised against common serious communicable diseases where vaccines are available'. To decide against this advice would leave you open to criticism from the GMC and colleagues. The best options are those that involve you having the flu jab (options B and C). The flu jab does not give you influenza but can cause low-grade temperatures and aching muscles for a few days. This should not be significant enough for you to take time off work, but you should not have to sacrifice your weekend to be unwell. Option B is therefore better than option C. The rest of the responses involve not having the flu jab, so they are not ideal. Option E is the best of those, since you are being proactive about what you believe; also contacting the management of the hospital will raise awareness that staff members may not agree with or understand the reasons behind staff vaccination, which could alert them to the need to address this issue. Option A is the next best response, in which you refuse the vaccination but are not untruthful about it, as in option D.

Recommended reading

General Medical Council (2013), *Good Medical Practice*, paragraphs 28–30.
NHS Choices, *Adult Flu Vaccine: Frequently Asked Questions*.

1.30 Out of practice

D A E B C

Medical careers are varied and when rotating from job to job you will need to be able to pick up new skills and recall old ones quickly. You will frequently find that you have forgotten how to do some things well, and in these circumstances, you need to take responsibility for your own learning and become competent again quickly. The best way to get help is to discuss retraining opportunities with your educational supervisor (D); by doing this, you can set goals and they will be able to support you in reaching them. The next best response is option A: your colleagues who practise these skills every day are excellent people to learn from, and it is in their best interests that you learn them well so that the work can be shared. Revising the procedure privately will help you (E), but learning face-to-face is much more effective when working on practical procedures than trying to remember it yourself by simulation. Option B is a fair response as you have learnt these procedures and performed them in the past, so – with sensible awareness of your limitations – having a go at a minor procedure such as cannulation is good for your learning. Option C is irresponsible and misses out on a vital learning opportunity as well as burdening your colleagues, so it is the most inappropriate response.

Recommended reading

General Medical Council (2013), *Good Medical Practice*, paragraphs 7–13.

1.31 Shooting

D B A C E

Injuries secondary to the use of a dangerous weapon need to be reported to the police. This question tackles how you balance your responsibility to protect your patient's confidentiality and your duty of care to the public by reporting this serious incident. Option D is the best response; the question doesn't contain a lot of detail as to why the patient doesn't want the accident reported, so if you can find this out you can better support your patient with these issues, and you will find it easier to explain why you need to report the matter to the police. Option B is the next best response since, as a junior doctor, it is unlikely that you have dealt with a situation like this before, and some advice and input from a senior colleague is valuable. It is also a good idea to inform senior colleagues as the patient may decide to leave untreated if he feels the police will be informed without his consent, and he could come to harm. Option A is the next best response; each trust will have a named Caldicott Guardian, who is available to give advice on patient confidentiality. However, when sharing of information is appropriate, a senior team member should ideally be involved first. Telling the patient that you will have to inform the police (C) is entirely correct since, in doing so, you are being open and honest with the patient. However, without knowing more information about the incident and without knowing how much to tell the police, this approach is likely to distress and worry the patient unnecessarily. Option E ranks last as you should always inform a patient if you have to break their confidentiality and explain why. You should also discuss the amount of information that you can safely share with a senior doctor or Caldicott Guardian to prevent sharing of unneccesary private information.

Recommended reading
General Medical Council (2009), Explanatory guidance, in *Confidentiality: Reporting Gunshot and Knife Wounds*.

1.32 Good Samaritan

C B D E A
In the UK a doctor has no legal obligation to offer assistance in a community-based emergency situation. However, the GMC states that, in an emergency, you must offer your assistance and provide a level of care that could reasonably be expected in the situation. You should, however, be aware of the limits of your own competence and warn the patient of those limits. Informing the staff of your alcohol consumption (C) is therefore the best response in this situation and preferable to simply giving your help (B). While giving the crew advice (D) offers some assistance, you would better serve the passenger by going to assist them. If you wait to see if someone else goes forward (E), the passenger may deteriorate while you wait, which is unacceptable. Failing to volunteer in an emergency situation (A), unless in exceptional circumstances, is entirely inappropriate and may risk your professional registration.

Recommended reading
General Medical Council (2013), *Good Medical Practice*, paragraph 9.
Shepherd B, Macpherson D, Edwards C. (2006), In-flight emergencies: Playing the good Samaritan, *Journal of the Royal Society of Medicine*, 99(12), 628–631.

1.33 Death certificate

A E H
According to the GMC: 'your professional responsibility does not come to an end when a patient dies'. As such you also have responsibility to a patient's relatives. A death certificate is important to relatives as it enables them to carry out a funeral and achieve a sense of closure over the death of their loved one. Death certificates should therefore be completed without unnecessary delay. In this scenario, while your shift has come to an end, you should still try to ensure that the certificate is completed. You should tell the bereavement office that your shift has ended, but you should also help in locating another appropriate doctor to complete the certificate. A doctor who made an entry in the notes prior to your last entry may be appropriate (H). You could also ask a colleague who knew the patient to complete it (A) and/or give the bereavement office the bleep number for an appropriate person for them to contact (E). This is in contrast to option G, which is inappropriate, since the person completing the death certificate should have known the patient when alive. It is not the responsibility

of the ward sister to find a doctor, as in option B. Simply declining to complete the death certificate is inappropriate as it does not offer a solution (D) and waiting until your next shift, as in option C, would cause an unnecessary delay. Option F would ensure that the certificate is completed in a timely manner; however, you should not be required to come back to work during your scheduled time off.

Recommended reading

General Medical Council (2010), Explanatory guidance, in *Treatment and Care Towards the End of Life: Good Practice in Decision Making*, paragraphs 83–85.

1.34 Near-miss event

C   E   B   A   D

'Near-miss' events are a valuable opportunity for learning and problem identification. Reviewing chest x-rays for NG tube placement is a very common task for junior doctors to be asked to undertake. Feeding through an incorrectly placed NG tube is a 'never-event' and has the potential to cause serious harm and even death. Your first priority is to ensure that the patient is out of danger (C). Following this, you must assess the situation and establish an action plan. The best course of action would be to seek help from a senior colleague (E). They will be able to offer advice; it may be that all the junior doctors in the trust require further support with the topic, in which case training could be scheduled. Ignoring the situation (D) is the least appropriate option as by doing so you are not preventing the issue from occurring again in the future, and you have not ensured that your patient is safe. Asking for a senior's opinion on NG tube placement chest x-rays in future (A) may be appropriate in the short term; however, you must develop as a doctor and take on a level of responsibility appropriate for your position by learning to do this yourself. Completing a personal learning program covering NG tube placement (B) could be an appropriate course of action; however, this would not help identify whether this issue was widespread or not.

Recommended reading

General Medical Council (2012), Explanatory guidance, in *Raising and Acting on Concerns about Patient Safety*, paragraph 11.

1.35 Advising friend

E   D   A   C   B

If you give advice to your friend you are accepting a duty of care towards them, which makes you responsible for any investigation or treatment that could be indicated. You should not make the decision that the mole is benign (B) as you are very vulnerable to both ethical and legal criticism, particularly if this is incorrect. Reassuring your friend that their lesion does not appear worrying and asking to re-examine further down the line (C) is a slightly better response because you are making an attempt to further evaluate the mole rather than simply making a one-off assessment. However, this still leaves the duty of care entirely with you. Although it is inappropriate to informally get an opinion from one of your seniors (A), and this colleague would probably be unwilling to be involved if they realised what you were doing, at least you would be trying to ensure that you are not the only professional who has seen the lesion. The best approach is to encourage your friend to see their own GP (options D and E), thus declining to have a duty of care towards them. It is safest not to give any opinion (E) as, if you reassure your friend, this may make them less likely to subsequently make an appointment to see their GP.

Recommended reading
General Medical Council (2013), *Good Medical Practice*, paragraph 16.

1.36 Consenting

A   B   E   D   C
This question highlights the importance of taking informed consent. General Medical Council (GMC) guidance states that you should only gain consent for procedures that you have either been trained to perform or that you have been trained to consent for. However, as there are local guidelines available for consenting and your consultant is unavailable, in this situation, it would be appropriate for you to consent the patient in your consultant's absence (A). Patient information leaflets can certainly be a useful aid to verbal explanations but should not be used as a substitute (E). For this reason, asking your SpR to help may be more suitable (B). While using information from a textbook can be useful (D), it is unlikely to have all the necessary information or be as up to date as local policies on the intranet. You should explain the risks and benefits of any procedure when gaining consent, and if you are unable to do this, you should endeavour to find out the information before the patient consents. It would therefore be inappropriate for the patient to sign his name before being fully informed. Obtaining consent is a requirement for any procedure, but in this particular case, it should be written and completed in a timely manner. Option C is therefore the least appropriate response as you are not being proactive in completing the task that may consequently delay investigation and future treatment.

Recommended reading
General Medical Council (2008), Explanatory guidance, in *Consent: Patients and Doctors Making Decisions Together*.
General Medical Council (2009), *Tomorrow's Doctors*, paragraphs 14, 20.
General Medical Council (2013), *Good Medical Practice*, paragraphs 17, 32, 68.
Medical Protection Society (2012), *MPS Guide to Ethics: A Map for the Moral Maze*, chapter 4: Duty of care.

1.37 Removing chest drain

D E B C A

It is absolutely imperative that you and your colleagues practise medicine within the boundaries of your competence to protect patient safety and to protect yourself from legal challenges if something goes wrong. The best response here is option D; if your registrar could come back to supervise you, you would be able to learn how to remove a chest drain and ensure that a competent doctor is present at the time to deal with any complications. Option E is the next best response as, when struggling to work with a specialist piece of equipment such as a chest drain, it is a good idea to get advice from the people who use it the most, in this case the respiratory or cardiothoracic team. They would also be able to tell you if they thought that removing it unsupervised was an appropriate thing to do. Option B is the third best response because although you would be showing a poor working relationship with your colleague by asking the nursing staff to 'guard' the patient for you, the patient is at least protected against an under-qualified doctor who could cause serious harm. Options C and A rank last because they involve your FY1 colleague going ahead with the chest drain removal. Option C is marginally less bad than A because you are not implicating yourself and supporting your colleague by removing it with them; however, you would still be doing nothing to stop them.

Recommended reading
General Medical Council (2013), *Good Medical Practice*, Duties of a doctor.

1.38 Poor teaching

B C G

The General Medical Council (GMC) states that 'you must keep your knowledge and skills up to date throughout your working life'. Your education is your own responsibility; therefore, in this scenario, you are obliged to act when the teaching you receive does not meet your expectations. Discussing your concerns with your educational supervisor (B) is a good response since their role is to support your learning. Option C is also an acceptable response since the issue is more likely to be resolved if a greater number of FY1s are raising a similar concern. If you feel that the current session topics are not useful, then a constructive approach would be to suggest topics that you and your colleagues do consider useful (G). Volunteering to lead a session (H) assumes that you will deliver a better standard of teaching and does not provide a long-term solution. While filling in an anonymous feedback form (D) may be appropriate, it is less likely to promote change than the previously discussed responses. You are expected to attend the scheduled FY1 teaching; therefore, avoiding the sessions, even if you do make constructive use of the time, is inappropriate (options E and F). Failing to address your concerns (A) is completely inappropriate and shows a poor attitude towards your work, your colleagues and your professional identity.

Recommended reading
General Medical Council (2013), *Good Medical Practice*, paragraph 12.
Medical Protection Society (2012), *MPS Guide to Ethics: A Map for the Moral Maze*, chapter 10: Competence.

1.39 Mentoring

E B A D C
Part of a doctor's role involves teaching as well as providing adequate supervision to those who are learning. The best way for the student to practise her skills is to learn through performing the cannulation. However, given the student's inexperience, this should be under your supervision, as in option E. Options A and B are also appropriate since they too give the student an opportunity to learn. Observing you (B), however, is a more favourable option than practising on a dummy (A). The student has already had experience with a dummy arm, and it is important to learn how to interact with and gain consent from patients for procedures such as cannulation. Putting the cannula in yourself without giving any teaching does not fulfil your role as a teacher, and sending an inexperienced student to cannulate alone may result in harm to the patient. Options D and C are therefore inappropriate.

Recommended reading
General Medical Council (2013), *Good Medical Practice*, paragraphs 39, 40, 42.
Medical Protection Society (2012), *MPS Guide to Ethics: A Map for the Moral Maze*, chapter 10: Competence.

1.40 Procedure confidence

B D C E A
If you do not feel completely confident in performing an examination or technique, it is useful to adopt the mentoring approach. This involves learning the scientific basis for a technique, then observing a competent mentor performing the technique and finally carrying out the technique yourself with a mentor who can give guidance and advice while you are building up your own competence. In this scenario, you have already successfully carried out the technique but feel out of practice. Therefore, the most appropriate option would be to talk through the procedure with another GP (a mentor) and then ask the GP to observe you while you perform the examination (B). Observing another GP performing the technique (D) may be useful if you feel that you could not perform the examination, but as you are simply lacking in confidence with the technique, it is likely that you only need some assistance and support. Booking an appointment with another GP (C) could result in a delay to the patient's treatment and would also be a missed learning opportunity for yourself. Performing a speculum examination without mentor supervision (E) may mean that the patient experiences pain or that you are unable to complete the examination if you do it incorrectly. This could also damage your confidence with this examination and impact your future practice. However, this is preferable

to option A, which would cause diagnostic delays, and if the patient returned to see you again, you would still have the same issues.

Recommended reading
Medical Protection Society (2012), *MPS Guide to Ethics: A Map for the Moral Maze*, chapter 10: Competence.

1.41 Time pressures and teaching

D F H

You should support the student to carry out cannulation. Although you are busy, your jobs are routine, and you have a responsibility to work with students. In addition, the student has already had teaching by simulation. Options E and G are therefore not the most appropriate as they avoid facilitating practical participation of the student. Option A is also avoidant, and it is likely that the FY2 is busy too. Handing responsibility for the student over to them may be seen as unfair team-working. It is important to inform patients of the level of skill of the person performing a procedure if you think that this information may affect their decision to consent. Option B is therefore not one of the most appropriate, whereas option F is one of the best answers. The student has not carried out the procedure before, so it is important for them to be supervised (H), which both ensures patient safety and supports the student to build their confidence. This makes option C inappropriate since it is an inadequate level of supervision for the first attempt at a skill. Delegating appropriately to team members is important in managing your workload. Asking the student to carry out the clerking for you prior to doing the cannulas together (D) is a deal which benefits both of you, especially as clerking is also educationally valuable for the student. Option D is therefore one of the best options.

Recommended reading
Foundation Programme Curriculum (2012), section 1.5: Leadership; section 12: procedures.

Medical Protection Society (2012), *MPS Guide to Ethics: A Map for the Moral Maze*, chapter 10: Competence, sections: Acquiring and developing new skills, mentoring.

1.42 Prescribing limits

D A B E C

FY1 doctors are not allowed to prescribe or transcribe cytotoxic or immunosuppressant drugs. The worst response is therefore one that involves prescribing the immunosuppressant (C). The best course of action is to prescribe acute antibiotics, which is within your competence and can be done following local protocol, and leave the prescription of the immunosuppressant to your registrar (D). This is better than prescribing nothing (A) as there is no reason why you shouldn't prescribe antibiotics and delaying this could be harmful. It would be advisable to get input from seniors within your team before consulting another team (B), but this response is a safe one and may be useful further down the line. Whatever you decide, you should not make the decision to discontinue the immunosuppressant (E). This response ranks second last because it makes no mention of alerting seniors, so the patient could miss doses of their immunosuppressant based solely on your decision, which would be dangerous. However, this is still safer than breaking the rules and prescribing the immunosuppressant (C).

Recommended reading
Foundation Programme Curriculum (2012), section 7.5: Safe prescribing.
UK Foundation Programme Guidance Note on Prescribing Cytotoxic and
    Immunosuppressant Drugs. Available from: http://www.rcoa.ac.uk/sites/
    default/files/TRG-AMRC-CHEMO.pdf.

1.43 Choosing training

D E B C A
It is important to choose training based on skills you need to develop, not just based on what you enjoy or find interesting. You will soon be in a position where you need good adult resuscitation skills. The options which include attending an ALS course therefore rank higher than options which do not. Option D is therefore the best response because it is better to be prepared ahead of starting the job. If you wait to organise training until starting cardiology (E), you will have to attend arrests prior to the course, when you may not be fully competent. Although your career path is focused on paediatrics, it is not a priority at this point in terms of competence; however, option B is better than C because it concerns resuscitation and therefore may include some transferrable skills. Option A is the worst option because it involves not taking responsibility for your training needs. Sometimes it is necessary to use your time off for training in order to maintain your competence.

Recommended reading
General Medical Council (2011), *The Trainee Doctor*, paragraph 37.
Medical Protection Society (2012), *MPS Guide to Ethics: A Map for the Moral
    Maze*, chapter 10: Competence, section: Maintaining basic standards.

1.44 Surgical error

B C E
Part of being a competent doctor is being able to admit when you have made a mistake, both to your colleagues and to the patient. In this case, the mistake was not made by you, therefore you should urge the registrar to own up to the mistake (options B and C) rather than informing others about it yourself. However, if the registrar does not wish to own up to their mistake, then option E is appropriate as the consultant should be made aware of what happened in the theatre since the overriding responsibility for the patient lies with them,

and the case will likely need to be brought up at a morbidity and mortality meeting. Option A is not appropriate as someone needs to be made aware of the mistake, particularly the patient. While discussing the case with your educational supervisor (D) would be a good idea, this will not lead to an improved outcome for the patient. Going over the registrar's head to their supervisor (F) is not a good idea, especially if you are questioning their abilities when you are junior to them and were not present at the initial operation. Options G and H are not appropriate responses as the mistake is not yours to explain and placing blame on the registrar in front of the patient will increase the likelihood of legal action being taken. As an FY1 you are also not qualified to perform this procedure and therefore are not the correct person to counsel the patient on this matter.

Recommended reading

General Medical Council (February 2013), 'Doctors make mistakes', in *GMC Student News*.

Medical Protection Society (2012), *MPS Guide to Ethics: A Map for the Moral Maze*, chapter 10: Competence, section: When things go wrong.

1.45 Performing new tasks

A   F   H

Suturing is one of the practical competencies set out in *Tomorrow's Doctors* that graduates are expected to have achieved; however, many people find it difficult the first time they perform it in a real situation. Options H and F are perhaps the most appropriate responses here as they involve you admitting your uncertainty to the consultant and either asking for supervision or allowing the consultant to make the decision themself. Although delaying the consultant from consenting other patients in his theatre list is not ideal, option A still ranks in the top three as it will hopefully enable you to perform suturing at some point in the future to improve your skills. While options D and G are good responses in that they are unlikely to cause the patient to come to harm, neither are in the top three because declining the opportunity will not allow you to improve your competence and having the consultant come back to check the sutures will delay the list. Option E also prevents the patient coming to harm but again results in you not having the chance to improve your skills. The two remaining responses (B and C) are not appropriate because simply performing the sutures if you do not feel competent is unprofessional, and scrub nurses are not trained in performing suturing and are therefore not appropriate supervisors.

Recommended reading

General Medical Council (2013), *Good Medical Practice*, paragraphs 9, 16d.

Medical Protection Society (2012), *MPS Guide to Ethics: A Map for the Moral Maze*, chapter 10: Competence, section: Maintaining competence.

1.46 Career progression

D C A E B

Maintaining the required training is important for all doctors. As an FY2 doctor you will still need to gain general medical experience regardless of your future career plans. While doctors may use their study leave days to attend extra training that may help their career progression, all doctors must attend basic training. Talking to the FY2 one-to-one is the best option here rather than immediately going to their educational supervisor, which is why options C and D rank higher than A. Option D ranks highest as successful completion of all mandatory training during the FY2 year is important for career progression. Option C comes next as it is important to keep up to date with medicine. Option E ranks higher than B as, even though attending extra training is useful, it is not appropriate to miss the core training to do this, and the FY2 should be told this.

Recommended reading

General Medical Council (June 2012), *Continuing Professional Development: Guidance for all Doctors.*

Medical Protection Society (2012), *MPS Guide to Ethics: A Map for the Moral Maze*, chapter 10: Competence.

1.47 Tourniquet

A F G

This question assesses your response when things go wrong at work. It is important first and foremost to own up to any mistake (G), to take steps to minimise further risk to the patient and then to report it through the correct local channels. This often takes the form of an incident report (F) which should be completed as soon as possible after the event takes place. In addition to the formalities, you must always maintain open and trustworthy relationships with your patients and, therefore, apologising to and reassuring the patient is another important task that should be completed imminently (A). Option C would not be incorrect; however, in this situation, a colleague has alerted you to the mistake, and it is arguably unlikely that you would need to check other patients. While FY1 colleagues can be useful sources of some information (B), in this instance there should be no need to consult colleagues as you should always own up to your mistakes. Denying blame (D) is dishonest and contravenes many of the duties of a doctor, in particular 'be honest, open and act with integrity'. This behaviour could lead to further disciplinary action. Option E is similarly dishonest, and despite apologising to the patient, it does not deal with the mistake in a professional manner. Discussing the incident with your educational supervisor (H) is certainly a good idea in the slightly longer term; however, it is not one of the first things you should do.

Recommended reading

General Medical Council (2013), *Good Medical Practice*, Duties of a doctor.

General Medical Council (2013), *Good Medical Practice*, paragraphs 19, 22, 23, 25, 32, 55, 65, 68.

Medical Protection Society (2012), *MPS Guide to Ethics: A Map for the Moral Maze*, chapter 10: Competence.

1.48 Ordering incorrect test

E D C A B

This question assesses how you deal with making mistakes in clinical practice, in particular with regards to communication with the patient, your colleagues and the steps you take to minimise harm. In this scenario, a CT scan may be very helpful in providing more information about the clinical condition of the patient; however, this should be balanced with the additional risk of radiation exposure from another CT scan. Option E is the most appropriate response initially as it is important to be honest with your colleagues about mistakes, and your consultant may wish to come and speak to the patient. You also need to check whether they would like another CT scan to be requested. This is possible on the phone; therefore, it is a more suitable response than option A. Option D is the second most appropriate as it demonstrates a proactive attitude and means that, when explaining the situation to the patient, you can reassure them that you are taking steps to rectify it. Option C is important as you must be open and honest with patients; however, there are other steps to take first. The least appropriate response would be to keep quiet about your mistake (B). This is unprofessional and does not show honesty or respect for the patient.

Recommended reading

General Medical Council (2013), *Good Medical Practice*, Duties of a doctor.

General Medical Council (2013), *Good Medical Practice*, paragraphs 15, 16, 17, 25, 31, 47, 49, 55, 65, 68.

Medical Protection Society (2012), *MPS Guide to Ethics: A Map for the Moral Maze*, chapter 10: Competence.

1.49 NG tube

B A C E D

Gaining competence in clinical skills through direct observation of practical skills (DOPS) is an important part of the foundation curriculum and is necessary in order to progress through your medical career. This question highlights the balance that is required between facilitating new learning opportunities and maintaining patient safety. Your initial response in this situation should be option B as this ensures both of these aspects and also courteously informs your senior that you are unhappy to work beyond the limits of your competence. The person observing needs to be trained in this skill, however, and it may be a more junior member of the team that is most suitable. Conversely, passing the NG tube without appropriate supervision (D) would be negligent, even if you do use a chaperone and check the position of the tube with a chest x-ray. Asking your SHO to supervise and using this situation as a learning experience (A) is the second best option. This is more proactive than asking your registrar to pass the NG tube (C) as you are capable of doing it but simply need to exercise the correct precautions. This response would not only waste a chance to expand your learning but would also unnecessarily impact a colleague's workload. Similarly, this would be the case in option E, which would delay patient care and fails to enact your consultant's request.

Recommended reading
General Medical Council (2009), *The New Doctor*, paragraphs 6, 7, 63.
General Medical Council (2009), *Tomorrow's Doctors*, paragraphs 6, 21.
General Medical Council (2013), *Good Medical Practice*, Duties of a doctor.
General Medical Council (2013), *Good Medical Practice*, paragraphs 9, 14.
Medical Protection Society (2012), *MPS Guide to Ethics: A Map for the Moral Maze*, chapter 10: Competence.

1.50 Audit

B A E C D
This question assesses your ability to facilitate your own learning and commitment to professionalism, while improving care for patients. Conducting an audit (B) is a proactive way of trying to improve the quality of service provision in your department and is an important activity that should be completed within your foundation years. Contacting your clinical supervisor (A) is also sensible and perhaps more appropriate than options E and C as, by doing this, you would still be working to benefit your team. They may also have good suggestions of how you can use your time to fulfil your training needs. Assisting in theatre can be a useful learning opportunity (E), but it would result in neglecting your commitment to the team in which you have been assigned. It is slightly more preferable to option C, however, in which you have not informed your team of your actions. Option D is inappropriate when there are many other opportunities for you to develop your learning and contribute to improving patient care; watching the news is a worthwhile activity but should be kept for leisure time.

Recommended reading
General Medical Council (2009), *The New Doctor*, paragraphs 7, 33, 63, 116.
General Medical Council (2013), *Good Medical Practice*, paragraphs 9, 13, 22.
Medical Protection Society (2012), *MPS Guide to Ethics: A Map for the Moral Maze*, chapter 10: Competence.

1.51 Unfamiliar with equipment

A C E D B
Once you have identified a gap in your knowledge or skill set, you should work to set this right. In this scenario, it is important to be proficient at this skill for future emergency situations; therefore, you should be proactive in

organising necessary training. The most appropriate action would therefore be A, asking a colleague to demonstrate the skill. Contacting your foundation programme director to arrange teaching on this skill (C) could result in training, but there could be a delay in arranging this teaching, and administering adrenaline during an arrest is a simple skill that shouldn't require structured training. Revising the BLS guidelines (E) may be useful for your general emergency knowledge, but it would be better to seek out practical teaching for this situation. Avoiding administering the drug in future cardiac arrests (D) is not a professional way of dealing with a lack of knowledge as it is important to learn and improve for the future. Filling in an incident form (B) would be unnecessary and irrelevant as the patient has not come to harm.

Recommended reading
General Medical Council (2013), *Good Medical Practice*, paragraphs 7–9.
Medical Protection Society (2012), *MPS Guide to Ethics: A Map for the Moral Maze*, chapter 10: Competence.

1.52 Confused patient pre-theatre

A C G
Patients' capacity can change and that can have an impact on the consent they have already given for procedures. In this scenario, a capacity assessment would need to be made to assess if the surgery should continue without the patient's consent. To get more information about her confusion, asking nursing staff is a good start (A) as they spend a lot more time directly with patients. New onset confusion can be a symptom of acute illness, so you should begin to investigate the cause appropriately, making option G an appropriate course of action. The final appropriate response here is option C: your registrar should be made aware of this patient's confusion and refusal to go to theatre as this could affect the day's list, and it would be wrong to send her to theatre without a full capacity assessment. The inappropriate responses in this scenario include: getting unnecessary reviews of the patient by psychiatry without first investigating the cause yourself (D); ignoring the situation (E): sending a patient to theatre when she refuses consent can amount to assault; cancelling the surgery before investigating the cause for the patient's confusion and her reasons for refusal (F), which is a bit rash; and waiting to see if the patient improves (H). This final response involves delaying a decision, and even if the patient does improve, your seniors should still be aware of their deterioration as it may be more appropriate to delay the surgery until a cause for the confusion has been found.

Recommended reading
Mental Capacity Act 2005 (2012), section 1. Medical Protection Society, *Consent to Medical Treatment* booklet, General advice on assessing capacity: Fluctuating capacity.

1.53 Coercion end of life

C D E B A

This question deals with the complicated ethical issue of patient coercion. If you feel that patients are behaving in a certain way because of pressures from others, such as family members, staff, or those with a financial interest, it is your duty to find out what the patient actually wants and to protect them from outside influences. In this question, it seems as if the patient had decided upon an end-of-life plan, yet, after only one meeting with an unfamiliar family member, he changed his opinion completely. The best response is to find out what actually happened during that meeting and ask the patient to clarify his new end-of-life wishes (C). The next best response is to speak to the palliative care team (D) who are very experienced in end-of-life ethical issues and will be able to offer support and advice regarding the potential coercion of this patient. Option E is the third best response since this is a complex end of life scenario, your registrar or even consultant should be involved to ensure that the patient is fully protected. Seeking legal advice (B) could also be considered if you believe that the patient has been persuaded by his son to withdraw from treatment. You will need to get some advice about how to act within the law, whether to leave this situation alone or go against the patient's new wishes and continue to hydrate him. However, this situation could potentially be resolved without involving external agencies, so escalating to your immediate seniors is more appropriate at this stage. Option A ranks last; you need to be careful when broaching the topic of coercion with his son as this is a serious accusation. It would be wise to leave this conversation to a senior doctor, if and when it becomes necessary.

Recommended reading
Mr Leslie Burke v GMC (2005), EWCA Civ 1003.

1.54 Needlestick

D A C E B

Needlestick injuries pose a difficult situation whereby you, as a doctor, become vulnerable to potential harm from a patient, and both parties require appropriate medical investigation and counselling. Option D is therefore the best course of action since by reporting this to your ward manager both you and the patient can receive the correct counselling. A risk assessment can also be undertaken and post-exposure prophylaxis can be given if necessary. It is always more favourable for an unexposed member of staff to approach the patient to gain consent (A), rather than the exposed one (C), so that the consenting doctor can remain impartial. It is inappropriate to test the patient for communicable diseases without their consent (E), and if a positive result were obtained, this would pose a further ethical and legal dilemma. To do nothing is irresponsible (B) since you put your own health at risk and pose a potential risk to your future patients if you unknowingly contract a serious communicable disease.

Recommended reading

British Medical Association (2009), *Consent Toolkit*, Card 12: Serious
    communicable diseases.
General Medical Council (2013), *Good Medical Practice*, paragraphs 17, 28.
Medical Protection Society (2013), *MPS Factsheet: Needlestick Injuries.*

1.55 Consenting

C B A E D

As your registrar will be performing the operation, it is his responsibility to
discuss the procedure with the patient and obtain consent (C). You are neither
trained nor qualified to consent the patient yourself, so options E and D are
unsuitable; however, in this situation, E would provide more accurate information to the patient and therefore ranks higher. The consultant from your
team would be your second choice (B) since, although he is not performing the
procedure, he has overall responsibility for the patient. The consultant from
the other team (A) would be qualified with specific knowledge of the proposed
operation, but it would be inappropriate to disrupt his activities before your
own consultant.

Recommended reading

General Medical Council (2008), Explanatory guidance, *Consent: Patients and
    Doctors Making Decisions Together*, paragraph 26.

1.56 Consent for student

D C E A B

As an FY1, it is common to have medical students attached to your team. While
it is part of the foundation programme curriculum to develop your teaching
skills, your priorities always lie with the patient. Although the patient has given
consent beforehand, they always have the right to withdraw the consent at any-
time. In this case the patient is complaining of feeling tired and dizzy. This could
be a symptom of progression in their illness or deterioration in their health, so a
full assessment by you is the most appropriate course of action (D). While your
registrar may need to see the patient as well (C), they will be busy with a number
of other tasks and should not be disturbed before you have assessed the patient
yourself. Completing the students' examination quickly (B) is entirely inappropriate because the patient has withdrawn consent to take part in teaching, and this
could make them feel worse. While leaving the bedside would prevent the students from harming the patient, this would not lead to you assessing the patient
(E). Option E is preferable to A, however, as this would provide the students with
education and yourself with an opportunity to practise teaching; however, it
would still not assess the patient, which should be your primary concern.

Recommended reading

General Medical Council (2008), Explanatory guidance, *Consent: Patients and
    Doctors Making Decisions Together*, paragraph 9h.

1.57 Dementia and consent

A D E

This question deals with the issue of a patient who may lack capacity. You must remember that you should always assume a patient to have capacity. In order to assess capacity, the patient needs to be able to understand, retain and weigh up the information given to them and then also be able to communicate a response to that information. Capacity is also decision-specific, meaning that every time a new decision is made, capacity must be reassessed. For this reason, in this situation, it is necessary for you to assess capacity (D) as it would be inappropriate to assume this without an assessment, as in options F and G. If a patient does lack capacity, it is advisable to contact those closest to the patient so that a decision can be made in the patient's best interests. Options A and E are also therefore the most suitable responses in this scenario. It would be inappropriate to simply inform the relatives/carers about the planned therapeutic course (H) as this would not demonstrate collaborative decision-making nor can you assume that this would be complying with the patient's wishes. Option B is not appropriate as you (and the ward sister) are unable to consent for a procedure that you are neither trained to carry out nor to consent for; in addition, this assumes capacity in a patient with severe dementia. You are also not involving those closest to the patient, which is equally important in difficult situations such as this. Asking a colleague to telephone the carers (C) is unnecessary because, as an FY1, you should be able to speak to the family on the phone, and it would be unnecessarily impacting another colleague's time.

Recommended reading

General Medical Council (2008), Explanatory guidance, *Consent: Patients and Doctors Making Decisions Together*.

General Medical Council (2013), *Good Medical Practice*; paragraphs 17, 21, 27, 31–34, 49, 60.

Medical Protection Society (2012), *MPS Guide to Ethics: A Map for the Moral Maze*, chapter 8: Patient autonomy and consent.

1.58 Disclosure after death

A D C B E

The best thing to do with phone calls from people whom you do not know is to take a number and call them back (A) so that you can verify that they are legitimate. In this case, you could ask which law firm they work at so that you can ensure that the number is real; this way you can have important conversations and be sure that they are with the correct person. Option D is the next best course of action as by remaining neutral, you would not accidentally disclose any confidential information. Option C is a good response if you are unsure what to do in this setting as nurses take phone calls far more commonly than doctors and so are often better at dealing with calls where the identity of the caller is uncertain. Confidentiality extends beyond death and therefore telling someone you do not know that Mrs Green died (B) would still be breaking her confidentiality. Option E is the worst response here as you would be confirming that Mrs Green has died and that you are the one signing the death certificate, therefore giving information out about both the patient and yourself.

Recommended reading

General Medical Council (2009), Explanatory guidance, *Confidentiality*, paragraphs 70, 71 and 72 (Disclosure after a patient's death).

Medical Protection Society (2012), *MPS Guide to Ethics: A Map for the Moral Maze*, chapter 9: Confidentiality.

1.59 Drug problems

A C D

In this situation, the best thing to do is to make your consultant aware of the difficulty you have with the situation as, by knowing the couple, you are personally involved and are at risk of breaking confidentiality, either by accident or on purpose to protect your friend and her child. The best responses here are therefore options A, C and D: to immediately remove yourself from the room and subsequently share with your consultant both your concerns and your personal difficulty with the situation. Option B is obviously a breach of confidence and, as an FY1, it would be inappropriate for you to counsel someone on child protection and drug rehabilitation. Discussing the situation again is an obvious breach of confidentiality, which therefore makes options E and G inappropriate. While informing their GP of the situation (F) is, of course, important, there are other people in the team who could do this, and you are much safer staying completely out of the case. The situation could be potentially dangerous for the child, but you shouldn't immediately try and remove the child from the father's care as this is potentially damaging for the entire family, and a social worker would be a much better person to liaise with the family around this. This is also the case for option H, so you should instead give the consultant all this information (A) and then be removed from the situation.

Recommended reading

General Medical Council (2009), Explanatory guidance, *Confidentiality*, paragraphs 12 and 13.

Medical Protection Society (2012), *MPS Guide to Ethics: A Map for the Moral Maze*, chapter 9: Confidentiality.

1.60 Friends with problems

A E B D C

In this scenario, the only correct way to act is not to allow your friend to know you have found out medical information about him and to try and treat him in exactly the same way as before. This is a difficult situation, especially when it concerns a mental health diagnosis. Unless your friend seeks your help regarding this problem, you cannot approach the subject with him. The best option from here on is to check all patients' names before you see their records (A), which would prevent you from finding out personal medical details about them. It would also be wise to discuss this with the GP (E) as they may have some helpful advice for you, and it would also make them aware that you may know other registered patients. Getting up and immediately leaving the room (B), while appearing strange initially, could easily be explained to the GP after the telephone consultation, and the GP is likely to be very understanding. Offering support to your friend (D) would be a caring thing to do, but it is not appropriate since this would alert him that you have discovered confidential information about him. Reading through his notes (C) is an obvious breach of confidentiality and is the worst option in this scenario.

Recommended reading
Medical Protection Society (2012), *MPS Guide to Ethics: A Map for the Moral Maze*, chapter 9: Confidentiality.

1.61 DVLA

C B E D A

In situations where a patient might put others at serious risk of harm or death, you can disclose their medical information to other organisations in the interests of protecting others. The responsibility for informing the DVLA lies with the patient; however, if a patient informs you that he fully intends to drive with a condition that could endanger the lives of others, you should intervene. The best response here is to sit with the patient and discuss the reasons why you think it is safer to abstain from driving and discuss with him his reasons for refusing (C). You could offer the advice and help of a social worker regarding the support he could claim while out of work. The second best response would be to talk to the patient's wife about your concerns (B). His wife would be well placed to advise the patient from a personal perspective, providing the patient consents to you sharing this information with his wife. Option E is the third best response; before disclosing medical information to others, a Caldicott Guardian can advise you on how much you need to share, which can prevent you breaking confidentiality unnecessarily. Every trust will have a Caldicott Guardian, whose role is to advise on the sharing of patient information. Option D is the fourth best response since breaking confidentiality is justified in this scenario; however, to ensure you approach the breach appropriately and only share what is necessary, you should discuss this with a senior, a Caldicott Guardian or your medico-legal malpractice insurer first. Calling the police (A) ranks last since this man has not committed a crime and may reconsider his reflex decision to continue driving. Additionally, informing the police will distress the patient and is not indicated at this stage. If you witnessed your patient subsequently driving with uncontrolled epilepsy, that might be an appropriate point at which to consider calling the police.

Recommended reading

General Medical Council (2009), *Confidentiality: Reporting Concerns about Patients to the DVLA or DVA.*

General Medical Council (2013), Explanatory guidance, *Confidentiality,* paragraph 53.

1.62 Fish and chips

C E A D B

Some particularly infectious diseases are 'notifiable' in the UK, which means they must be reported to a public health official. A list of these can be found on the website of the Health Protection Agency. The General Medical Council (GMC) views disclosures of serious infectious diseases in the interests of public safety; therefore, this is one of the scenarios in which confidentiality can and should be broken. The best response is to spend time with Mr Green and explain that only medical staff and those involved in investigating the cause of this infection will know about his illness (C). The second best option is E, asking one of the doctors who will be directly involved in the investigation to speak with Mr Green may alleviate some of his fears and answer his questions about the depth and publicity of the investigation. Informing the public health officers of his infection behind his back without his consent (A) is the next best option in this list. You do not need Mr Green's consent to disclose this information to the public health team, but you should always try and gain it first. Option D should rank after this: to give Mr Green some public health advice regarding staying off work while he is unwell is part of being a responsible doctor. This option is similar to advising patients with epilepsy to abstain from driving in order to protect the health of the wider public. Mr Green's confidentiality should only be broken to those who need to know in the public interest, so breaking it to the general public is both unnecessary and damaging to Mr Green's business. Option B is therefore ranked last.

Recommended reading

General Medical Council (2013), *Confidentiality,* Public interest: Disclosures in the public interest.

The Health Protection Agency (2010), Health Protection Regulations.

1.63 Lost patient list

B C A D E

As an FY1 doctor, confidentiality is central to the doctor–patient relationship. You should take care to avoid unintentional disclosure. Human error unfortunately means that this cannot always be avoided. Option B is the most appropriate course of action: you should apologise and inform the patient that the list is confidential and ask them not to divulge any information from it. Option C should be considered next. This is difficult as it may result in a negative effect on yourself, but you should remember that, as a doctor, you have a duty to put patients' interests first. It should also be noted that early recognition of an adverse event can allow issues to be tackled and problems to be put right. As a doctor, you should be able to reflect on events and provide alternatives, which may avoid the same mistakes in the future. Option A is an example of this as it would anonymise patient information; however, in this situation, this would not change the fact that your patient has already read your list. You may find option D useful, but it is not as important as options B, C and A. Option E is the least appropriate response as this prevents a concern being raised, discourages a culture of openness and would be unprofessional.

Recommended reading
General Medical Council (2009), Explanatory guidance, *Confidentiality*, paragraphs 12, 13, 16.
General Medical Council (2012), Explanatory guidance, *Raising and Acting on Concerns about Patient Safety*, paragraphs 2, 7, 9, 10, 11.

1.64 Driving against medical advice

B D E A C
Confidentiality is an important aspect of the doctor–patient relationship. However, it is important to note that confidentiality is not absolute, and there are a few exceptions. One such exception is disclosure in the public's best interest. After a first generalised unprovoked seizure, the DVLA states that the patient should have six months off driving from the date of the seizure. The patient should be informed that, firstly, the condition may affect their ability to drive, and secondly, it is the patient's legal responsibility to inform the DVLA. General Medical Council (GMC) guidance states that 'if a patient continues to drive … you should make every reasonable effort to persuade them to stop'. Option B is therefore the most appropriate response. The patient should be contacted to rediscuss their condition and the legal obligations associated with it. The GMC also says that you could talk to family, friends or carers if the patient agrees. After making reasonable effort and if the patient is still driving, you should contact the DVLA (D), and you should also inform the patient that you are doing this. Option E might be perceived as confrontational, unprofessional and beyond 'reasonable effort'. Option A is inappropriate as it is not the correct way of informing the authorities; however, it is better than option C, which would be neglecting your duties as a doctor.

Recommended reading
Driver and Vehicle Licensing Agency (2013), *For Medical Practitioners: At a Glance Guide to the Current Medical Standards of Fitness to Drive*, introduction: Notification to DVLA; chapter 1: Neurological disorders.
General Medical Council (2009), Explanatory guidance, *Confidentiality: Reporting Concerns about Patients to the DVLA or the DVA*.

1.65 Transferring computer files

D A C B E

The use of hospital computer systems is common during the foundation years and information is often transferred between devices. Patient confidentiality must be ensured at all times and maintaining the anonymity of images and text, while following local trust guidelines, is essential. In this case the best way to transfer images would be to send them over the dedicated trust network to the lecture theatre (D), which would ensure confidentiality. For this reason the least appropriate response would be to transfer the images to your personal memory stick (E). In general, this should never be done as memory sticks can be lost and could result in a breach of confidentiality. If you were unsure of how to transfer the images, the IT department would be willing to offer advice (A); however, that would take valuable time that could be spent completing other tasks. While rewriting the presentation would ensure confidentiality, it would not be a good use of your time (C). Leaving the images out of a presentation (B) would be detrimental to the learning of your colleagues and would therefore be unsuitable.

Recommended reading

General Medical Council (2009), Explanatory guidance, *Confidentiality*, paragraph 14.

1.66 Food poisoning

C A D E B

This is a difficult case because while gastroenteritis is not a notifiable disease, your patient is a takeaway chef and could therefore potentially put the public at risk. Agreeing with the patient after further discussion that he will stay away from work is the best course of action (options A and C). However, the patient is clearly anxious about keeping his job. In this case it would be courteous and helpful for the patient if you were to have a short discussion with his manager to inform them of the situation (C). While legally the patient can self-certify for his illness (A), in option C you would be responding to the patient's concerns by telephoning his place of work, and therefore this ranks higher. Contacting the public health authorities (D) would be appropriate if the patient refused to stay away from work and would ensure the safety of the public; however, this would be better left until after attempting to tackle the problem yourself. Giving the patient some extra antibiotics (B) would be clinically inappropriate and would still put the public at risk if he returned to work. Option E would prevent him from going to work; however, it would be a highly inappropriate admission for such a minor illness.

Recommended reading

General Medical Council (2009), Explanatory guidance, *Confidentiality*, paragraph 39.

Health Protection Agency (2010), *Health Protection (Notification) Regulations*; List of notifiable diseases.

1.67 Domestic violence and children

C   A   B   E   D

In this scenario, there are two parties involved, the patient in front of you and the children at home. This changes the scenario because there are vulnerable individuals at risk who may come to harm if you don't take action. The General Medical Council's *Confidentiality* guidelines suggest that 'you should usually abide by a competent adult patient's refusal to consent to disclosure, even if their decision leaves them, but nobody else, at serious risk of harm'. In this case, the children are potentially at risk so this can be ignored as disclosure would be necessary to protect them from a risk of serious harm. This therefore means that attempting to persuade the patient to inform the police herself (D), although both polite and empathetic to the patient, ranks last as in practice, it is unlikely to lead to this matter being brought to the attention of the appropriate bodies. Option C would be the first response as good communication would hopefully build rapport with the patient at this difficult time. This is quite a serious case, so involving senior colleagues early (A) would be appropriate. While treating the patient and then phoning social services (E) would hopefully ensure the patient and her children's safety, it does not demonstrate good communication and would be likely to harm the doctor–patient relationship. Telephoning the police immediately (B) could help to protect the children and would involve the patient in the process; however, further discussion with senior colleagues would be appropriate before escalating the situation.

Recommended reading

General Medical Council (2009), Explanatory guidance, *Confidentiality*, paragraphs 51, 63.

1.68 Coffee house discussion

E   D   A   B   C

Breaking confidentiality in a situation like this is relatively easy because when you are surrounded by your team, you can easily slip into discussing patients and then disclose confidential information. It is important to remember other potential breaches in this situation as well, for example leaving your list visible for people to see. Option E is clearly the best response here as it is important to make sure that the other doctor is aware of his mistake, but there is no need to highlight this in front of the team in a public place (D). However, it is better to mention the mistake in public than simply ignoring it completely (C) or changing the subject (A) as the doctor may then not realise his error and do it again. It is not appropriate to inform the patient (B) as it is not up to you to point out someone else's mistake. In this scenario, it appears that no one overheard the confidential information, so there is no need to push things further and risk a complaint against the doctor and the team, although this is perhaps better than saying nothing at all (C).

Recommended reading

General Medical Council (2009), Explanatory guidance, *Confidentiality*, paragraphs 12, 13.

Medical Protection Society (2012), *MPS Guide to Ethics: A Map for the Moral Maze*, chapter 9: Confidentiality.

1.69 Case note security

B D F

Confidentiality is intimately related to information governance, which is what this case concerns. Patients' notes contain a lot of personal information and therefore need respecting and protecting to ensure that people who are not concerned with their care cannot look at them. Option B would be a good response as this would discuss confidentiality in a non-confrontational way. Reminding your consultant about the importance of confidentiality would also be appropriate (D), but it would need some courage to take this line with your consultant. Suggesting that a trust-wide notice is distributed (F) would be a good response as well since it will prompt not only your consultant but also others within the trust to consider the confidentiality of case notes. Even if it were true that the consultant was out of the office for a very brief time only (G), this response doesn't involve doing anything about the potential breach in confidentiality. Waiting outside the office (A) is also appropriate as you shouldn't enter your consultant's office without permission when they are not there, which also means that option H is not a suitable course of action. Assuming that no non-staff will come across the notes within the consultant's office (C) may be true but is a very blasé approach to take.

Recommended reading

General Medical Council (2009), Explanatory guidance, *Confidentiality*, paragraphs 12, 13.

Medical Protection Society (2012), *MPS Guide to Ethics: A Map for the Moral Maze*, chapter 9: Confidentiality.

1.70 Food poisoning

A D B C E

This question requires you to break patient confidentiality in the interests of wider society. You must remember that food poisoning (if suspected to be caused by a public eatery) is a notifiable disease and must be disclosed to the relevant local health authority. In this scenario, as an FY1, it is probably wise to get advice from a senior with regard to notifying the relevant bodies (D); however, the first priority should be patient care, and therefore, you need to ensure timely, appropriate treatment is given first (A). If there is a delay in seeking senior help, however, the next most appropriate action to take would be to speak to the local authority yourself (B). It would also be sensible to let your colleagues know of the link between these cases (C), both as a matter of courtesy and to maintain good communication within the team. Sampling the restaurant's food (E) would be entirely inappropriate, and in this option, you risk both yourself and others contracting and passing on an infection as you fail to notify the authorities.

Recommended reading

General Medical Council (2013), *Good Medical Practice*, Duties of a doctor.
General Medical Council (2013), *Good Medical Practice*, paragraphs 11, 12, 22, 23, 50, 73.
Medical Protection Society (2012), *MPS Guide to Ethics: A Map for the Moral Maze*, chapter 9: Confidentiality.
Public Health (Control of Disease) Act 1984, chapter 22.

1.71 Discussing patients

D   B   E   C   A

This question focuses on the importance of maintaining patient confidentiality both inside and outside the hospital. When you are not in your professional capacity as a doctor, it is still your duty to maintain respect and confidentiality for your patients. Your colleague's behaviour in this scenario is inappropriate, both because he has written details about patients in public view and because he is discussing them. It is therefore your duty to stop your colleague before he reveals any more information. Option D is more appropriate than B as it is also necessary to remember that you should respect your colleagues and talk to them in a polite manner. Talking to them in private would be a less aggressive way of voicing your concerns. Reporting the FY1 to his educational supervisor (E) may be appropriate if you saw this repeatedly happen and he appeared to disregard patient confidentiality multiple times. It is always best to talk to your colleague first, however, before involving seniors. This is more sensible than options C and A though, in which you are ignoring the issue. As a doctor, your first priority should be the care and respect of your patients. In no circumstances should you actively follow your colleague's behaviour, as in option A, and even though in option C you are not divulging confidential details yourself (which makes this mildly preferable to A), it would be unprofessional to encourage this behaviour; instead, you should try and prevent it from happening again.

Recommended reading

General Medical Council (2009), Explanatory guidance, *Confidentiality*.
General Medical Council (2013), *Good Medical Practice*, Duties of a doctor.
General Medical Council (2013), *Good Medical Practice*, paragraphs 20, 23, 36, 47, 50.
Medical Protection Society (2012), *MPS Guide to Ethics: A Map for the Moral Maze*, chapter 9: Confidentiality.

1.72 Disclosing to a third party

A B E

This question highlights the importance of maintaining patient confidentiality regardless of your personal connections with a patient. In this scenario, you should therefore discuss with the patient what he would be comfortable with his relatives knowing (options A and B) and then explain politely to his brother that you cannot divulge any information without express permission from the patient (E). As you have not had any prior instruction from the patient to tell your brother about their admission (not to mention the fact that your brother has said that his friend is refusing to say what is wrong), it would be unprofessional to break this trust, as in options F and G. Similarly, asking a colleague to do this is inappropriate as well (D). Directing your brother to his friend (H) is not necessarily wrong as this would not break confidentiality; however, by doing this you would also not be explaining to your brother why you are unable to say anything and the patient may not want to see any visitors. Calling security (C) seems like an overreaction as your brother has shown no signs of aggression, and this would be an inappropriate use of the security team, who may be required elsewhere.

Recommended reading

General Medical Council (2009), Explanatory guidance, *Confidentiality*.
General Medical Council (2013), *Good Medical Practice*, Duties of a Doctor.
General Medical Council (2013), *Good Medical Practice*, paragraphs 20, 31, 47, 50.
Medical Protection Society (2012), *MPS Guide to Ethics: A Map for the Moral Maze*, chapter 9: Confidentiality.

1.73 Diabetes and driving

A D C E B

This question presents a situation in which you need to balance your professional duty to respect confidentiality with the need to protect the public. If you are aware that a patient is driving illegally, you should do your best to persuade them to inform the DVLA themselves (A); this would mean that you did not need to break confidentiality. It would be unprofessional to inform the DVLA yourself (B) without first giving the patient the opportunity to do this. Reassuring the patient is a good idea (D) as it may help to alleviate any anxieties and hopefully help to persuade them that honesty is the best policy, while also showing both compassion and good communication skills. Written information can be a helpful adjunct to this (C), but it should not be used to replace a verbal discussion. You should also remember to provide information in a way that the patient can understand. Obtaining advice from a senior (E) would be appropriate if you are unsure how to handle the situation; however, a senior house officer (SHO) or specialist registrar (SpR) is likely to be more accessible to provide support (as would diabetes nurse specialists) and could potentially therefore be a more practical source of advice than your consultant.

Recommended reading

Diabetes UK (2009), *Driving and Diabetes.*
General Medical Council (2009), Explanatory guidance, *Confidentiality.*
General Medical Council (2013), *Good Medical Practice*, Duties of a doctor.
General Medical Council (2013), *Good Medical Practice*, paragraphs 11, 12, 23, 32, 34, 47, 50, 51, 71, 73.
Medical Protection Society (2012), *MPS Guide to Ethics: A Map for the Moral Maze*, chapter 9: Confidentiality.

1.74 Media

A G H
You need to be careful how you share information with the press so as not to be misquoted or be persuaded into giving your opinion on something you cannot back up. As an FY1, you should not feel pressured into giving information; if you do have concerns about the care in the hospital, it is better to try internal reporting routes before speaking to the press. The best answers in this scenario are those that are helpful to the journalist by directing them to someone more senior who is able to provide more accurate and less subjective information. This could be the hospital management (A), your foundation programme director (G) or one of the senior clinical doctors (H). It is important to remember that, if you are making comments in the public realm in your capacity as a doctor, you should also declare yourself by name and therefore remaining anonymous is not an option here (B). Lying or falsely embellishing the real picture to the press (C) is unprofessional, and there have been examples in the press of trusts, hospitals and staff who have augmented reports and subsequently experienced adverse consequences. Hanging up the phone (D) is rude and gives the journalist a poor picture of the behaviour of staff at the hospital. Offering a private interview to the journalist (E) is risky; if you really felt strongly about the matter, you should first seek advice from your medico-legal insurer, your seniors and perhaps a medical union such as the British Medical Association (BMA) about the limits of what you wish to discuss. Deferring the call to a colleague (F) is unprofessional, discourteous and again would give a false impression to the journalist of your opinion regarding the matter.

Recommended reading

General Medical Council (2013), Explanatory Guidance *Doctors' Use of Social Media*, paragraph 17.

1.75 Interpersonal relationships

D C B E A
This is a serious matter as the consultant is responsible for the training and well-being of the staff working in their team, and it is therefore inappropriate for them to be entering into sexual relationships with their junior colleagues, especially not within the hospital grounds. The best thing therefore would

be to report this matter to your foundation programme director and allow them to take the matter further (D). Option C is preferable to B, as your FY1 colleagues may be able to give you more objective advice than the nursing staff working on the ward. It should, however, be respected as a private matter, and therefore, advice should be sought as opposed to simply gossiping about it. Ignoring the situation (E) is better than option A, since accusing the consultant of rape when you do not know the full story is a very serious allegation.

Recommended reading
Rughani G. (2012), When I kissed the consultant, *BMJ Careers*. http://careers. bmj.com/careers/advice/view-article.html?id=20007623.

1.76 Raising concerns

D   A   C   B   E
As this is an issue of patient safety, the worst choice would be to do nothing (E). It would be best for the SHO to raise their concerns themselves (D) as you were not directly involved in the incident. Despite this, you can still raise concerns yourself and indeed should do if you are not confident that the SHO has done so. Your clinical supervisor, as your line manager, is the most appropriate source of guidance (A) and can escalate the matter if necessary. You should seek to address the issue within your organisation before going to external bodies such as the GMC (C). However, it would be inappropriate for you to contact the radiologist directly as this will seem confrontational, particularly as you do not have a professional relationship with them, and your concerns are based entirely on the reports of others (B). This option is worse than those that involve using more formal channels to investigate and address the problem. However, it would still be preferable to contact the radiologist than to do nothing (E) as it shows you are taking some action towards improving safety for future patients.

Recommended reading
General Medical Council (2013), *Good Medical Practice*, paragraphs 43–44.
Medical Protection Society (2012), *MPS Guide to Ethics: A Map for the Moral Maze*, chapter 11: Relating to colleagues, section: Raising concerns.
The UK Foundation Programme Curriculum (2012), section 7.1: Makes patient safety a priority in clinical practice.

1.77 Acting on hearsay

A   D   C   B   E
Foundation doctors often spend a lot of time teaching medical students on the wards and should be willing to do so. Additionally, medical students will often need clinical skills and history-taking exercises to be 'signed off' by a doctor. General Medical Council (GMC) guidelines explain that you must be honest and objective when completing such assessments. In this case, it seems likely that your colleague has not followed these guidelines. However, you should not

act on your suspicions without first asking your colleague about what you have heard. Option A is therefore the most appropriate course of action. Your clinical supervisor will also be able to offer support as to what you should do (D). Asking the students to repeat all of their clinical skills (C) may be putting patient safety first, but it would not address the underlying issue that your colleague is signing paperwork incorrectly. Informing the medical school dean (B), without first addressing the issue with your colleague or supervisor, would be inappropriate in this scenario. Conversely, ignoring the situation (E) could be potentially dangerous and could lead to the students performing clinical skills unsupervised and incorrectly.

Recommended reading
General Medical Council (2013), *Good Medical Practice*, paragraphs 41 and 42.

1.78 Inappropriate requests

A D E B C
Treating friends and family should be avoided if at all possible when practising as a doctor. In this scenario, offering an appointment for your friend and his wife with another GP is the most appropriate response (A). This not only allows them to be correctly investigated and managed but also prevents you from treating a friend, which could create a conflict of interest. Threatening to inform the GMC (C) is the most inappropriate response in this scenario as your friend has not made a dangerous request, and this is somewhat melodramatic and potentially inflammatory. Informing the GMC would not help the situation and could prevent your friend and his wife from receiving necessary treatment. Taking an accurate history and referring the case to your trainer is another appropriate course of action (D), but it is highly likely that they will both need appointments to see a GP in person regardless of whether he has a further conversation with your trainer. Prescribing pain relief and asking him to take his wife to the emergency department is the next best response (E) as in doing so at least his wife will be properly assessed in person. Prescribing antibiotics over the phone (B) is not appropriate as you do not have enough information to know whether the prescription is warranted (or whether the patient has any drug allergies) without having seen and clinically assessed the patient yourself.

Recommended reading
British Medical Association (2010), *Ethical Responsibilities in Treating Doctors Who are Patients.*

1.79 Newspaper cutting of colleague

A C D E B
The GMC offers advice about openness with legal or disciplinary procedures. GMC guidelines outline that you must inform the organisation without delay if you have either accepted a caution, been charged with or been found guilty

of a criminal offence. In this situation, the best course of action would be to privately ask your colleague about the incident (A). Your colleague may have already raised the issue with your seniors and the GMC without your knowledge and approaching him privately could avoid any unnecessary distress. Informing the GMC (C) would be the second best response as this would raise the issue with the appropriate body, while not causing unnecessary distress or embarrassment. Taking the article to work and confronting your colleague on the ward round (D) would be an inappropriate way to raise your concerns. However, waiting for a court verdict determining whether or not he is found guilty (E) is not in line with guidance as the GMC must be informed even if an individual is only charged with a criminal offence. Finally, ignoring the issue could be potentially dangerous and is not in line with GMC guidance, so option B is the least appropriate course of action.

Recommended reading
General Medical Council (2013), *Good Medical Practice*, paragraph 75.

1.80 Phony thank you's

E   B   C   A   D

Medicine is a competitive field, and doctors are always under pressure to be the best. However, lying on your CV or fabricating qualifications or experience to get a job is viewed very seriously by the GMC and is likely to result in disciplinary action. The best response here is to advise your colleagues against writing fake thank you letters (E), reminding them of the duties of a doctor to be 'honest about your experience, qualifications and current role'. In this way, you take steps to prevent your colleagues acting dishonestly as well as taking a step back from this situation yourself. The next best response is to decline to be involved in writing the letters for each other (B), which means that you are protecting yourself from dishonest practice. Your educational supervisor would then be the next appropriate port of call (C) as they will be able to help you to improve your CV honestly, although this response does little to prevent your colleagues from potentially going ahead with their plan. Nevertheless, it is better than jumping to conclusions and informing the GMC of their dishonest practice (A) without any evidence since your colleagues may decide not to go ahead with the letters. The worst response is to go along with the plan and get involved in writing the letters yourself (D), which both goes against the guidance of the GMC and means you commit professional misconduct.

Recommended reading
General Medical Council (2013), *Good Medical Practice*, paragraph 66.

1.81 Sexism

E   B   A   C   D

This scenario concerns workplace sexism and its effects on your colleagues. It also tests your integrity since, as you are not the direct victim here, it would be easy to stand by and do nothing. The best response is option E, to discuss this issue privately and outside of the clinical team with a person who is likely to give impartial advice. Your educational supervisor would be able to show you the correct channels if you decided to take this issue further and how to do it tactfully. Speaking with another consultant in the team (B) could be sensible, but there is a risk of partiality. Ideally, they should respect and consider your point of view, but it could result in them automatically defending their colleague. Option A, speaking directly to the consultant about their poor conduct, may seem intimidating and outside the role of an FY1; however, if you approached the subject carefully and respectfully, you may find that the consultant hadn't realised that their comments were offensive, and subsequently, they begin to treat your colleague better. Option A therefore ranks third. To encourage your colleague to raise this issue with the BMA (C) is the fourth most appropriate response because although your union may be able to give you advice on how to proceed with a complaint about sexism, it does little to deal with the issue at hand, and you should attempt some measures yourself to rectify the situation first. The least appropriate response is to do nothing and advise your colleague to avoid your consultant to evade his sexist comments (D). This shows a lack of integrity and respect for your colleague as a doctor. By doing nothing it also implies that you are accepting this behaviour as normal and condoning your consultant's actions.

Recommended reading
General Medical Council (2013), *Good Medical Practice*, Duties of a doctor.
General Medical Council (2013), *Good Medical Practice*, paragraphs 56–80.

1.82 Breast exam

E   B   D   C   A
This question focuses on the importance of gaining informed consent before any type of procedure and asking whether a patient would like a chaperone present for intimate examinations. Option E is the most appropriate initial response as it is important that the patient understands why you wish to examine the breasts and what it will involve. This should happen before you find a chaperone (B), which should always be offered. Clear, accurate documentation in medicine is vital, particularly in these types of situation (D). If a patient declines a chaperone, it is even more important to state this. All documentation should be done as soon as possible after the event. Leaving this task for your SHO (C) would be unprofessional and shows a disregard for clinical duties. However, it would not be as inappropriate as performing the examination without informed consent or a chaperone (A).

Recommended reading
General Medical Council (2008), Explanatory guidance, in *Consent: Patients and Doctors Making Decisions Together*.
General Medical Council (2013), Explanatory guidance, in *Maintaining a Professional Boundary Between You and Your Patient*.

General Medical Council (2013), *Good Medical Practice*, Duties of a doctor.
General Medical Council (2013), *Good Medical Practice*, paragraphs 15, 17, 19, 21, 32, 36, 47, 57.
Medical Protection Society (2012), *MPS Guide to Ethics: A Map for the Moral Maze*, chapter 5: Morality and decency.

1.83 Doctor harassing nurse

A B E
This situation requires a balance between maintaining respect for colleagues and not jumping to make accusations with the duty to act if you suspect that a colleague's behaviour may be inappropriate or jeopardising the safety of staff or patients. In this scenario, it is therefore important that you give your colleague a chance to explain their behaviour (E) but that you don't ignore what potentially could be harassment (D). Reporting the FY1 before hearing his side of the story (options F and H) would be unfair and should only be resorted to if there were subsequent causes for concern. You may, however, wish to speak to a senior in confidence, and your educational supervisor would be best placed to discuss this (A). The subject should not be shared with the other members of your team (G) as this is unprofessional and is unlikely to help to solve the dilemma. Offering support if the nurse wishes to talk in confidence may be a sympathetic approach (B); however, if she does not wish to talk, you should not force her (C).

Recommended reading
General Medical Council (2013), Explanatory guidance, in *Sexual Behaviour and Your Duty to Report Colleagues*.
General Medical Council (2013), *Good Medical Practice*, Duties of a Doctor.
General Medical Council (2013), *Good Medical Practice*, paragraphs 23–25, 35–37, 59, 65, 68.
Medical Protection Society (2012), *MPS Guide to Ethics: A Map for the Moral Maze*, chapter 5: Morality and decency.

1.84 Embarrassing colleague photos

C D E A B
This question focuses on the balance between a doctor's right to a private life and their duty to maintain the public's respect and trust in the profession. This is ever more important with the advent of social media. You should advise your colleague to remove the photos from her public online profile (C) because if they were seen by the wrong people, this could prove detrimental to her career and the respect of the profession. She should also read the new guidance on the use of social media (D) so that she is suitably able to maintain her professional responsibilities alongside her right to a social life and online social interaction. It may be appropriate to seek advice from a colleague if you are unsure as to what to do (E); however, you should not spread this news among other

ward staff as a means of entertainment (B). Similarly, doing nothing would not be conducive to upholding your professional duties nor maintaining good working relationships (A). If you are in a position to give advice or to support colleagues, you should do so.

Recommended reading

General Medical Council (2012), Explanatory guidance, in *Raising and Acting on Concerns About Patient Safety*.

General Medical Council (2013), Explanatory guidance, in *Doctors' Use of Social Media*.

General Medical Council (2013), *Good Medical Practice*, Duties of a doctor.

General Medical Council (2013), *Good Medical Practice*, paragraphs 25, 34–37, 43, 59, 65.

Medical Protection Society (2012), *MPS Guide to Ethics: A Map for the Moral Maze*, chapter 5: Morality and decency.

1.85 Patient–doctor relationship

D   B   C   E   A

This question deals with the relationship between doctors and their patients and the duty to make the care of patients the first priority. A romantic relationship between doctors and their patients may be seen as a breach of the natural trust that exists in this kind of relationship, especially if the patient in question is vulnerable. In this situation, it would be wise initially to ask your colleague if he has any feelings towards the patient or whether the attraction is one-sided (D). If not, he should be the one to talk to the patient about the reasons why a relationship would be inappropriate (B). You should not encourage such a relationship (A), particularly as you have no evidence that both parties like each other. Talking to the patient yourself (C) may be appropriate in some situations, for example if you had good cause to believe that the patient liked the doctor, but the doctor refused to acknowledge the situation. Regardless, it is important to be open and honest with patients. Disclosing this information to other colleagues (E) when you are unsure of the facts would be premature. Ideally, you should talk to your colleague first and then if you have cause to require further advice, a senior opinion may be appropriate at that stage.

Recommended reading

General Medical Council (2013), Explanatory guidance, in *Ending Your Professional Relationship with a Patient*.

General Medical Council (2013), Explanatory guidance, in *Maintaining a Professional Boundary Between You and Your Patient*.

General Medical Council (2013), *Good Medical Practice*, Duties of a doctor.

General Medical Council (2013), *Good Medical Practice*, paragraphs 16, 25, 31, 36, 43, 46–48, 53, 59, 62, 65.

Medical Protection Society (2012), *MPS Guide to Ethics: A Map for the Moral Maze*, chapter 5: Morality and decency.

1.86 Gynaecology complaints

B C E

The most important matter here is that, if the patient was upset by an event, those involved must apologise and explain their behaviour to the patient; most complaints to the National Health Service (NHS) are the result of poor communication. Therefore, the actions that you should take must ensure that your consultant is aware of the problem (B) so that they can apologise personally. You should also make sure that the registrar is aware of the problem (E) as they too were involved and should discuss the matter with the consultant . While you were not personally involved, as a member of the team, you can talk to the patient and try and understand how they feel (C). Passing the issue on to one of the nursing staff (A) is not very professional, although it may be useful to have a member of the nursing staff present (as a chaperone) when you talk to the patient. Leaving the matter (D) or telling the patient they are mistaken (H) will not help to alleviate the patient's anxieties and may make matters worse. Raising the matter at the next M&M meeting is important (F), but the matter should be mentioned to the staff involved first. Recommending that the patient make a complaint (G) may be appropriate if your consultant subsequently refused to acknowledge the situation; however, they may not thank you for recommending that a complaint be made about them before they have chance to remedy the situation. As healthcare professionals, complaints should be advocated only if all relevant bodies have been informed of the situation and have neglected to take action to remedy the issues.

Recommended reading

Handling complaints poorly makes problems worse, says NHS ombudsman (2010), *BMJ*, 341.

Medical Protection Society (2012), *MPS Guide to Ethics: A Map for the Moral Maze*, chapter 5: Morality and decency.

1.87 Alcohol and misdemeanours

C D G

It is important to talk to the FY1, and this conversation should be conducted in private to avoid embarrassing them (G). You should be kind and explain why you are worried (C) rather than taking an accusatory approach (H). In addition, it is important that you involve others in order to get support for the FY1 if needed and to ensure that there are no concerns over their fitness to practice. The FY1's educational supervisor (D) is a better choice than the foundation programme director (E) as an initial contact. You should avoid discussing the situation with the other FY1s (B) as there is no issue here that you need to clarify with peer support, and it is more sensitive to avoid spreading knowledge of the FY1's potential difficulties. It would be an overreaction to contact the GMC at this stage (A). Observing them at the next social event (F) would be irrelevant as you already know that the FY1 is getting into trouble with their binge drinking.

Recommended reading

General Medical Council (2013), *Good Medical Practice*, paragraph 65.
Medical Protection Society (2012), *MPS Guide to Ethics: A Map for the Moral Maze*, chapter 5: Morality and decency, section: Personal behaviour.

1.88 Sexist consultant

A C D E B

This scenario is difficult, given that it takes a fair amount of courage to challenge a senior colleague about his behaviour. The best approach would be to get advice from your educational supervisor (A) as they can advise you from outside the immediate clinical team. This is a sensitive issue and their support may be important. In challenging the consultant's sexually inappropriate behaviour, it is better for this to be done in private by a member of his peer group (C), than in public by you as a junior (D). Option D could lead to an escalating confrontation and have a lasting negative impact on your working relationship. You should try to address the problem from within the organisation before consulting external bodies (E), except where there are serious concerns over fitness to practice. The behaviour of the consultant is indecent and unacceptable as it constitutes sexual harassment, so the worst option would be to take no action at all (B). As you are aware of these issues regarding the consultant's behaviour, you have a responsibility to raise and address these concerns.

Recommended reading

General Medical Council (2013), *Good Medical Practice*, paragraph 59.
Medical Protection Society (2012), *MPS Guide to Ethics: A Map for the Moral Maze*, chapter: Morality and decency, section: Employment.

1.89 Inappropriate comments in mortuary

A B D

This situation is perhaps not common, but it does have implications on a range of other potential scenarios. The important factor here is to act with discretion and to put the comments into context. Despite the comments being inappropriate, it is unlikely that any harm has been caused. However, if your colleague is making unacceptable comments in the mortuary, this could be a sign that they are acting unprofessionally in other situations. It is therefore important to flag your concerns but to do this correctly and diplomatically. Discussing this with the people who were involved (options A and D) would be most appropriate and hopefully lead to this not happening again. Asking senior colleagues for advice without mentioning the names of the people involved (B) could provide you with valuable advice without inadvertently escalating the situation. Ignoring the comments would potentially let this behaviour continue without challenge and would therefore be unsuitable (E). Reporting the situation to the consultant in charge (G) or completing an incident form (C) would probably be reacting excessively to a situation that could be dealt with more discretely.

Informing the patient's family (H) would create unnecessary distress and not be of any benefit in this scenario. Raising the comments in a large group and implicating your colleague (F) would lead to uncalled-for conflict and distress for your colleague.

Recommended reading
General Medical Council (2013), *Good Medical Practice*, paragraphs 47, 48 and 50.

1.90 Recommending illegal substances

D   A   E   B   C

The priority in this situation is to provide help and support for your patient's symptoms, while maintaining professional standards and practising within the law. In this scenario, your patient is clearly experiencing severe pain that is not currently under adequate control. The best course of action would be to acknowledge your patient's request for information, inform her that cannabis is illegal and offer more conventional alternative medications to help with her pain (D). This option would ensure that you are not breaching the law, while helping to control your patient's symptoms. Booking the patient in for a further consultation (A) would delay the issue temporarily, but this could equip you with some valuable advice and a plan from your educational supervisor. Your educational supervisor could also offer advice on alternative pain relief that could help your patient. Booking the patient into a specialist pain clinic (E) could eventually help the patient with her symptoms; however, in the primary care setting, you should attempt a wide range of medications before referring her to secondary services. Refusing to talk about the situation (B) ensures that you have not provided unprofessional advice, but it does not address the patient's symptoms and offer any ways to alleviate them; therefore, this is an inappropriate response. Advising the patient to take illegal substances (C), even for medicinal purposes, is not professional behaviour and should be discouraged.

Recommended reading
General Medical Council (2013), *Good Medical Practice*, paragraph 1.

1.91 Smart phone pictures

A   C   E   D   B

This is a common scenario, where you are asked to perform a task by a senior doctor which may not be best practice. In this situation, the ideal course of action would be for the hospital photographer to take the images (A), which would ensure both that patient confidentiality is maintained and that the images are of a suitable quality with adequate patient consent. Not dressing a large, open wound is potentially very dangerous and could risk introducing infection, therefore this is the least appropriate option (B). Taking a photograph of any part of a patient with or without consent on personal photographic equipment is not advised, therefore options E and D are both inappropriate. However, transferring images via secure email servers (E) is more appropriate than sending the images to a personal smart phone (D). Refusing to take the image may delay the operation (C), but with an appropriate dressing, the patient will not be at risk of infection, and the wound could be assessed personally by the surgeon on arrival at the hospital.

Recommended reading
General Medical Council (2011), Explanatory guidance, in *Making and Using Visual and Audio Recordings of Patients*, Principles.

1.92 Gift

C   B   D   A   E
The General Medical Council's (GMC) stance on this situation is perhaps surprising: you may accept unsolicited goods from patients or their relatives (C) as long as it does not affect or appear to affect the way you practise medicine, for example your prescribing and referring practices. The guidance also states that you should not use 'your influence to pressurise or persuade patients or their relatives to offer gifts'. Accepting the card alone (B), however, may be appropriate if you feel uneasy about accepting a gift. The next best response is not to accept either (D), but this is likely to be perceived as rude and ungrateful. The GMC states that 'you must not put pressure on patients or their families to make donations to other people or organisations', so option A would be inappropriate. Asking the family to take you out for a meal (E) would be rude and could be perceived as not maintaining a professional boundary between yourself and your patient and is clearly the least appropriate response.

Recommended reading
General Medical Council (2013), Explanatory guidance, in *Financial and Commercial Arrangements and Conflicts of Interest*.
General Medical Council (2013), *Good Medical Practice*, paragraphs 77–80.

1.93 Termination of pregnancy

B   D   E
During your time as a doctor, you may be asked to carry out or give advice about procedures that conflict with your religious/moral beliefs. The General Medical Council (GMC) advises that you do two things in this situation: 'explain to patients if you have a conscientious objection' (E) and 'tell them about their right to see another doctor' (B). You must make sure that they can see another one of your colleagues soon, who can give impartial advice, so option B is the most appropriate response. If this may cause undue delay or is not possible, you should make the referral to a tertiary centre so that they can have access to TOP services. In this case, you should also discuss

the reasons why your patient wants to end her pregnancy (D), which would show that you are not dismissing her decision. Advising her to take alternative options, such as adoption (A), is not appropriate as in doing this you would be using your beliefs to influence her decision. Asking her to take another week to consider her options (C) would delay her abortion if she should choose to go ahead with the TOP, especially if this would mean that another colleague would have to make the referral. The Royal College of Obstetricians and Gynaecologists (RCOG) guidelines state that 'the earlier in pregnancy an abortion is performed, the safer it is'. Refusing to refer the patient (G) would deny the patient her right to access abortion services. Giving the patient written information about TOP (F) may be useful, but in the first case, she should be given access to services and the opportunity to discuss with a colleague without a conscientious objection to abortion. It is unclear in the RCOG guidance whether signing the abortion certificate (H) is covered by the 'conscientious objection' clause but not signing the certificate is unlikely to be an issue as long as your patient has access without delay to TOP services.

Recommended reading
British Medical Association (2007), *The Law and Ethics of Abortion – BMA Views*, Part 1: Legal considerations.
General Medical Council (2013), *Good Medical Practice*, paragraph 52.
Royal College of Obstetricians and Gynaecologists (2011), *The Care of Women Requesting Induced Abortion, Evidence-based Clinical Guideline Number 7*, sections 3.3, 4.3 and 4.7.

1.94 Aggressive patient

C D G
While this is not your patient and your shift has finished, you still have a professional responsibility to ensure the safety of both the patient and the public. It would therefore be irresponsible to continue walking to your car (F). It is unlikely that you are going to be able to manage the situation alone, so it is reasonable to call both the police and the hospital security (options C and D). You do not know why the patient is behaving in such a way, so it would be inappropriate to call the psychiatric team at this point (E), although they may require psychiatric input in the future. You should not try to approach the patient (A) as you risk provoking him and putting yourself at risk, and similarly, you should not ask passers-by to help you restrain him (B). Telling the patient to stop damaging the cars may also worsen the situation (H). You should instead try to prevent others from approaching him (G).

Recommended reading
General Medical Council (2013), *Good Medical Practice*, paragraph 65.
Medical Protection Society (2012), *MPS Guide to Ethics: A Map for the Moral Maze*, chapter 3: Professionalism and integrity, chapter 5: Morality and decency.

1.95 Racist comments

B A E D C

Racial discrimination is unacceptable in any walk of life and should not be tolerated. In this scenario, you should therefore make it clear to the registrars that their behaviour is unacceptable (B). This is a difficult situation, particularly since it involves an issue with your senior, so it would be a good idea to ask your educational supervisor for their advice (A). Printing some GMC guidance (E) does not properly address the problem, but it is preferable to doing nothing (D). Informing the consultant of the comments made about them (C) is inappropriate. Knowing about the comments will only serve to upset or anger them and does not improve the situation.

Recommended reading

General Medical Council (2013), *Good Medical Practice*, paragraphs 36, 59.
Medical Protection Society (2012), *MPS Guide to Ethics: A Map for the Moral Maze*, chapter 5: Morality and decency.

1.96 Child protection

C B E D A

This question deals with the issues surrounding child protection but is complicated by issues of confidentiality. The abuse outlined in the question is severe, including burns and head injuries. Sending this patient back into such a dangerous environment would be irresponsible, and it is your duty as a doctor to protect children from harm. The confidentiality of children should be respected and given the same weight as that of adults. However, *Good Medical Practice* states that you should 'disclose information if this is necessary to protect the child or young person, or someone else, from risk of death or serious harm', and this is the case here. Getting advice from an expert on how to protect this child from danger is the best response (C). Offering support for the child while he makes the disclosure to his parents (B) is the next best response; this keeps the parents informed and also allows you to ensure appropriate safeguards are put in place. Option E is the next best course of action since social services may be able to give help and advice to this child, but it would be best to discuss the breaking of confidentiality with a senior Caldicott Guardian before doing so. A Caldicott Guardian is a senior person responsible for protecting the confidentiality of patient information, and each NHS organisation is required to have one. Calling the police (D) is a rash decision to make, and you should not jump to this conclusion without using the proper channels of support first; however, it would be better than doing nothing (A) and allowing a child to return to a knowingly violent situation which may result in serious harm.

Recommended reading

General Medical Council (2013), *0–18 Years: Guidance for all Doctors*, paragraphs 44–52, 56–63.

1.97 Relationships

F G H

This question raises the issue of personal relationships with patients, particularly romantic relationships. Using your professional position to gain a romantic relationship goes against many of the duties of a doctor. The main issue in starting a relationship with an ex-patient is the implication that you may have acted dishonestly during your professional relationship in order to develop a personal one. There is also the wider implication of patients not being able to trust their doctors if doctors view patients as potential partners. The GMC's *Good Medical Practice* (2013) states: 'If a patient pursues a sexual or improper emotional relationship with you, you should treat them politely and considerately and try to re-establish a professional boundary.' Accepting a phone number with the intention of developing a relationship with this patient (E) is absolutely inappropriate as you have a strong professional responsibility for this patient. Accepting the number with the hope of making other personal gains, such as publications (C), is similarly dishonest and inappropriate. Accepting the number with no intention to call (options A, B and D) is also dishonest, as well as not trying to re-establish a professional boundary, and these responses are therefore inappropriate. The only appropriate responses involve refusing the phone number (options F, G and H). This should be done with the utmost respect and a clear explanation of why a personal relationship cannot occur (G), but it is still better to refuse the number honestly and bruise the patient's feelings somewhat (F and H) than to be dishonest with them.

Recommended reading

General Medical Council (2013), Explanatory guidance, in *Maintaining a Professional Boundary Between You and Your Patient.*

Medical Protection Society (2012), *MPS Guide to Ethics: A Map for the Moral Maze*, chapter 5: Morality and decency.

1.98 Colleague missing teaching

C E B A D

This question requires you to act professionally and not to judge colleagues based on hearsay, while also remembering that you have a duty of care to your patients. Participating in training courses is a necessary GMC requirement in order to keep your skills up to date. Asking your colleague for an explanation would be the most appropriate first step (C), followed by some polite advice to come in if at all possible (E), which shows compassion for your colleague and a genuine consideration for their learning. Seeking advice from colleagues is good practice when dealing with professional dilemmas (B) and is more appropriate than telling the programme director before you have spoken to the FY1 in question (A). Spreading rumours about your colleague is unprofessional and seeks to achieve nothing except embarrass the individual (D).

Recommended reading

General Medical Council (2012), *Continuing Professional Development; Guidance for All Doctors.*

General Medical Council (2013), *Good Medical Practice*, Duties of a doctor.

General Medical Council (2013), *Good Medical Practice*, paragraphs 1, 8–10, 12, 24, 25, 36, 43, 59, 65.

Medical Protection Society (2012), *MPS Guide to Ethics: A Map for the Moral Maze*, chapter 3: Professionalism and integrity.

1.99 Prescribing error

D   A   B   E   C

Making mistakes is inevitable in medicine, and this question assesses your ability to respond to such a situation in a professional manner. It is firstly important to own up to your mistake and to prevent any further harm to the patient by ensuring that the drug is crossed off the drug prescription chart (D). It is then also courteous to reassure and apologise to the patient (A). Informing the nurses (B) is not as important a priority as both of these actions since crossing the drug off the prescription chart should prevent the antibiotic being given. While it may be important to explore and reflect upon your mistake with other members of your team and to come up with ways to ensure it doesn't happen again (E), this is not a priority at the moment. Denying knowledge of the mistake (C) is dishonest and unprofessional, even if you do prevent the antibiotic from being subsequently administered. One should always own up to mistakes.

Recommended reading

General Medical Council (2012), *Continuing Professional Development: Guidance for all Doctors.*

General Medical Council (2013), *Good Medical Practice*, Duties of a doctor.

General Medical Council (2013), *Good Medical Practice*, paragraphs 1, 16, 22, 23, 25, 32, 36, 37, 55, 61, 65, 68.

General Medical Council (2013), *Good Practice in Prescribing and Managing Medicines and Devices.*

Medical Protection Society (2012), *MPS Guide to Ethics: A Map for the Moral Maze*, chapter 3: Professionalism and integrity.

1.100 Receiving a gift

E   A   B   D   C

The GMC recognises that doctors are sometimes given gifts by patients as a thank you for the care they have received. It is not inappropriate to accept these gifts, so long as you are honest and open about it and do not let it influence the care you provide. It is wrong, however, to ask for inducements in return for an altered standard or programme of care. Option E is therefore most appropriate as you are declaring the gift to your supervisor. This may well be a good course of action as a more junior doctor. You may want to share it with the team (A) if you feel uncomfortable about keeping it to yourself, but you should declare this to the patient. If you feel unable to accept the gift, you should politely decline (D), but you could suggest that the hospital charity may be a more suitable recipient (B). It would be inappropriate to take the patient out for a meal with the money (C) as this would be breaching the professional doctor–patient relationship and may potentially lead to a conflict of interest.

Recommended reading

General Medical Council (2013), Explanatory guidance, *Financial and Commercial Arrangements and Conflicts of Interest*.

General Medical Council (2013), Explanatory guidance, *Maintaining a Professional Boundary Between You and Your Patient*.

General Medical Council (2013), *Good Medical Practice*, Duties of a doctor.

General Medical Council (2013), *Good Medical Practice*, paragraphs 16, 46, 53, 56, 59, 62, 65, 77–80.

Medical Protection Society (2012), *MPS Guide to Ethics: A Map for the Moral Maze*, chapter 3: Professionalism and integrity.

1.101 Colleague's appearance

A   F   G

Appearance is an important part of being a doctor and ensuring that people trust you as a professional. It is difficult to address these things with your colleagues, so you should bear in mind how you would like to be told if this were the case for you. Therefore ensuring someone discusses the matter privately and diplomatically with the FY2 is appropriate. Since the nursing staff are unhappy with the situation, they or their immediate senior (the sister in charge) will be the best placed to bring up their concerns (options A and G). The other thing to ensure is that the FY2 doesn't have any problems at home distracting him from his professional appearance (F). If these responses did not solve the issue, then it may be appropriate for you to intervene (H). The other options here involve talking about the colleague with others (options B and C), which is not ideal and may be seen as gossiping. Simply leaving the matter (D) is not good for your colleague as looking unprofessional affects the trust of the doctor in the eyes of the public. Telling the consultant about the nurses' thoughts is a possible course of action (E), but it is a bit drastic and also isn't likely to help the situation.

Recommended reading

Medical Protection Society (2012), *MPS Guide to Ethics: A Map for the Moral Maze*, chapter 3: Professionalism and integrity.

1.102 Keeping promises

B   A   D   C   E

This scenario has to do with keeping your promises to patients. It is very easy to make promises to patients and often very difficult to keep them! Option B is ranked the highest in this case as it involves an apology to the patient. This is always the most important thing to do when you fall short in people's expectations. In addition, you need to remember to have boundaries from letting your work impact your private life, so it is appropriate to wait until the morning to give the patient her results (B). For the same reason, calling the night-time FY1 (A) ranks higher than going back into work to give the patient her results (D) because your shift has ended. Completely dismissing the patient's concerns and disregarding your promise (E) ranks lowest here as this is unprofessional. However, lying to the patient to make you seem like you are keeping your promises (C) is very inappropriate, so it must also be ranked low.

Recommended reading
General Medical Council (2013), Explanatory guidance, in *Delegation and Referral.*
Medical Protection Society (2012), *MPS Guide to Ethics: A Map for the Moral Maze*, chapter 3: Professionalism and integrity.

1.103 Hungover

E C D A B

If you know that you are going to be unfit for work the next day, you should be honest about this so that alternative arrangements can be made (options E and C). It is best for you to try to make up for your mistake by arranging for cover so that you have not let your colleague down (E). Option C leaves your colleague with the stressful job of trying to find someone else to work. The lower ranking responses (options D and A) involve not dealing with the problem that evening, but they at least include the proviso that you will not work if it is not safe to do so. However, if you do not communicate this decision to the hospital until the morning, the hospital may be left with inadequate cover, or the night FY1 could have to stay until a locum can be brought in. Option D is preferable to option A because if you do end up calling in sick, at least you have been responsible enough to go home and try to be well for work (D) than to give up entirely (A). The worst response is to go to work when you are hungover (B) as this is both a risk to patient safety and likely to undermine patients' trust in the medical profession if you look unwell or smell of alcohol.

Recommended reading
General Medical Council (2013), *Good Medical Practice*, paragraph 25.
Medical Protection Society (2012), *MPS Guide to Ethics: A Map for the Moral Maze*, chapter 3: Professionalism and integrity, section: Unprofessional.

1.104 Train late

C E A D B

If you know that you are going to be late for work, you should let your colleagues know that there is a problem as soon as possible (options C and E). This is polite and responsible and allows for them to plan around your absence. It is better for you to follow official channels and inform the registrar (C) than to pass the message through one of your peers (E). Leaving it until you get to work to apologise in person (A) means that, until you arrive, your team will have been left wondering whether you were coming in at all. Emailing your supervisor is an attempt at being open about the problem (D), but you have no idea whether they will see the message, and it is therefore useless to the team who are expecting you. It is this ward team predominantly that you need to apologise to, which is why option D ranks lower than option A. The worst approach is to be dishonest and take the day as a sick day (B) as you are perfectly capable of working and would just be joining the team slightly later in the morning. It is an attempt to make up an excuse and avoid criticism, which is unprofessional and brings your integrity into question.

Recommended reading
General Medical Council (2013), *Good Medical Practice*, paragraph 68.
The UK Foundation Programme Curriculum (2012), chapter 1: Professionalism.

1.105 E-learning certificate plagiarism

E G H
E-learning is a key part of the foundation programme, with most hospital trusts running comprehensive induction modules online. These modules must be completed within the deadline set and not only improve personal knowledge and skills but also help to boost patient safety. In this scenario, it is unlikely that completing the equality and diversity module will affect your colleague's patient care in the short term, but it would be unprofessional to allow him to pass your work off as his own. The best course of action in this scenario would be to offer your colleague several solutions to his problem without acting unprofessionally yourself. Offering the use of your own laptop to a close friend would be entirely appropriate (G), and it is good practice to offer help to colleagues in difficulty. If your colleague contacted his foundation programme director and explained the situation (H), it is probable that they would be understanding and offer an extension to the deadline in these extenuating circumstances. While attending work out of hours should not be done regularly, in this scenario, completing the module in your colleague's own time before his morning commitments would also be suitable (E). Part of the specifications of a foundation doctor is being able to judge when it is appropriate to report incidents that may affect patient safety and when a private conversation would suffice. In this case, contacting your colleague's educational supervisor would be rather extreme and unlikely to help the situation (C). Similarly, contacting a senior colleague (B) is not necessary, when you can easily suggest solutions to the problem yourself. Allowing a colleague to copy work or certificates (A), regardless of their perceived importance, is poor practice and is unacceptable under any circumstances. Reprimanding your colleague (D) wouldn't help the situation and would be more likely to damage your relationship with him. Equality and diversity are extremely important factors in the modern NHS, and knowledge of NHS policy is a prerequisite for practising as a doctor in the United Kingdom; therefore, not completing the module (F) is not an option.

Recommended reading
General Medical Council (2013), *Good Medical Practice*, paragraph 56.
Medical Protection Society (2012), *MPS Guide to Ethics: A Map for the Moral Maze*, chapter 3: Professionalism and integrity.

1.106 Illegible colleague signature

C D A B E

General Medical Council (GMC) guidance suggests that: 'You must be familiar with your GMC reference number … (and) … make sure you are identifiable to your patients and colleagues. All entries in medical notes must include a date, time, signature, full name, GMC number and contact number'. This information allows fellow healthcare professionals to easily contact one another to discuss cases. In this scenario, your colleague has clearly not been documenting the necessary information. The simplest and most appropriate course of action is to ask your colleague to document the required information in the notes (C). Using a rubber stamp is a quick and easy way of documenting this, and it is offered by many NHS trusts. It is always best for your colleagues to take responsibility for their own behaviour, and therefore, it would be better for them to contact human resources (D) rather that you do (A). Offering to carry out all the writing tasks on the round (B) would solve the problem of documentation, but this would not confront the central issue of your colleague's poor documentation, so this is the second last appropriate option. Retrospectively documenting your colleague's details in the notes yourself would be unacceptable (E) and therefore this response ranks last. This is because the entry has been signed by your colleague and any additions, regardless of their content, should be completed by your colleague. Adding to the documentation of others without their permission is both unprofessional and could lead to medico-legal difficulties.

Recommended reading
General Medical Council (2013), *Good Medical Practice*, paragraph 13 and 35.
Medical Protection Society (2012), *MPS Guide to Ethics: A Map for the Moral Maze*, chapter 3: Professionalism and integrity, section: Unprofessional.

1.107 Diarrhoea and vomiting

D B E A C

The symptoms of acute diarrhoea and vomiting indicate an infectious gastro-enteritis episode, for example rotavirus or norovirus. If you attend work with these symptoms, you pose an infectious risk to hospital patients, which could result in adverse health outcomes for your vulnerable patients or in the worst case scenario the closing of some hospital wards, which would negatively affect patient flow and the general efficiency of the hospital. Many, if not all, trusts have an infection policy whereby staff are required not to attend work until 48 hours after diarrhoea and vomiting have resolved, if it is suspected to be due to infection. Therefore, the most appropriate course of action would be option D: calling into work that evening to inform the appropriate member of staff that you will not be able to attend work the following day. This gives the hospital a chance to try and find a replacement for your working role for the weekend; postponing the call till the next morning (B) will decrease the chance of finding a replacement. Informing the HPA (E) is inappropriate as you have no evidence of infectious disease; on the other hand, if symptoms continue, you may have to provide a stool sample to your GP or occupational health department. Going into work and avoiding patient contact (A) is unlikely to be feasible or practical, and this would also pose an infectious risk to your colleagues. Option C is the least appropriate option as good hand hygiene and medication are not fail-safe measures in stopping the spread of infectious gastroenteritis.

Recommended reading
General Medical Council (2013), *Good Medical Practice*, paragraph 28.

1.108 Prescribing for a friend

B C D

Prescribing for yourself, your friends or your family is something that should be avoided if at all possible. In this scenario, however, there is little other option because not prescribing the antibiotic (E) may result in a more severe, systemic infection. The correct answers are to gain a more thorough history (B), including any allergies to medicines, so as to exclude anything more serious, to prescribe the antibiotic (D) and to inform her GP on Monday (C). The General Medical Council (GMC) states that, if you prescribe medication for someone close to you, you need to make a record at the time, which includes your relationship to the patient and why it was necessary for you to prescribe the medication. Then you are required to tell the patient's GP which medicines you have prescribed and any other necessary information. Option A, advising your friend to take on lots of fluids, is unlikely to treat the infection and may risk the infection becoming systemic. Option F, taking a urine sample to the laboratory, is not the first priority in a simple UTI, and it would be logistically difficult to chase the results. Taking her to the emergency department (G) is likely to result in an antibiotic prescription but would be an unnecessary use of resources as this is neither an accident nor an emergency. Option H, making her wait until Monday to see her GP, may be appropriate but runs the risk of her infection becoming more systemic.

Recommended reading
General Medical Council (2013), *Good Practice in Prescribing and Managing Medicines and Devices*, paragraphs 14 and 17–19.

1.109 Dress code

D B A E C

A doctor should epitomise respectability and part of this involves adhering to a smart dress code. Dressing professionally encourages trust and respect from both patients and colleagues. Jeans are unlikely to look smart in a hospital environment and are therefore not advisable. In this scenario, it is appropriate to suggest to your colleague that she considers wearing something other than jeans (D). Option B, doing nothing, is the next best response. While this does not address your concerns, it is better than the remaining options which have the potential to cause problems. It is, after all, your colleague's responsibility rather than yours to maintain her own appropriate attire. You should not seek the opinion of other team members (A) since this could be seen as gossiping and does not improve the situation. Similarly, it is not your place to criticise your colleague in front of your consultant (E); if the consultant has a problem with a team member's dress, then they will deal with it of their own accord. The most inappropriate option would be to wear jeans yourself simply because someone else does, especially as you feel that this is an inappropriate dress code (C).

Recommended reading
Medical Protection Society (2012), *MPS Guide to Ethics: A Map for the Moral Maze*, chapter 3: Professionalism and integrity.

1.110 Other commitments

A F G

Commitment to a specialty and an ambitious character are valuable and admirable traits in a junior doctor; however, your primary commitment should be to your current clinical job. The correct responses in this question are those that mean your day job is covered safely. Option G, trying to swap shifts, is sensible; swaps can frequently be made within the on-call rotas of specialties without difficulty, although the rota coordinator should be informed of this. Option F, asking for a few hours off, is also appropriate as your registrar will know how busy the day is likely to be and may be able to cover your absence safely for a couple of hours. Sharing the work with your supervisor (A) is also an appropriate course of action as it will allow you both to have a proper night's sleep so that you are capable of working tomorrow and able to give your personal input into the project. Sacrificing your sleep to complete the project and going to work tired (H) puts patient safety at risk and is therefore inappropriate. Calling in sick when you are well (B) is dishonest and means that the shift is understaffed, so it is therefore unacceptable. However, while your day job is important, you should not sacrifice important career-progressing events without trying out other options first, so abandoning your project (C) is unsuitable. Turning off your bleep while at work (D) is dangerous and puts patient safety at risk. Finally, but perhaps most importantly, it should not be forgotten that fabricating study data (E) is dishonest, risks your professional General Medical Council (GMC) licence and shows a complete lack of integrity.

Recommended reading
British Medical Association (updated 2013), *Medical Ethics Today* (3rd ed.), chapter 21: Reducing risk, clinical error and poor performance.
General Medical Council (2013), *Good Medical Practice*, Duties of a doctor.

1.111 Domestic violence

E   B   D   C   A

If a competent adult does not consent to a disclosure, you must respect their decision even if it leaves them at risk of harm. This is providing that nobody else (such as a child) is at risk of harm. You should therefore reassure the patient that you do not intend to break her confidentiality (E). In doing so, you may improve her trust in you and in turn promote a more open discussion about her situation. Whilst you should not pressure the patient into consenting to a disclosure, you should provide encouragement (B). Giving information about further support, such as a charitable organisation is also appropriate (D). Contacting the police without the patient's consent is a breach of confidentiality and particularly inappropriate if you have not informed the patient of your intention to do so (C, A).

Recommended reading
General Medical Council (2009), *Confidentiality*, paragraph 51.

1.112 Patient discrimination

A   D   E   C   B

This scenario presents a potential conflict of interests: that of ensuring that you attempt to remain impartial and not judge the behaviour of your colleagues whilst ensuring the best standard of care for patients, free from the risk of discrimination. Ideally in this situation, you should tell the nurse that she should speak directly to the FY1 in question (A). You should not immediately act as a third party between the two colleagues. However, it is also important to get both sides of the story, and therefore, it might be courteous to speak to the FY1 in person if you feel that their behaviour poses a threat to the quality of patient care (D). It would be unfair to go straight to their educational supervisor with a report based on hearsay and no actual evidence of wrongdoing, and therefore, option B is the least appropriate. Speaking to the patient may be a sensible option if the nurse was very worried about the FY1's conduct (E) and if you felt that there was a potential case of discrimination; however, likewise, you should encourage the nurse to act upon her concerns directly. Speaking to a senior in confidence for advice before making any decisions (C) may be one of the last resorts if you are really unsure how to proceed.

Recommended reading
General Medical Council (2013), *Duties of a Doctor*.
General Medical Council (2013), *Good Medical Practice*, paragraphs 23–25, 31, 35, 36, 48, 54, 56, 57, 59.
General Medical Council (2009), *The New Doctor*.
Medical Protection Society (2012), *MPS Guide to Ethics: A Map for the Moral Maze*, chapters 7 and 11.

1.113 Criticising collegues on hearsay

A B D

This question focuses on balancing your responsibility to raise concerns if you believe patient safety is at risk, to maintain the public's trust in the profession and to not judge colleagues unfairly on the basis of hearsay. In this situation, as you have overheard his comments firsthand, it would be appropriate to speak to your colleague about his conduct (A); however, it would be unprofessional to interrupt the consultation (E). You have a duty to raise the issue, and monitoring the situation as it evolves (C) would therefore neglect your professional responsibility. Explaining your concerns (D) and suggesting that he apologises to the patient, thereby maintaining good communication whilst acknowledging a mistake, would also be suitable (B). Reporting your colleague to seniors before speaking to him and giving him the chance to rectify the situation would be premature (options F and G). If you saw this behaviour repeated, it may be appropriate to then speak to your supervisor for advice. Speaking to the A&E doctor in question is not appropriate at this stage (H) as your behaviour would amount to adverse judgement based on hearsay, and it is not your place to get involved.

Recommended reading

General Medical Council (2012), *Raising and Acting on Concerns About Patient Safety.*

General Medical Council (2013), *Duties of a Doctor: Maintaining Trust.*

General Medical Council (2013), *Good Medical Practice*, paragraphs 24, 25, 35–37, 54–56, 59, 61, 65, 68.

Medical Protection Society (2012), *MPS Guide to Ethics: A Map for the Moral Maze*, chapters 7 and 11.

Chapter 2

COPING WITH PRESSURE

QUESTIONS

2.1 Forgotten patient review

You are an FY1 in general surgery. A nurse calls you to ask you to review a patient whom she is concerned about. You agree but tell her that you are very busy and that you'll have to come later. As you arrive into work the next day, you realise that you completely forgot about it and have not reviewed the patient.

Choose the **THREE most appropriate** actions to take in this situation.

A Apologise to the nursing staff.
B Claim that you did review the patient and that the nursing staff must have lost the documentation.
C Create a jobs list.
D Do nothing; the nursing staff will contact you if they need you again.
E Go to the ward and check that the patient is alright.
F Inform your consultant of your error.
G Tell the nursing staff that they should have bleeped the on-call doctor if they were concerned.
H Write your review and time it as yesterday.

2.2 False statement

A colleague approaches you to tell you that a patient's relative has made a complaint against her for the way that she spoke to him on the phone. You have found her to be a hardworking, professional and polite colleague, and you are aware of this relative and know that he is very difficult. She asks you to make a statement to say that you were witness to her making the phone call even though you weren't present.

Rank in order the following actions in response to this situation (1 = Most appropriate; 5 = Least appropriate).

A Make a complaint against your colleague to a senior.
B Make the statement that you heard the conversation.
C Refuse to make the statement.

D   Refuse to make the statement but offer to submit a general report about her professional behaviour.
E   Speak to the relative and tell them that their complaint is inappropriate.

2.3 Nursing pressure to refer

You are the FY1 doctor working in a busy emergency department, and you have just arrived for the morning shift. There are ten patients to see from the night shift who are going to breach in less than 30 minutes. As you pick up the notes before going to see the most urgent patient, the sister in charge approaches you and says 'can you refer them to the surgeons quickly please, it's where all the patients with abdominal pain need to be referred to'.
   Choose the **THREE most appropriate** actions to take in this situation.

A   Approach the patient, apologise for the delay in seeing a doctor and take a history and examination before referring the patient to the surgeons.
B   Document that the sister has behaved inappropriately.
C   Ignore the remark and go to assess the patient.
D   Immediately inform the consultant in charge that the sister is behaving inappropriately.
E   Inform the consultant in charge that you are unlikely to be able to safely see and refer this patient in time because the night shift was busy, and the patient has already been here for three and a half hours.
F   Politely inform the sister in charge that you need to take a proper history and examine the patient before referring them to ensure the safest and most appropriate care for that patient.
G   Refer the patient to the surgeons and then quickly take a history.
H   Refuse to see the patient as they are likely to breach anyway and you could try and prevent others breaching by seeing them first instead.

2.4 Audit presentation

You are an FY1 working at a large teaching hospital. You have carried out an audit with one of your FY1 colleagues and have been invited to present your findings at the large annual departmental audit afternoon. You are working nights the week of the presentation, so you had agreed with your colleague that she would attend and deliver the presentation so that you could go home and rest. On the morning of the presentation she sends you a text message explaining that she doesn't feel well and is unable to present the audit that afternoon.
   Rank in order the following actions in response to this situation (1 = Most appropriate; 5 = Least appropriate).

A   Reply to your friend that you don't feel it is fair for her to leave you in this situation and that if she is at all able to she should come in as planned.
B   Go home, and email the meeting chair saying that you are both unwell and won't be able to give the presentation.

C Go home, and if you bump into the meeting chair in the future, say that you had forgotten about the presentation.
D Find the meeting chair and ask if you can be moved to the end of the meeting so that you can rest longer during the day.
E Keep your assigned slot for the presentation and ensure that you are able to get a few hours rest either side of it.

2.5 Prioritization

You are an FY1 currently working in a general medicine job. One evening you are on call, covering all of the medical wards. You are seeing a patient who has a temperature and whose blood pressure has dropped. You receive a bleep from the ward you are usually based on about a patient under your day team. The patient's family is asking to speak to a doctor for an update. You are aware that there have been some difficulties with this family who are unhappy about how long it is taking to reach a diagnosis for the patient.

Rank in order the following actions in response to this situation (1 = Most appropriate; 5 = Least appropriate).

A Tell the nurse that you are on call dealing with emergencies and cannot come to see the family.
B Ask the nurse to explain to the family that you would be happy to speak to them, but as you are on call, you cannot guarantee how soon you will be free, but they are welcome to wait if they wish.
C Ask the nurse to apologise to the family and explain that you are on call and cannot speak to them this evening. Suggest a time the following afternoon for a scheduled family meeting.
D Call your senior house officer (SHO) and tell them that you need them to take over looking after the sick patient so that you can go speak to the family.
E Call the registrar on call and ask them to go and speak to the family.

2.6 List of jobs

You are an FY1 on call over the weekend in general medicine. It is very busy, and you have a list of tasks to complete. There is a patient who needs their bloods checking over the weekend, a task which was handed over by a ward doctor on Friday. A nurse has called you because they are worried about a patient who is deteriorating rapidly. Another nurse calls you to tell you that their patient does not understand the rationale behind a new medication that they have started and wants to discuss it with a doctor.

Rank in order the following actions in response to this situation (1 = Most appropriate; 5 = Least appropriate).

A Do all the jobs as quickly as possible.
B Tell the nursing staff to bleep the on-call senior house officer (SHO).

C Ask the nursing staff for more information on the patient who requires their bloods checking and see if anyone else would be able to do this.

D See the patient who is deteriorating as soon as possible.

E Inform the nurse that speaking to patients about their new medication which has already been started before the weekend is inappropriate and not an on-call job.

2.7 Seeking help

It is your first week of a job in paediatric surgery. You are on call in the evening when you are asked to see a boy who is bleeding heavily after a tonsillectomy. You call your registrar who is at home, and they advise you to try conservative treatment. You do this, but it does not stop the bleeding, and you are concerned that he is losing a lot of blood and will soon become haemodynamically unstable. When you call the registrar back and explain that you think the boy needs to go to theatre, they refuse to come in and review the child and instead advise you to continue your conservative management. You do not feel experienced enough to manage the patient alone and remain concerned that he needs to go to theatre urgently.

Rank in order the following actions in response to this situation (1 = Most appropriate; 5 = Least appropriate).

A Ask the medical registrar for help.

B Ask the on-call anaesthetist for help.

C Call the consultant and ask him to come and review the patient.

D Call the registrar back, explain the situation again and insist that he come in and review the child.

E Continue conservative measures and wait to see if they have an effect.

2.8 Coping with pressure

You are the FY1 working on a surgical unit covering patients on three different wards. The other FY1 in your team has phoned in to let you know that they are unwell and will be away from work for the next two days. This has therefore left you alone on the wards to cover the jobs. There are also two senior house officers (SHOs) on the firm: one who is working night shifts, the other who is scheduled to be in theatre sessions both today and tomorrow. You note that the other surgical team in the hospital have the same number of patients and both FY1s are present. You are struggling to manage seeing both unwell patients and to complete discharge letters for patients and feel that you will need to stay late both days to complete all the jobs.

Choose the **THREE most appropriate** actions to take in this situation.

A Ask the FY1s on the other team if they can help you to complete some of your jobs.

B Ask the night FY1 to stay late to help you clear the discharge letters.

C Ask the SHO if they would be able to leave theatre and help you with the jobs.

D Call the FY1 at home and let them know that they need to come into work regardless of their health.

E Call the rota coordinator and request that they call in a locum to help.

F Leave the discharge summaries for the night team to complete.

G Prioritise seeing ill patients over the discharge letters.

H Stay late for the two days.

2.9 FY1 on call

You are the FY1 on evening call for surgery at a district general hospital, covering both the wards and the admission unit. You have been made aware that there are three admissions waiting to be seen, but you are caught up looking after sick patients on the ward. Your registrar and senior house officer (SHO) are in theatre, and consequently, you are not sure how to safely manage all of these patients.

Choose the **THREE most appropriate** actions to take in this situation.

A Admit the waiting patients to the surgical ward as they may be unstable.

B Ask the theatre staff to get the SHO to ring you in between their cases as you are very busy and would appreciate their help.

C Call the admissions unit and ask the nurse in charge to perform baseline observations on the waiting patients and let you know if any patient is scoring on the 'early warning scores' system.

D Call the medical team to see if they could spare one of their juniors to help you.

E Call the ward nurses and ask if any of the day team doctors are still around to look after their patients because you are too busy.

F Call the ward nurses and ask if any of the patients they have asked you to see are stable and can wait a while before a review.

G Continue to see patients on the ward and see the admissions when the ward jobs are complete.

H Go to theatre and demand the SHO be released to help you.

2.10 Coping with work

You are an FY1 working on a busy surgical firm. You have been struggling with stress and anxiety over recent weeks. You are tearful most days when you get home from work but so far have been managing to keep calm around your colleagues. You do not feel that your problems have been affecting the care of your patients, but they are having a negative impact on your life and relationships outside of work.

Choose the **THREE most appropriate** actions to take in this situation.

A Arrange to meet with your educational supervisor.

B Arrange to take annual leave as soon as possible.

C Call in sick until you feel better.
D Call the General Medical Council (GMC) for advice.
E Discuss with your FY1 friends outside of your team.
F Discuss with your team to let them know that you may need extra support.
G Do more regular exercise.
H Make an appointment with your GP.

2.11 Stressed and overworked

You are an FY1 working in general surgery. It is a busy job, and a senior house officer (SHO) whom you work with is currently off sick, so you are a team member short. You often do not have time for lunch, and you feel exhausted and stressed. You speak to your registrar who tells you that it is all part of the 'journey', and it will make you a better doctor in the end.

Choose the **THREE most appropriate** actions to take in this situation.

A Ask another SHO on your team to help you with your workload.
B Ensure that you are getting regular exercise.
C Have a couple of glasses of wine when you get home in the evening.
D Inform your supervising consultant.
E Make sure that you are getting regular breaks.
F See your own GP.
G Take a day off sick.
H Tell the nursing staff not to bleep you to give you a break.

2.12 On call prioritising

You are working as an FY1 on a busy on-call weekend shift with the surgical team. You have a long list of tasks to complete and are holding the on-call bleep. You receive two bleeps from nurses within a few minutes of each other, each informing you of a patient who is unwell. The first patient has a tachycardia and is experiencing some chest pain. The second patient has a low blood pressure and is feeling dizzy. Each nurse is concerned about their patient and wants an immediate review.

Choose the **THREE most appropriate** actions to take in this situation.

A Inform the nursing staff of your situation and ask one of them to bleep the on-call senior house officer (SHO) about their patient.
B Perform a brief review of each patient and write down a quick management plan.
C Place both patients on your list and see them after you have completed your other tasks.
D Place both patients on your list and see them in the order the nurses contacted you.
E Take details of both patients and their clinical condition and bleep the on-call SHO to ask them to review one of the patients.

F   Take details of both patients and their clinical condition and make your own assessment as to whether you can see the patients in succession.
G   Take details of both patients and their clinical condition and request one of the nurses to bleep the on-call SHO and then to get back to you if she doesn't receive a reply.
H   Write an email to the director of surgery informing her that your workload is too heavy at the weekend.

2.13 Escalating concerns for patient safety

You are working as an FY1 in a busy teaching hospital. You have just started your second rotation on a care of the elderly ward. Over the first few weeks, you notice that your new ward is consistently under-staffed. The nurses appear to be looking after too many patients, and there are not enough healthcare assistants. At lunchtime you have seen patients who are unable to feed themselves being left without enough support to eat their food or have a drink.

Rank in order the following actions in response to this situation (1 = Most appropriate; 5 = Least appropriate).

A   Contact your local newspaper with your concerns.
B   Discuss the situation with the General Medical Council (GMC).
C   Discuss with your consultant the possibility of helping at lunchtime, by feeding patients and providing drinks yourself.
D   Document your concerns in writing by completing an incident form.
E   Raise your concerns with the ward manager or charge nurse.

2.14 Using guidelines

You are an FY1 working on a surgical ward. One of your patients develops palpitations, and you diagnose atrial fibrillation from the trace present on the electrocardiogram (ECG). You realise that you don't know how to treat this condition acutely. When you ask your registrar for advice, they say that they are busy in theatre and that they don't know how to manage the condition anyway. The patient's vital signs are currently stable, but you need to deter-mine the initial steps for managing the situation.

Rank in order the following actions in response to this situation (1 = Most appropriate; 5 = Least appropriate).

A   Ask the other FY1 on the ward for advice as you are aware that they worked on a cardiology ward on their last rotation.
B   Bleep the medical registrar on call.
C   Look for a guideline on the internet from the National Institute for Health and Care Excellence (NICE).
D   Look for a trust guideline on the intranet.
E   Put out a medical emergency team (MET) call.

2.15 Prescribing warfarin

You are the FY1 doctor on a busy general surgical ward. Your shift was supposed to finish two hours ago, but you have still not completed the tasks from the morning's ward round. The sister on the ward approaches you about a patient, recently diagnosed with atrial fibrillation, who has not had his warfarin prescribed. Glancing at the patient's notes, you realise that he has not had his international normalised ratio (INR) checked today. There is no one else available on the ward who is trained in venepuncture.

Rank in order the following actions in response to this situation (1 = Most appropriate; 5 = Least appropriate).

A As the INR had previously been within range, don't prescribe the warfarin.
B Pass the job over to the night medical team for them to complete.
C Prescribe the same dose that the patient received the day before as you do not have time to check the INR again.
D Take the blood yourself, send an urgent INR request to the laboratory and ask the night team to chase the results and prescribe the warfarin.
E Tell the nurse that you are very busy but will ask another doctor to take the blood and request the INR.

2.16 Skills unsupervised

You are reviewing a patient with a severe laceration to their head after a fall. After a full examination, you are satisfied that their neurological status is normal, and you ask your senior house officer (SHO) to supervise you suturing the wound as you haven't practised this skill since medical school. Your SHO says they are too busy to supervise you and says that a competent FY1 should be able to suture alone. They ask you to suture the patient quickly so you can continue with other jobs as it is very busy on the ward at the moment.

Rank in order the following actions in response to this situation (1 = Most appropriate; 5 = Least appropriate).

A Ask a doctor who is working in the emergency department (ED) if they would come and suture your patient.
B Ask an FY1 colleague who has an interest in surgery and performs suturing frequently to supervise you.
C Ask your registrar if they can supervise you
D Delegate this task to a fellow FY1 colleague who is more confident than you.
E Suture the patient to the best of your ability.

2.17 Learning from mistakes

You are having a busy day and accidentally prescribe a penicillin-based antibiotic to a patient who reports having an allergic reaction to penicillin. The nurse drawing up the drug checks the allergy section of the drug card and notices the reported reaction. They do not deliver the antibiotic and contact you to prescribe an alternative antibiotic. You are worried that this may happen again.

Rank in order the following actions in response to this situation (1 = Most appropriate; 5 = Least appropriate).

A   Add an additional column to your handover sheet for allergies to help avoid this situation in future.
B   Discuss your workload with your consultant and the serious errors you are making because you are so stretched.
C   Fill in an incident form.
D   Prescribe an alternative antibiotic and think no more of the event.
E   Reflect on this event in your e-portfolio.

2.18 Not coping

You are having some problems in your personal life. You are finding it difficult to get to work on time, and when you are at work, you find it difficult to concentrate on your patients. You are aware that you have been making mistakes that you would not normally have made.

Choose the **THREE most appropriate** actions to take in this situation.

A   Ask an FY1 colleague to check your work.
B   Ask an FY1 colleague to take some of your shifts.
C   Call in sick for a few days while you try to resolve the problems in your personal life.
D   Continue working but make an effort to be on time.
E   Discuss your situation with your clinical supervisor.
F   Go and see your GP for help.
G   Inform your consultant of your situation.
H   Take some annual leave.

2.19 Mistake

You are looking after an elderly lady who has been vomiting for the past two hours. She was admitted with an extradural haematoma. This is your first time looking after a patient with a head injury. You therefore do not realise that her continued vomiting is a sign that her condition may be deteriorating. Instead you prescribe an anti-emetic. When your senior house officer (SHO) comes up to the ward, he explains to you that you have made a mistake and arranges an urgent computed tomography (CT) head scan for the patient. The CT scan shows that there has been no further bleed, and the patient is unharmed by your mistake.

Rank in order the following actions in response to this situation (1 = Most appropriate; 5 = Least appropriate).

A   Ask the SHO not to tell anyone about your mistake.
B   Ask your consultant to arrange a teaching session on head injuries for you and your colleagues.

C Discuss your mistake with your educational supervisor.
D Read the guidelines from the National Institute for Health and Care Excellence (NICE) on the management of head injuries.
E Reflect on the incident in your e-portfolio.

2.20 Failing to do arterial blood gas

You are an FY1 on a very busy medical on-call night shift and are asked to see a patient who is suffering from breathlessness and a productive cough. She has a high respiratory rate and a widespread wheeze. You notice that she has a history of chronic obstructive pulmonary disease in her notes. As you are talking to her, she becomes increasingly drowsy. You complete your history and examination and decide on your management plan. Part of this is to carry out an arterial blood gas (ABG) test. You have done several before, but unfortunately, you have failed the last four attempts you made on previous patients.

Rank in order the following actions in response to this situation (1 = Most appropriate; 5 = Least appropriate).

A Ask the on-call senior house officer (SHO) to come and watch you perform the procedure, giving advice on technique.
B Ask the on-call SHO to complete the ABG while you order a chest x-ray and document your findings.
C Attempt the ABG yourself and bleep your SHO if you are unsuccessful.
D Attend the clinical skills department for further teaching on ABGs.
E Perform a venous blood gas (VBG) instead.

2.21 Challenging a senior

You are an FY1 in breast surgery, and you are assisting a specialist registrar (SpR) in theatre. You notice that he has contaminated his sterile field, but he continues with the operation as though he has not noticed.

Rank in order the following actions in response to this situation (1 = Most appropriate; 5 = Least appropriate).

A Inform the SpR of his mistake and suggest that he re-familiarises himself with theatre infection control procedures.
B Ensure that the patient receives appropriate post-operative antibiotics to lessen the risk of infection but do not challenge the SpR.
C Point out to the SpR that he has contaminated his sterile field.
D Ask the theatre sister to tell the SpR.
E Make a complaint about the SpR to his consultant.

2.22 Incorrect consent

You are an FY1 on a surgical ward and receive a phone call from a member of the theatre nursing staff asking you to bring a patient's consent form to theatre, which has been accidentally left on the ward by the hospital porters. You are unfamiliar with the procedure the patient is going to have but understand that they will be having a general anaesthetic. The patient left the ward with the porters 20 minutes ago, and you are informed that the patient is in the anaesthetic room, about to have the anaesthetic. While you are checking that you have the correct form, you notice a section of the consent form that has not been completed correctly. On the first page of the form the 'risks of the procedure' section is blank. The remainder of the form has been completed and signed by your consultant and the patient.

Rank in order the following actions in response to this situation (1 = Most appropriate; 5 = Least appropriate).

A   Complete the blank section on the form using your knowledge of the general risks of operations and take the form to theatre.
B   Presume the operation has no risks and walk to theatre, taking the form with you.
C   Telephone the anaesthetic room and ask the anaesthetist not to undertake the anaesthetic until you have spoken to your consultant.
D   Telephone the theatre coordinator and inform them to stop the operation.
E   Telephone your consultant in theatre to inform him that the consent form has been incorrectly completed and ask him to stop the anaesthetic until the form is completed.

2.23 Patient control of discharge summary

You are an FY1 working on an acute medical unit. You are preparing the discharge paperwork for a patient. When you reviewed her earlier in the day, she explained that she was under a lot of stress and struggling with her mental health. She also mentioned that she was not currently able to live at her registered address so was staying with a friend. You record what she has told you in the notes and mention these facts in her discharge letter. The patient becomes angry, accuses you of abusing her trust and asks for the details of her mental health and living situation to be removed from her notes and all other paperwork.

Rank in order the following actions in response to this situation (1 = Most appropriate; 5 = Least appropriate).

A   Ask the senior nurse in charge to speak to the patient with you, and explain that you must record information you are aware of accurately on all medical documents.
B   Call your registrar to ask for advice and support when speaking to the patient.
C   Change the discharge address back to her registered address only.
D   Refuse to change anything on the discharge letter and leave.
E   Remove the relevant page from her medical notes and change the address on the discharge summary.

2.24 Absent without leave (AWOL)

You are on call working with a registrar whom you have worked with before. You find him quite difficult to work with as he does not answer his bleep promptly, and when he does, he is very short with you and talks over you when you try to give him patient information. You are worried that his lack of listening is compromising patient care as he does not give you enough time to finish telling him about sick patients.

Rank in order the following actions in response to this situation (1 = Most appropriate; 5 = Least appropriate).

A Ask the switchboard operator if there is another registrar you can talk to.
B Conclude that he is a registrar and more experienced than you, so you should trust his judgement; if he was really worried, he would listen.
C Persist in calling the registrar because you should call for help if you are concerned for a patient and feeling out of your depth.
D Ring the on-call consultant and ask them to come and review your patients.
E Talk to the senior house officer (SHO) on duty with you and ask them to review your patients for the rest of the shift.

2.25 Bullying registrar

You are the FY1 on a surgical team. You are having difficulty getting on with one of the new registrars. You feel that they constantly undermine you in front of other colleagues, are patronising when delegating jobs and overly critical when you have been unable to complete all of your tasks due to a high workload. This problem is making you dread coming to work.

Choose the **THREE most appropriate** actions to take in this situation.

A Challenge the registrar next time they make a critical comment on the ward.
B Contact the hospital staff counselling and conflict resolution service.
C Discuss the issue with your clinical supervisor.
D Make an appointment to see your GP.
E Talk to the registrar in private to let them know that you are upset.
F Telephone the General Medical Council (GMC) to report the registrar's behaviour.
G Try to swap the weekend you are supposed to work on call with the registrar.
H Warn the next group of FY1s that this registrar can be a bully.

2.26 Understaffing

You are an FY1 working on a busy medical ward, which you struggle to manage on your own when your junior colleagues are away. Your FY2 is part time and so only works two days a week. However, during those two days she insists on attending optional off-site teaching leaving you to manage the ward alone for the afternoon.

Rank in order the following actions in response to this situation (1 = Most appropriate; 5 = Least appropriate).

A Ask your educational supervisor for advice.
B Discuss the issue with your FY2 colleague.
C Raise the issue with your consultant.
D Raise your concerns about understaffing at the next ward meeting.
E Talk to your FY1 colleagues and ask them to hint to the FY2 that she should spend more time on the ward.

2.27 Absent colleague

You are working in plastic surgery with another FY1 who wishes to pursue a career in that specialty. You aspire to work in general practice. On the days that you are scheduled to work together on the wards, you often don't see them because they attend theatre to gain experience, leaving you on the ward to cope alone. They often don't tell you where they are going or turn up for ward round in the morning, assuming that you will do the work in their absence. They get along very well with your seniors due to their dedication to the specialty.

Rank in order the following actions in response to this situation (1 = Most appropriate; 5 = Least appropriate).

A Speak to your clinical supervisor about how to get fair help on the wards.
B Speak to your registrar about your colleague's lack of support on the ward.
C Speak to your colleague about needing them to help out on the wards more often.
D Keep covering for your colleague so that they can gain more experience.
E Arrange with your colleague for them to cover your shifts sometimes so that you can gain experience in what you would like to do.

2.28 Mean registrar

You are working as an FY1 in general surgery at a busy teaching hospital, and the job is notoriously hard work. You are managing the long hours and large patient load to the best of your ability, but your registrar is constantly berating you. He expects you to know all the day's blood tests by heart, get tests done the same day and have completed a mini ward round yourself before he starts at 7 am. When you fail at any of these tasks, he shouts at you publicly on the ward and threatens to talk to your clinical supervisor about your incompetence. His demands mean that you feel you have to come to work hours early and stay hours late to complete all the tasks, and it is wearing you down.

Choose the **THREE most appropriate** actions to take in this situation.

A Call in sick for work when you become too tired.
B Discuss with your registrar ways by which you can achieve his objectives without having to stay hours late every day.

C Inform the trust of the registrar's unfair behaviour.
D Refuse to carry out your registrar's unreasonable demands and complete the tasks that you think are appropriate.
E Speak to the British Medical Association (BMA) about how to handle workplace bullying.
F Speak with your registrar privately to discuss your working relationship.
G Talk with your consultant about the unfair demands of your registrar.
H Work as hard as you can to achieve your registrar's demands.

2.29 Shredding nurse

You are an FY1 working on a surgical ward. You have a challenging working relationship with one of the nurses on your ward. She is very competent and good at her job, but she can be very sharp and demanding of you at times and is very critical when you make mistakes. On a busy weekend day shift, you are working alone covering all of the surgical wards and have come to review a sick patient. You leave your handover sheet with the day's jobs on it on the nurses' station while you assess the patient. On your return you cannot find your handover sheet, and this nurse informs you that she has shredded it as it is confidential information and should not be left lying around. You now do not know what jobs you have left to complete.

Rank in order the following actions in response to this situation (1 = Most appropriate; 5 = Least appropriate).

A Shout at the nurse for her inconsiderate behaviour.
B Speak to the ward sister or charge nurse about the nurse in question and her inconsiderate actions.
C Speak privately with the nurse in question about shredding your list and discuss your working relationship.
D Complain to your consultant about this nurse who is making your job difficult.
E Calmly leave the ward, print out a new list and spend some time methodically trying to remember all of your jobs that are outstanding.

2.30 Interpreters

You are the FY1 on call on the admissions unit for the evening. A young woman, looking very unwell, comes in with her sister. The patient does not speak English, but her sister can speak some. You are quite worried about the patient.

Choose the **THREE most appropriate** actions to take in this situation.

A Ask another doctor who you think speaks the same language as the patient to see her.
B Ask her sister to act as a translator for you.
C Ask the nurse to come and help you take the history.
D Contact the local interpreter service and ask them to send someone in.

E   Decide to see another patient waiting to be seen instead.
F   Instead of taking a history, examine the patient to get a better idea of what may be causing her clinical picture.
G   Order some tests and send the patient for those while trying to find an interpreter.
H   Use a phone interpreter.

2.31 Demanding patient

You are the FY1 working in a clinical decision unit. You have two unwell patients on the ward. One is a middle-aged man who has suffered an acute myocardial infarction. The other is an elderly woman with a urinary tract infection causing her to be confused. However, you are called frequently regarding another patient, a young man who has been admitted for observation after being brought to hospital intoxicated. This patient is demanding that you come to see him and threatening to self-discharge if you do not.

Rank in order the following actions in response to this situation (1 = Most appropriate; 5 = Least appropriate).

A   Assess the young man and discuss his concerns.
B   Prescribe initial treatment for the patient with the myocardial infarction.
C   Decline to see the young man.
D   Prescribe antibiotics for the patient with a urinary tract infection.
E   Organise the transfer of the patient with the myocardial infarction to a hospital providing definitive management.

2.32 Nurse–patient breakdown

You are an FY1 in general surgery doing a night shift. A nurse tells you that she is struggling with a demanding patient who has recently had an operation. The patient is complaining a lot and requesting frequent doses of strong opioids. The nurse also says that the pain is 'all in her head'. You notice that the nurse is not attending the patient for a long time when the patient pushes the button to call her. You feel that their relationship has broken down.

Rank in order the following actions in response to this situation (1 = Most appropriate; 5 = Least appropriate).

A   Speak to the lead nurse on the ward about the issue.
B   Ask the patient to stop being rude and demanding.
C   Decrease the patient's analgesia.
D   Suggest that the nurse changes the care of the patient to another nurse.
E   Leave the nurse and the patient to resolve their issues.

2.33 Patient error

You are an FY1 on a care of the elderly ward. You review a patient's chest x-ray, which shows consolidation that is consistent with pneumonia.

You inform the patient, prescribe an appropriate antibiotic and insert a peripheral cannula. After the patient has received a dose of the antibiotic, you realise that you have looked at the wrong patient's chest x-ray and have therefore given the wrong patient antibiotic treatment.

Rank in order the following actions in response to this situation (1 = Most appropriate; 5 = Least appropriate).

A   Leave the patient to complete the course of antibiotics.
B   Ask your senior house officer (SHO) to inform the patient of your error and stop the antibiotic.
C   Cross the antibiotic off the prescription chart without informing the patient.
D   Fill in an incident form.
E   Inform the patient of your mistake, apologise and stop the antibiotic therapy.

2.34 Unable to get chaperone

As a male FY2 working in a GP surgery, you see a woman with dyspareunia in your clinic. You explain that you need to do an examination of her external genitalia and a vaginal examination with a chaperone present. She agrees to the examination, but you cannot find a member of staff who is trained to be a chaperone. You feel uncomfortable doing the examination without a chaperone.

Rank in order the following actions in response to this situation (1 = Most appropriate; 5 = Least appropriate).

A   Ask her partner who is in the waiting room to be a chaperone.
B   Perform the examination without a chaperone present.
C   Ask her to come to see you tomorrow when you can arrange for a chaperone to be present.
D   Make a diagnosis and treat the patient on the basis of your history.
E   Ask your patient to see one of your female colleagues.

2.35 Chaperones

You are an FY1 working a busy weekend night shift in an emergency department. A young woman with known alcoholism has attended due to an episode of bleeding per rectum. You suspect rectal varices and wish to examine the anus and perform a digital rectal examination. The young woman smells of alcohol and has obviously been drinking. She consents to the examination, but when you offer her a chaperone she declines on the basis that it will take a few minutes to find a chaperone, and she has already been waiting to be seen for four hours and wants to go home as soon as possible.

Rank in order the following actions in response to this situation (1 = Most appropriate; 5 = Least appropriate).

A   Perform the examination and document fully in the notes the patient's refusal of a chaperone.

B Explain to the patient the reasons for having a chaperone present during intimate examinations and refuse to undertake the examination until one is present.
C Explain to the patient the reasons for having a chaperone present during intimate examinations but that because of her long wait to be seen you will bypass this protocol this time.
D Decide not to undertake the examination at this time.
E Ask the advice of the emergency department registrar regarding the need for a chaperone in this case.

2.36 E-portfolio

You are working as an FY1 on a busy surgical ward, and your department is struggling with the workload since one consultant is off on long-term sick leave. You have not been able to meet with your clinical supervisor because of this, and you are finding it difficult to complete the mandatory aspects of your FY1 e-portfolio. Every time you approach your consultant, they say that they are far too busy to be dealing with junior doctors' paperwork.

Rank in order the following actions in response to this situation (1 = Most appropriate; 5 = Least appropriate).

A Inform your educational supervisor of this problem.
B Inform the foundation programme director at your trust and ask to switch clinical supervisors.
C Come in to the hospital during your annual leave to try and meet with your supervisor.
D Ask another consultant to meet with you and sign off your paperwork.
E Write a letter of complaint to the clinical lead of the department about your consultant's failure to meet your educational needs.

2.37 Educational supervision

You are an FY1 working on a medical ward. You are running late one evening and are still on the ward after the end of your shift. You have previously arranged a meeting with your educational supervisor, which is due to begin in 10 minutes. You are asked by one of the nurses on your ward to see a patient who is scoring on the 'early warning scores' and whom she is quite concerned about. You call the on-call doctor who tells you they are currently with another sick patient.

Rank in order the following actions in response to this situation (1 = Most appropriate; 5 = Least appropriate).

A Ask the on-call senior house officer (SHO) to come and see the patient on your ward when they are done.
B Call the on-call registrar and ask them to see the patient.
C Go and quickly review the patient to alleviate the nurse's worries.
D Go and perform a full review of the patient knowing it will make you late for your meeting.

E   Ring your educational supervisor and let them know the situation, ask
if they can come and observe you seeing the patient as a mini-clinical
evaluation exercise (CEX).

2.38 Clerking responsibilities

You are an FY1 doctor working on call in the medical assessment unit of a
teaching hospital. Your duties are to clerk patients and present them to the
medical registrar or the consultant on call. You are looking at the long list of
patients to be seen, and you notice that in the few hours you have been on your
shift you have seen four patients, and your FY1 colleague has only managed to
see one patient. There are many patients waiting to be seen, and you feel that
you are under significant pressure.

Rank in order the following actions in response to this situation (1 = Most
appropriate; 5 = Least appropriate).

A   Contact the medical registrar and voice your concerns about your
colleague.
B   Continue to see the patients on the list and hope your colleague can catch
up with you later on.
C   Inform the medical registrar that you feel you are under too much pressure
to work through such a long list of patients.
D   Offer to take over the clerking of the patient your colleague is seeing as
they are taking too long.
E   Politely ask your colleague why they have only seen one patient during
the day.

2.39 Emergency in the community

You are driving to meet a friend for a meal; you haven't seen them for a while,
and you are late. You see a person lying slumped on the pavement – you cannot
see any signs of life, and there are people crowding around looking concerned.

Rank in order the following actions in response to this situation (1 = Most
appropriate; 5 = Least appropriate).

A   Tell the people to call an ambulance, but don't stop to help.
B   Make a quick assessment and perform cardiopulmonary resuscitation
(CPR) if necessary, ensuring emergency services are informed.
C   Do nothing as you don't have an obligation to help outside of work.
D   Phone for an ambulance yourself, but don't stop to help.
E   Ask if anyone there has first-aid training; if they do, phone for an ambu-
lance and then leave.

2.40 Unsafe on call

You are an FY1 working a medical weekend on call. You are extremely busy
and receive many calls to see deteriorating patients. Your senior house officer

(SHO) has asked you not to contact him in the morning as he will be doing a post-take ward round with a consultant. You are struggling to keep up with the workload and feel that some deteriorating patients are being left for a long time before a medical review. Before the weekend, you had spoken to a few of your FY1 colleagues who all feel that the workload is unmanageable.

Choose the **THREE most appropriate** actions to take in this situation.

A   Ask one of your friends who is also a doctor to come in to work and help you.
B   Ask the nurses to contact you only when they are very worried about a patient.
C   Inform the medical registrar on call.
D   Inform the SHO that you are not coping with the workload.
E   Prioritise your workload, seeing the most unwell patients first.
F   See all the unwell patients as quickly as possible and do not stop for lunch.
G   Speak to your consultant about your concerns after the weekend.
H   Write a letter to the medical director highlighting your concerns.

2.41 Complaint

You are a male FY1 working in medicine. Your educational supervisor informs you that one of the female patients on the ward has lodged a complaint against you. The patient had originally presented with symptoms consistent with raised intracranial pressure. You had therefore performed fundoscopy but had done so in a room alone with the patient. The patient has complained that they felt uncomfortable during the examination. Your educational supervisor has therefore arranged for you to work on a different ward until the patient is discharged.

Rank in order the following actions in response to this situation (1 = Most appropriate; 5 = Least appropriate).

A   Approach the patient and explain that there must have been a misunderstanding.
B   Ask a colleague to approach the patient and explain that there must have been a misunderstanding.
C   Ask the patient to drop the complaint as it may damage your career.
D   Contact your medical defence organisation and seek their advice.
E   Do nothing and allow the hospital to continue resolving the complaint.

2.42 Coroner statement

You return to your ward after a week of annual leave to find a letter waiting for you in your letter tray. It is a letter from the coroner's office regarding a patient who died on your ward a couple of weeks ago. The letter explains that there are some concerns regarding the circumstances of the patient's death and asks you to make a statement about your involvement with their care. You have never written a statement for the coroner before, and you remember little about the patient since you only met them briefly.

Choose the **THREE most appropriate** actions to take in this situation.

A   Ask the nurses about their recollection of the case.
B   Ask to see what another doctor involved in the case has written in their statement.
C   Consult your educational supervisor for advice regarding how to write a statement.
D   Decide that as you only met the patient briefly, there is no need to write a statement.
E   Locate the patient's notes, re-familiarise yourself with the case and subsequently write a statement.
F   Put off writing the statement until you have time to think about it properly.
G   Ring a medical defence organisation for advice.
H   Write the statement as soon as possible based on your memory of the case.

2.43 Angry registrar

You are an FY1 in surgery, and you are on a busy ward round. The registrar has asked you to prescribe a medication, but you didn't hear what dose was required, so you ask for clarification. The registrar turns around and shouts at you in front of the nursing staff, patients and other juniors for not listening and being incompetent in your role on the ward round.

Rank in order the following actions in response to this situation (1 = Most appropriate; 5 = Least appropriate).

A   Loudly defend yourself: the registrar is making you look bad in front of all of your co-workers.
B   Apologise to the registrar, explaining that you wished to be careful in your prescribing and ask him how you could better help on the ward round in future.
C   Apologise to the registrar, explaining that you wished to be careful in your prescribing and then avoid working with that registrar in future.
D   Apologise to the registrar, explaining that you wished to be careful in your prescribing and ask to speak with them later to discuss your working relationship.
E   Apologise to the registrar and then speak to your consultant about the incident.

2.44 EWTD breach

You are an FY1 working on a busy surgical team, and you are understaffed because a fellow FY1 is off on long-term sick leave. Although you have locum FY1s on a regular basis, they do not know the ward or the patients, and you and your FY1 colleagues find yourself staying extra hours beyond your contracted finishing time almost every day. When you mention this to your registrar, they say that when they were a junior, they had to work much harder than you do and that you should just get on with it.

Rank in order the following actions in response to this situation (1 = Most appropriate; 5 = Least appropriate).

A Continue working as normal; you will change jobs in a few months and then things will be easier.
B Speak to your foundation programme director.
C Speak to your consultant about such extreme hours.
D Take some days off 'sick' to pay yourself back for the extra hours.
E Send an email to the chief executive officer (CEO) of your trust informing them of the breach of hours.

2.45 Responding to colleague's request

It is a busy morning on the medical admissions unit (MAU). One of the staff nurses approaches you and asks how long it will be before you see Mrs Clark. She says that the patient has already been waiting two hours with a lot of pain and she can't give any analgesia until you have clerked them and prescribed their medicines.

Rank in order the following actions in response to this situation (1 = Most appropriate; 5 = Least appropriate).

A Approach the patient and apologise for their wait; explain that you are very busy but are aware of them and will be with them as soon as you can.
B Explain calmly to the nurse that you are aware of the patient and will get to them as soon as you can.
C Prescribe some morphine without seeing the patient to keep the nurse happy.
D Make sure that you leave Mrs Clark until last on your list, just to annoy the nurse.
E Ask your senior house officer (SHO) whether they have time to see Mrs Clark.

ANSWERS

2.1 Forgotten patient review

A C E

It is very easy to forget about jobs when you are busy. When you make a mistake, you must firstly be honest and admit your error and then apologise (A). As well as acknowledging your mistake, you should try to prevent the same incident from occurring again, which could be achieved by creating a jobs list (C). You should also check that the patient is stable and not deteriorating (E). Claiming that you did review the patient and that the nursing staff must have lost the documentation (B) or writing a review and timing it as yesterday (H) are both dishonest and immoral. The Medical Protection Society (MPS) warn against altering entries in records or creating entries made after an event. These are called non-contemporaneous records and are taken very seriously by courts of law and regulatory bodies (Medical Councils and Medical Boards). Doing nothing (D) is likely to damage your relationship with the nursing staff because they will be less likely to trust you in the future. Informing your consultant of your error (F) is unnecessary as you should be able to resolve this incident yourself. Telling the nursing staff that they should have bleeped the on-call doctor if they were concerned (G) is appropriate but less so than the other three options because it also shifts the blame onto the nursing staff.

Recommended reading

Medical Protection Society (2012), Honesty, in *MPS Guide to Ethics: A Map for the Moral Maze*, chapter 6.

2.2 False statement

D C A E B

This is a difficult scenario as you would want to support your colleague. It would, however, be immoral to submit a fabricated and false statement (B), so that is the least appropriate response. Your colleague is likely to be frightened about the complaint and has therefore asked you to do something that is unprofessional, without thinking about the possible implications for you; you should refuse to make the false statement but offer to submit a general report about her professional behaviour to support her (D). Simply refusing to make the statement (C) would be completely moral but is not ideal as it does not offer the support that your colleague requires. Making a complaint against your colleague to a senior (A) is also less appropriate for the same reasons. Speaking to the relative (E) is inappropriate since this is not likely to result in the relative withdrawing the complaint, and the relative still has a right to complain even if you find the issue unfounded.

Recommended reading

Medical Protection Society (2012), Honesty and Personal conduct, in *MPS Guide to Ethics: A Map for the Moral Maze,* chapters 6 and 12.

2.3 Nursing pressure to refer

A E F

This question assesses your ability to cope under pressure while ensuring that you always put the care and safety of your patients first. Sometimes in medicine, pressures that are outside your control will affect your behaviour. However, it is important that you deal with them in a calm, safe and professional manner. In this scenario, you may disagree with the sister's instruction, and it is therefore imperative that you use your communication skills to respond politely to the sister while doing your job to the best of your ability. It would be appropriate to explain your stance diplomatically (F), which would both show respect for your colleague and ensure that the care and safety of the patient takes priority. Apologising to the patient is also a courteous gesture and one that demonstrates empathy with their situation; therefore option A would also be sensible. In situations where you feel that patient safety is being compromised, it is important to alert your seniors, which is why option E is also appropriate; however, this should be done without trying to lay blame on other colleagues without evidence (options B and D). Options C and G, while involving an assessment and/or referral of the patient, do not concurrently demonstrate a safe approach to assessing a sick patient and do not show respect for your colleague. Refusing to see the patient (H) is wholly inappropriate as this behaviour could have a negative impact on a sick patient.

Recommended reading

General Medical Council (2012), *Raising and Acting on Concerns About Patient Safety.*

General Medical Council (2013), *Good Medical Practice,* paragraphs 15, 23, 25, 35–37, 55–57, 68.

2.4 Audit presentation

D E A B C

You have made a commitment to delivering the presentation and should therefore endeavour to do so even though you are tired (options D and E). You have put time and effort into the audit, and this is a valuable learning opportunity that it would be a shame to pass up. It is sensible and reasonable to ask to move the time to allow you to get home to rest adequately (D). Options B and C rank lowest because they are both dishonest. You are not unwell (B), but at least in option B, you will have informed the chair of your absence rather than just failing to show (C). Insisting that your friend comes in is not professional: it is likely to start an argument, and it may well be that she really is incapacitated (A). Nevertheless, this would be preferable to options B or C because it does not involve deceit, and it attempts to ensure that the presentation is delivered.

Recommended reading

General Medical Council (2013), *Good Medical Practice,* paragraphs 65–80.

The UK Foundation Programme Curriculum (2012), section 3.2: Quality and safety improvement.

2.5 Prioritization

C   B   A   D   E

Your priority when you are on call is to be available to attend emergencies on the wards. Option C is therefore the best option because it declines politely and makes a proactive suggestion for an alternative meeting, which will hopefully satisfy the family. Option C is better than B because your workload is unpredictable when you are on call, and you may struggle to get there and leave the family more frustrated. Informing the nurse that you will be unable to attend (A) is realistic but sounds somewhat rude and offers no alternative to placate the family, which is likely to leave the nurse feeling fobbed off and stuck with angry relatives. It is reasonable to defer the family meeting until in-hours, and the two options that involve other members of the on-call team therefore rank lowest (options D and E). If you are going to take up the time of other on-call doctors, it is better for you to ask the SHO to attend to the emergency and go to see the family as you know them and the case already. It will use up more time for the on-call registrar to read and find out about a patient they don't know, and they are likely to be busy with sick patients themselves (E).

Recommended reading

General Medical Council (2013), *Good Medical Practice*, paragraphs 31–34.
The UK Foundation Programme Curriculum (2012), section 1.4: Team-working.
The UK Foundation Programme Curriculum (2012), section 8.1: Promptly
    assesses the acutely ill, collapsed or unconscious patient.

2.6 List of jobs

D   C   B   E   A

Being on call is a key part of being a doctor, and your workload can be very heavy at times. In these situations you need to be able to prioritise effectively. The most appropriate option is D: seeing the patient who is deteriorating as soon as possible as a quick response could prevent a critical situation. The next most appropriate course of action would be to find out more information about the patient requiring bloods checking and see if someone else would be able to take the bloods, for example a phlebotomist (C). In times of increased workload, you may need more information to effectively prioritise jobs, and you should be able to delegate work when appropriate. Telling the nursing staff to bleep the on-call SHO (B) is a reasonable response, but it would be preferable to gather more information about the jobs required and subsequently bleep the SHO yourself so that you have more information to hand over. It may be true that speaking to patients about medication which has already been started before the weekend is an inappropriate job when on call at the weekend (E), but had you been less busy you may have been able to do this. This attitude is also unlikely to help your working relationship with the nurse. Doing all your jobs as quickly as possible (A) is the least appropriate action because you should not rush reviewing unwell patients, and you are more likely to make errors working in this way.

Recommended reading
General Medical Council (2013), *Good Medical Practice*, paragraphs 14–16.

2.7 Seeking help

D C B A E

While challenging situations are helpful to aid your learning, you should never feel unsupported. Help should always be available, particularly once you feel that you have reached the limits of your competency. In this scenario, the registrar has a responsibility to aid you and a responsibility to ensure the safety of the patient. It is therefore appropriate to insist that they come in to review the patient (D). When seeking help, it is advisable to work up the chain of seniority within your team. The consultant should therefore be your next option if the registrar is unable or, in this case, unwilling to assist (C). There may be occasions where the rest of your team are genuinely unable to attend due to other emergencies, and you should therefore be aware of other people who may be able to assist. In this scenario, it would be appropriate to call the anaesthetist for help if your team was unavailable (B). While the medical registrar (A) may also be able to provide help, the anaesthetist is a more favourable choice since they will likely have more experience with surgical patients. In addition, they will ultimately be involved with the patient if or when he goes to theatre. The least appropriate option is E: you are struggling to manage this patient alone and you risk his condition becoming worse if you continue unaided. Even if you have been refused help once, it is your responsibility to continue seeking help if needed.

Recommended reading
General Medical Council (2013), *Good Medical Practice,* paragraphs 14, 15c, 16d.

2.8 Coping with pressure

A C G

This is a difficult, but common scenario and most of the listed options could in reality be considered; however, you need to determine how you can manage the workload to the best of your ability as an FY1. If the other team is better staffed than you, asking them to help is appropriate (A). Asking your SHO to help (C) is also sensible as they too are on the team and are required to help supervise you, provided that there are enough people in theatre to safely operate. As always when working, it is crucial to prioritise assessing ill patients (G). Option E will already be in hand as the FY1 will have to call the rota coordinator to notify them of their absence, and they should already be trying to improve the situation. Unfortunately, it may be likely that you will need to stay later than your contracted hours (H), but you should not use this as your only management plan. The other three options are not appropriate: asking the night team to stay out of hours is unfair and will leave them tired for the next shift (B), calling an ill FY1 into work puts patients and them at risk (D) and discharge summaries are not a job for the night team, so it is unfair to ask them to do this (F).

Recommended reading

Medical Protection Society (2012), Professionalism and integrity, in *MPS Guide to Ethics: A Map for the Moral Maze,* chapter 3.

2.9 FY1 on call

B C F

This is a difficult but common scenario which you must become adept at managing. The most important thing is to ensure that all the patients are safe while they wait for your review. Therefore, this makes options C and F both good choices as finding out from the nursing staff if anyone is haemodynamically unstable will help you triage which patient is sickest. Option B is also in the top three because, while demanding the SHO be released to help (H) is not professional as the SHO is likely needed in theatre, asking if the SHO could help between cases is useful as there is usually a significant time period at this point where they could help you with your workload. Simply admitting the patients and ignoring the wards (A) or vice versa (G) is not safe as you do not know what the other patients' presenting problems are. Calling the medical team (D) is not appropriate, and they will likely have their own list of patients to see, nor is option E because if you are on call out of hours, the day team should be able to leave on time in order to adhere with their rota as per the European Working Time Directive.

Recommended reading

https://www.gov.uk/maximum-weekly-working-hours/overview
http://www.juniordr.com/index.php/mps-advice-centre/the-stress-factor.html

2.10 Coping with work

A F H

It is important to recognise times when you might be struggling and to seek appropriate help through official channels. As you are managing to cope at work, there is no immediate need for you to remove yourself from the hospital (C). While you may find it helpful to take some annual leave (B), this is not one of the best options as it is more important to take active steps to get more support while you are at work. Your educational supervisor is the most important person to arrange to meet with (A). They can advise and provide support as well as link into other sources of help. It would also be proactive to speak to members of your team (F) as they can keep an eye on you on a day-to-day basis and could raise any patient safety concerns if the situation deteriorated. This is more useful than discussing with other FY1s (E) because, although peer support is valuable, they are not in a position to provide support to you directly on the job. You do not have any concerns about your fitness to practise, so you do not need to call the GMC (D). It is important to see your GP (H) for several reasons. First, it is useful to talk to a professional outside your work environment. Second, your GP can assess the extent of your mental health difficulties and consider medication or talking therapies if appropriate. Although it may well help to increase your levels of physical activity (G), this is an adjunct to seeking help and is not as important as the three most appropriate answers.

Recommended reading
General Medical Council (2013), *Good Medical Practice,* paragraphs 28–30.
The UK Foundation Programme Curriculum (2012), section 3.1: Risks of fatigue, ill health and stress.

2.11 Stressed and overworked

A D E
Coping with pressure is a necessary skill for doctors; however, it is also important to recognise when this pressure is too much and you need help. Unfortunately, your registrar does not seem to have understood your situation and has not provided you with helpful advice. In this case, it would be best to inform a more senior colleague who is approachable, such as your supervising consultant (D) or your educational supervisor. In the meantime, you need to make sure that you are reducing your stress levels at work. Asking another SHO to help you (A), and thereby admitting that you are struggling, could be difficult but your team should be made aware of this so that changes can be made. Making sure you are getting regular breaks (E) should also help your performance levels and give you the chance to eat something and recuperate. Not only will this help your well-being, it should also improve your concentration and thereby improve patient safety.

Ensuring that you are getting regular exercise (B) is useful for some people to de-stress, but it does not deal with the immediate problem as effectively as options A, D and E. Having a couple of glasses of wine when you get home (C) may be helpful as a 'one-off' but it is not a long-term solution! Seeing your GP (F) is important if you notice that your mental health is significantly impacting your life; however, hopefully that is not the case at this stage. Taking some time off (G) may be necessary in some instances, but again this is not a long-term resolution and the issues should be addressed before reaching this stage. It would also leave the remaining staff in your team with even more work. Telling the nursing staff not to bleep you to give you a break (H) is not a good solution as nurses may subsequently be discouraged from contacting you in an emergency.

Recommended reading
General Medical Council (2013), *Good Medical Practice,* paragraph 25.

2.12 On call prioritising

E F G
This is a very common scenario to be placed in while working on-call shifts. The most important factor to consider is patient safety. You do not know the

full details about the patients who, in this scenario, could be suffering from a myocardial infarction and sepsis respectively. The most important thing to do is to take details about each patient as this will allow you to make an informed decision. Option F is appropriate as, with more information, you may be able to prioritise your workload and/or decide whether one patient needs to be seen by one of your colleagues. Option E is also valid as this would personally ensure that the message has been relayed to your SHO colleague. Option G includes a 'safety net' and is therefore advantageous. This means that if the nurses do not get a reply from the on call SHO you will be made aware of it and can arrange for a review yourself. This is the reason why option H is preferable to simply asking one of the nurses to contact the SHO themselves (A). Performing a brief review of each patient (B) may lead to inappropriate management plans and incomplete reviews. If you feel your workload is too heavy (H), it may be prudent to raise it with the relevant people; however, this should be done at a time that doesn't endanger patient safety. Non-urgent jobs can be completed in the order that they were referred to you; however, prioritising an unwell patient should encompass a range of other factors rather than just time (D). Option C is unacceptable as this involves prioritising non-urgent tasks over potentially unwell patients.

Recommended reading
General Medical Council (2013), *Good Medical Practice,* paragraphs 14, 15, 16.

2.13 Escalating concerns for patient safety

E   D   B   C   A

This is a difficult and very topical scenario. The Francis Inquiry Report into the events at the Mid-Staffordshire NHS Trust between 2005 and 2009 led to the introduction of 'duty of candour'. This requires staff to disclose information to their employer in cases where they believe that poor care has resulted in death or serious injury to a patient. In this scenario, while the issues may not seem a priority, poor nutrition and hydration can ultimately lead to death or serious injury, especially in elderly patients with multiple co-morbidities. In practice, the best way to tackle this scenario would be first to discuss your concerns with the ward manager or charge nurse as they may not be aware that this has been happening (E). They may be able to find a solution, and the problem could be rectified. However, following this, your concerns should be documented in writing to your employer (D). There is good guidance available to advise when you should escalate the issue to higher governing bodies. You should discuss concerns with the GMC (B) in cases where you cannot discuss your problems locally, or you have raised your problem locally without success or there is immediate serious risk that must be addressed. Offering help yourself (C) is inappropriate as you should not be taken away from your own duties, and this would not help to solve the issue in the long term. Your responsibility as a doctor is not to nurse your patients; this is the role of the nursing staff, and if they are unable to provide adequate care, the issue should be raised with the appropriate higher body. The least appropriate option here would be to contact your local newspaper directly (A). A concern should only be made public when you have done all you can do to deal with it within the organisation or have good belief that patients are still at risk of harm.

Recommended reading
General Medical Council (2012), Explanatory guidance, in *Raising and Acting on Concerns About Patient Safety,* paragraphs 11–17.

2.14 Using guidelines

A D C B E

In this scenario, the patient is stable, so there is some time for you to try to solve the problem yourself. The most readily available source of advice is from your FY1 colleague on the ward (A) who, given their previous experience, should be able to help you with the initial steps you should take, including whom you may need to call. It will be slightly slower to search by yourself for guidelines that you are unfamiliar with (options D and C); however, these are still a good source of advice. Where they are available, local guidelines (D) are preferred over national ones (C). It is appropriate to do some investigatory work yourself to ensure that, if necessary, you refer in the correct manner and make prompt early decisions rather than jumping straight into calling for help (B). However, if you are worried or uncomfortable with a situation, it is never wrong to escalate to others with more experience than yourself. The patient is not acutely unstable, so it would be entirely inappropriate to call the MET or peri-arrest team (E).

Recommended reading
Foundation Programme Curriculum (2012), section 6.2: Evidence, guidelines, care protocols and research.

Medical Protection Society (2012), *MPS Guide to Ethics: A Map for the Moral Maze,* chapter 4, Duty of care, section: Current thinking.

2.15 Prescribing warfarin

D E B A C

This scenario requires you to act safely and in the best interests of the patient while under pressure. Option D is the most appropriate response because patient safety and duty of care should be your first concern, even when you are busy. This response ensures that the patient gets the optimum dose of their medication, but by delegating some of the job to the night staff, you are looking after your health needs as well. Option E is the second most acceptable response as the job would be completed; however, it is unfair to burden colleagues with simple tasks on patients who are not their own, especially as they may be very busy as well. Similarly, passing the job over to the night staff (B) should result in the task being completed but after much delay, and it is a job that the day team should be completing during their shift. The least appropriate response is option C because your actions could potentially harm the patient. Option A is slightly more appropriate (although still not advised) as there is less chance, given the patient's INR history, that omitting one dose will cause harm. However, you are failing to provide the basic standard of care that this patient's condition requires.

Recommended reading
General Medical Council (2009), *The New Doctor,* paragraphs 6, 10.
General Medical Council (2013), *Good Medical Practice*, Duties of a doctor.
General Medical Council (2013), *Good Medical Practice*, paragraphs 15, 16, 45.
Medical Protection Society (2012), *MPS Guide to Ethics: A Map for the Moral Maze,* chapter 4, Duty of care.

2.16 Skills unsupervised

C   B   A   E   D

Senior supervision is not always readily available in practice on the wards and, as an FY1, you need to determine whether you should wait for them or if you are competent enough to undertake skills on your own. Where possible, you should try to develop your practical skills, so getting someone to supervise you both protects patients and facilitates your learning. These responses are the most highly ranked in this question. Option C is the best response because your registrar is the next port of call if your SHO is busy and they could even sign off a direct observation of practical skills (DOPS) section of your e-portfolio. Option B is the next best response as your colleague who has sutured many times before can easily show you a good technique, but it is often better to ask a senior first. Option A is safe so it ranks third: asking an ED doctor to suture your patient. In specialties where suturing is an unusual skill to practise, it is common to request another doctor to attend to suturing, and although they may not be able to attend immediately, an ED doctor is well suited for this. The two worst responses involve suturing without confidence and delegating the task to a colleague to get you out of the difficult situation. If you have been taught this skill properly at medical school and had supervision before, you have had adequate teaching, even though you do not feel confident. For this reason, if you attempt suturing, you are not acting outside your competence, and so option E ranks fourth. Passing the buck to a colleague will not win their favour and doesn't reflect good team-working, so option D is the least appropriate.

Recommended reading
General Medical Council (2013), *Good Medical Practice*, paragraphs 7–13, 35–38.

2.17 Learning from mistakes

C   A   E   B   D

Drug errors are common and some can be lethal. It is important to try and learn from every mistake you make to prevent it happening again. In this question, an incident form (C) is a good way of ensuring this incident is formally looked at by ward management. There may be a pattern in this mistake that you are not aware of, and you shouldn't feel like you are 'turning yourself in' by reporting it. Option A is the second best response: adding another column to your handover sheet is a proactive and resourceful solution and will help you and your FY1 colleagues by having a patient's allergy status to hand at all times. To achieve satisfactory sign-off for the FY1 year, you need to reflect on various situations of your choice. The aim of this being that a dedicated period of time to think about the cause and effect of a situation enables you to tackle it better in future. Therefore, reflecting on the event in your e-portfolio (E) ranks third. Option B is fourth as if the incident occurred because you were too busy to make basic checks, it is important that the team leaders are aware of it; however, it would be difficult to attribute not checking a patient's allergy status solely to being too busy. Not doing anything to prevent the error occurring again (D) is inappropriate and so comes last.

Recommended reading
General Medical Council (2013), *Good Medical Practice,* paragraphs 22–23.

2.18 Not coping

E F G
In this scenario, you are not maintaining your performance as an FY1, and this may be a risk to patient safety. It is important to both recognise and act upon this concern. You should inform your clinical supervisor that you are struggling so that they can provide the support that you need (E). Similarly, you should make your consultant aware of the situation (G). It is also appropriate to see your GP as they may be able to provide the help that you need in order to better cope at work (F). Now that you have recognised a problem with your ability to work, it would be inappropriate to continue trying to resolve the issue (D). Taking annual leave or calling in sick (options H and C) do not properly address this issue. You should not ask an FY1 colleague to check your work (A), and although it may seem like a responsible option, it is not your place to reallocate your workload (B). This is better left to your consultant once you have spoken to them.

Recommended reading
General Medical Council (2013), *Good Medical Practice,* paragraphs 7, 13, 14, 24, 25, 28, 30.

2.19 Mistake

B D C E A
Making mistakes is an inevitable part of being a doctor. While we should always strive to avoid mistakes, when they do happen, they can be used as a valuable learning opportunity. In this instance, option B is most appropriate since it enables both you and your colleagues to learn from your mistake.

Reading the NICE guidelines on head injuries is also important for your own learning (D). Discussing the event with your educational supervisor is also appropriate (C). They may be able to help you to further analyse your actions as well as provide advice on how you can improve your practice. You should continually reflect on your own practice, particularly where you have identified a weakness. Your e-portfolio is a useful way to document those reflections (E), and indeed all doctors are required to keep a record of their reflections. While you would not expect your SHO to talk about your mistake extensively, he may feel it necessary to discuss the events with a supervisor. You should respect that decision; therefore, option A is inappropriate.

Recommended reading
General Medical Council (2013), *Good Medical Practice*, paragraphs 7–15, 22.
Medical Protection Society (2012), *MPS Guide to Ethics: A Map for the Moral Maze*, chapter 10, Competence.

2.20 Failing to do arterial blood gas

C A B D E
A patient with shortness of breath is a common reason for an on-call FY1 to be bleeped. Part of your investigation plan in most cases will include an ABG, and you will be expected to be able to perform this. It is often difficult to practise this skill as a medical student as it is a painful procedure that patients do not like to have to undergo. In this scenario, though, you have clearly been competent at the skill in the past. Occasionally failing at various clinical skills is to be expected when working as a doctor. It is inevitable that, with the workload and the number of procedures you are asked to carry out you will fail at some. In this scenario, the option that would fulfil the patient's needs and not waste any time would be to attempt the procedure yourself (C). Asking the SHO to attend may be appropriate if you either failed to get the required blood or were not working a busy on-call shift. The next most appropriate response would be to ask the SHO to watch you perform the technique (A). This will inevitably prevent your SHO from reviewing other patients, but it would mean that your learning needs are met. Asking the SHO to perform the task themselves (B) would ensure that the patient gets the test they require; however, you would not benefit from the potential learning opportunity. Performing a VBG (E) may be appropriate in some situations (e.g. diabetic ketoacidosis or hyperkalaemia); however, in this scenario, a VBG would not provide the information you require (whether the patient is in type 2 respiratory failure or acidosis). This makes option E the least appropriate. Attending the clinical skills department may lead to you improving your skills and ultimately your confidence (D); however, in this scenario, your patient has an immediate need.

Recommended reading
Foundation Programme Curriculum (2012), section 8.2: Responds to acutely abnormal physiology.

2.21 Challenging a senior

C D A B E

Challenging a senior colleague is difficult but necessary at times, especially if patient safety is at risk. Therefore the most appropriate response is C, pointing out to your SpR that he has contaminated his sterile field, followed by other options that involve alerting him to his mistake. If you do not feel confident doing this, you could ask the theatre sister to tell the SpR (D). Informing the SpR and suggesting that he looks at infection control guidelines (A) is unnecessary since it is likely to be a mistake and saying this to the SpR could be perceived as being rude and unnecessarily abrasive. Option A, however, is preferable to option B: giving the patient post-operative antibiotics and not challenging the SpR. Junior doctors should feel that they can challenge a senior, thereby promoting a culture of openness in the NHS. Making a complaint about the SpR to his consultant (E) would be unwarranted, unless this was an ongoing issue, and also would not involve dealing with the current safety risk to the patient.

Recommended reading

Medical Protection Society (2012), Competence and Relating to colleagues, in *MPS Guide to Ethics: A Map for the Moral Maze,* chapters 10 and 11.

2.22 Incorrect consent

C E D B A

This is a difficult situation for an FY1 to find themselves in; however, it is important to remember that the patient is always the first priority. The least appropriate response is to complete the consent form yourself (A) as this would be illegally adding information that the patient potentially has not been informed of to a document that has already been signed by them. Without a correctly completed consent form, the operation would not be allowed to go ahead; therefore, your priority is to prevent the patient from undergoing an unnecessary general anaesthetic. Stopping the anaesthetist (C) is therefore the most appropriate response as this would provide you with time to discuss the situation with your consultant. Telephoning the consultant, who is likely to be in theatre, would be the next course of action (E) as he would be able to arrange for the form to be completed by the patient before the anaesthetic; however, this is less preferable than option B as it will not necessarily prevent the patient being anaesthetised. Telephoning the theatre coordinator (D) would not be an efficient use of time as they would have to discuss this with the theatre staff anyway. Walking to theatre (B) is not advisable as the patient may already have undergone the anaesthetic by the time you arrive; in addition, it is inappropriate as all operations and procedures have risks and patients must be informed of these risks beforehand. General Medical Council guidance suggests that risks can take a number of forms: side effects, complications or failure of an intervention to achieve the desired aim.

Recommended reading

General Medical Council (2008), Explanatory guidance, in *Consent: Patients and Doctors Making Decisions Together,* paragraphs 28–36.

2.23 Patient control of discharge summary

A   B   D   C   E

When a patient has become angry, it is always a good idea to get some support from a colleague. This is important for your safety and so that someone else witnesses the proceedings. The key message in this question is that the patient's accusation of breach of confidentiality is entirely wrong. Recording the information patients tell you accurately is an important part of your job. The sharing of information between professionals is vital in order to provide high-quality care. The best two responses therefore involve explaining to the patient that you will not change their records. A senior nurse will be more readily available to help with this and will most likely be experienced in managing conflict (A). Your registrar would be the next best choice (B). Option D respects the principles of medical record-keeping but is confrontational and will not repair the doctor–patient relationship. Option C is better than E because it involves only changing a small detail on the discharge letter rather than tampering with important clinical details in the medical records, which is illegal.

Recommended reading

General Medical Council (2013), *Good Medical Practice,* paragraph 50.
Medical Protection Society (2012), *MPS Guide to Ethics: A Map for the Moral Maze,* chapter 9, Confidentiality, section: Maintaining patients' trust.

2.24 Absent without leave (AWOL)

C   D   E   A   B

It is important to ask for help if you think you need it, and a difficult registrar should not put you off. If you are concerned about the health of your patient, then you need to be persistent with the registrar to come and see your patient (C); such persistence will usually work, which is why this is the best response. If you are still concerned, then you need to escalate higher than your registrar, which would involve contacting the consultant on call (D). Talking to the SHO and asking them to review your patients instead (E) is a good next response as they may have more success in contacting the registrar if they too are concerned about the patient. However, the SHO is likely also to be busy, and therefore, they may not be happy for you to call them for the rest of the shift. It would also be appropriate to ensure that your patients are reviewed by physicians more senior than your SHO and therefore options C and D rank higher than E. Again, if you are acutely concerned about your patient, you need to get the best help you can, and therefore asking the switchboard operator for the contact details of another registrar (A) is better than pushing aside your concerns (B); however, there is unlikely to be another registrar on call for your specialty, especially if you are working in a district general hospital.

Recommended reading

General Medical Council (2013), *Good Medical Practice,* paragraphs 35–38.

Medical Protection Society (2012), *MPS Guide to Ethics: A Map for the Moral Maze,* chapter 11, Relating to colleagues.

2.25 Bullying registrar

B C E

The registrar's undermining behaviour is seriously affecting your working life. It is therefore important that you seek support. The hospital counselling service (B) can provide advice to help you cope with the situation and help to support a dialogue between the registrar and yourself if you are struggling with this independently. At the same time as seeking help, you should let the registrar know that you are finding your working relationship difficult and that this is something you wish to work on together (E). Your clinical supervisor should be aware (C) so that they can ensure you have the support you need and also because it is an issue that could have a large effect on their clinical team if it is not addressed. Given that the issue purely occurs at work, you do not have to go see your GP at this stage (D). Although this is always a reasonable source of seeking support, there are better answers for this question. Furthermore, local sources of support should be accessed at this stage rather than contacting the GMC (F) as patients are not at risk. You should avoid having this conversation in public and being confrontational (A) as this can undermine patients' trust in your team and the medical profession. It is not constructive to try to avoid the registrar altogether (G) and will mean that other FY1s have to spend more time working with a senior who they too may find stressful dealing with. It would be inappropriate and unprofessional to say negative things about the registrar to their future FY1s (H) and could be seen as intentionally discrediting them or even as a way of seeking revenge.

Recommended reading

Medical Protection Society (2012), Relating to colleagues, in *MPS Guide to Ethics: A Map for the Moral Maze,* chapter 11, section, Conflict.

NHS Choices. Bullying at work. http://www.nhs.uk/Livewell/workplacehealth/Pages/bullyingatwork.aspx.

2.26 Understaffing

B C A D E

Attending regular teaching and developing your knowledge is of obvious importance, but your primary responsibility is always to ensure the safety of patients you are responsible for. In this scenario, the FY2 is continually leaving the ward understaffed in order to attend optional teaching. This has the potential to compromise patient safety. It is most appropriate to discuss your concerns with the FY2 (B) so that she is aware and has the opportunity to act. It would also be a good idea to discuss the issue with your consultant (C) so that they can try to resolve the issue. Seeking advice from your educational supervisor is appropriate (A), but it would be better to first discuss the issue with your consultant since they have a direct responsibility over staffing within your team. Raising the issue of understaffing at the next meeting (D) does not directly tackle the problem in this scenario and so is less suitable. It is inappropriate to ask your FY1 colleagues to make hints to the FY2 (E) since this is an unprofessional approach to solving the problem.

Recommended reading
General Medical Council (2013), *Good Medical Practice,* paragraphs 24, 25, 35–38.
Medical Protection Society (2012), Relating to colleagues, in *MPS Guide to Ethics: A Map for the Moral Maze,* chapter 11.

2.27 Absent colleague

C E B A D
The aim of the FY1 year is to become a competent junior doctor in managing patients with both acute and chronic illnesses as well as achieving the FY1 competencies outlined in the foundation programme curriculum. In addition to these commitments, you will work for a trust and be expected to perform clinical duties. If you can gain experience in other ways, such as attending clinics and theatre sessions, this is of additional benefit but should always come second to your primary commitments which tend to be to the patients on the ward. This scenario describes a colleague who is putting their own personal objectives ahead of their usual jobs and expecting you to pick up the pieces. Importantly, if two doctors are scheduled to be on the ward, this is because there is enough work to require two juniors. Taking on all this work alone means that you will be seriously overworked. The best response is option C, to speak with your colleague directly as they might not realise how much of a burden they are putting on you or whether you mind them being absent. Talking together you can work out a better way of working between you. Option E ranks second: arranging a fair amount of time for both of you to do something you're interested in seems reasonable as long as the wards are always adequately and safely covered. Your registrar might not realise they are putting you in difficulty on the wards by taking your colleague to theatre and so speaking to them would also be appropriate (B). Once the registrar understands the situation, in future they could check with your colleague to make sure that the ward is quiet before allowing them into theatre. Speaking to your clinical supervisor about how to address this situation (A) is a sensible response, but the wording of this option suggests that you are requesting additional help rather than help from the FY1 who should be working on the ward anyway, which is why it is ranked fourth. Option D is the least appropriate response as taking on extra work can leave you dangerously overstretched, and you shouldn't have to feel like you have to work extra hard to cover for your colleague's absences.

Recommended reading
General Medical Council (2013), *Good Medical Practice,* paragraphs 35–38.
The UK Foundation Programme Curriculum (2012).

2.28 Mean registrar

B F G
As a doctor, you will work with many different people, and some of those will
have different expectations of you and ways of working. Having said that,
the demands of the registrar detailed in this question seem unnecessary, and
his response when you don't achieve them over the top. The best responses
here involve speaking to your registrar privately to discuss how you can both
achieve your objectives together (options B and F). If your registrar doesn't
respond to your efforts to maintain a positive working relationship, you have
at least tried to deal with the problem directly and can then escalate this issue
if nothing changes. Option G, to discuss your registrar's demands with your
consultant, is the next most appropriate response. As well as informing them
of your registrar's difficult behaviour and how his demands are forcing you
to work many hours over your contract, you could ask your consultant what
they think is really important regarding care on the wards and what should
be prioritised, and then act accordingly. The inappropriate responses in this
question include continuing to work until you burn out (options A and H). You
need to ensure that you work healthy hours as a junior and look after yourself
to enable you to better care for your patients; nobody works well when they
are tired. Informing the trust about your registrar's behaviour (C) is a drastic
step, so you should escalate this issue to your consultant and supervisors first.
Refusing to carry out tasks that you see as unreasonable (D) is potentially dangerous. As a junior doctor, you are not yet experienced enough to decide what
is appropriate, and you could make a serious mistake. Getting information
from your union (E) may give you some useful advice. It is perhaps worth considering; however, it is not included among the three most appropriate options
because it doesn't involve any direct action.

Recommended reading
Carter M., et al. (July 2013), Workplace bullying in the UK NHS: A question-
    naire and interview study on prevalence, impact and barriers to reporting,
    BMJ Open, 3.
NHS Employers guidance (April 2006), Bullying and harassment.

2.29 Shredding nurse

C B D E A
As an FY1, you will work with a large number of different people from different specialties and seniority. It is very likely that you will find some of these
relationships challenging. Despite this, it is important to remember that we are
all working towards the same aim: helping our patients. The situation outlined
earlier sounds very frustrating, and the nurse seems to have acted hastily and

unfairly to teach you a lesson about the importance of patient confidentiality. The best response would be to speak to the nurse privately to explain how difficult her hasty shredding has made the rest of your day, and to work out a way you can prevent this happening again with a bit more tolerance of each other (C). The second best response would be to speak to the nurse's immediate manager, the sister on the ward, about this situation and how to prevent it happening again (B) while remembering that it is not the role of doctors to discipline or tell nursing staff how to do their jobs. Option D ranks third as complaining about this to your consultant isn't likely to do much to improve your working relationship with the nurse, and as mentioned earlier, it is not the role of doctors to discipline allied health professionals. It may, however, help you with the rest of your day's planning as they could remind you of the most important tasks of the day. Deciding to do nothing to help your working relationship and leaving the ward to make a new handover sheet (E) will at least help you with the rest of the day but ignores the main issue in the scenario, and so this option ranks fourth. The most inappropriate course of action here is option A: shouting at anyone at work is unprofessional. You should not need to raise your voice to get your point across, and this could also upset patients and further disrupt your working relationship.

Recommended reading
General Medical Council (2013), *Good Medical Practice,* paragraphs 35–37.

2.30 Interpreters

A D H
In this situation, you need to put the care of the patient first. This means you need to try and find a way to communicate with the patient. The best ways of doing this are to see if there is another doctor available who speaks the same language as the patient or to find an interpreter (options A, D and H). Asking the interpreter service to send someone in may be appropriate (D), although it depends on how unwell you think the patient is, but this may take some time. However, phone interpreters (H) can be very helpful in allowing you to get the history without waiting for an interpreter to be present in person. Family members should not be used as interpreters (B), unless it is an emergency. Taking a nurse with you (C) is not going to be particularly helpful in this case, if they are unable to communicate with the patient any more than yourself. Seeing another patient instead (E), when you are clinically concerned about the patient in front of you, is not acceptable, neither is simply examining the patient without the context of a clinical history (F). Similarly, ordering tests blindly is not going to help your clinical decision-making (G).

Recommended reading
BMJ Careers, Medical interpreters, http://careers.bmj.com/careers/advice/view-article.html?id=20000223.
General Medical Council (2013), *Good Medical Practice,* Duties of a doctor.

2.31 Demanding patient

B   D   E   A   C

It is important to prioritise the patient in the most life-threatening situation regardless of how demanding other patients may be. Myocardial infarction is the condition requiring the most urgent treatment; therefore, you should ensure that emergency management is prescribed to this patient first (B). Arranging the transfer to a specialist unit (E) is also vital to ensure definitive management of this patient and must happen in a timely fashion. However, option D, prescribing antibiotics for the patient with a urinary tract infection, ranks before option E because it is a relatively quick job, and potential sepsis in the elderly is also a very serious condition which should be treated promptly. Although he should be assessed (A), the young man is your lowest priority because he is not as acutely unwell as the other two patients, and you must address their problems in order of clinical need. Option C is the worst response because you should not refuse to see a patient, even if their behaviour is challenging, until you have attempted to assess the situation. It may be that there is an underlying pathology that needs to be treated. There are a number of steps that can be taken to ensure staff safety if a patient becomes aggressive, including involving security, but they should still receive care whenever possible. However, the threat of self-discharge should not alter how you prioritise the needs of the patients.

Recommended reading

General Medical Council (2013), *Good Medical Practice,* paragraph 9.

The UK Foundation Programme Curriculum (2012), Recognition and management of the acutely ill patient, chapter 8.

2.32 Nurse–patient breakdown

D   A   E   B   C

Conflicts between patients and nursing staff are difficult. You must appreciate the opinions of the nursing staff while also ensuring that patient care is not compromised. In this case, you could try to resolve the issues between the nurse and the patient, but if you feel that their relationship has broken down this is unlikely to work. The most appropriate response in this case is therefore option D, to suggest that a different nurse looks after the patient. The General Medical Council (GMC) states that a professional relationship with a patient can be ended only when 'the breakdown of trust means that you cannot provide good clinical care to the patient'. The next most appropriate response is speaking to the nurse in charge about the issue (A). It is a good idea to involve the senior members of nursing staff, but this may be perceived as complaining about the nurse, unless the nurse is involved in or aware of the discussion. Doing nothing (E) would not help the situation but does not damage the situation further and therefore ranks next. The two remaining responses, asking the patient to stop being rude and demanding (B) and decreasing the patient's analgesia (C), fail to address the conflict between the nurse and the patient and are likely to exacerbate the situation further. To leave a patient with less analgesia following an operation is the worst course of action as this would be immoral and would deny the patient one of their basic rights in hospital.

Recommended reading
General Medical Council (2013), *Good Medical Practice,* paragraphs 57, 59 and 62.

2.33 Patient error

E B D C A
After realising that you have made a mistake relating to a patient's management that can cause harm or distress, the General Medical Council (GMC) states that you should do three things: put matters right if possible, apologise and explain the situation, including the likely short-term and long-term effects. In this situation, the patient may experience side effects from the antibiotic and has unnecessarily been cannulated. Therefore, the most appropriate course of action would be to inform the patient of your mistake and apologise (E). Asking your SHO to discuss with the patient (B) is less appropriate as this is your mistake, and you should not need senior input, but at least in doing this, the patient will receive an explanation about the abrupt changes to their management. Filling in an incident form (D) may be useful to prevent a further incident, but this would not deal with the current situation in hand. Stopping the antibiotic course without informing the patient (C) would be tempting as a dose of antibiotic is unlikely to cause the patient harm, but you should be honest to the patient to maintain openness and trust. The least appropriate response in this question is allowing the patient to complete the antibiotic course (A). This would be unnecessary and may result in side effects or adverse events for the patient, for example making them susceptible to a *Clostridium difficile* infection.

Recommended reading
General Medical Council (2013), *Good Medical Practice,* paragraph 55.

2.34 Unable to get chaperone

C E D B A
Chaperones are used to protect both yourself and your patient, and it is important to offer one for any intimate examination regardless of the patient's or your gender. Option C is therefore the most appropriate response as you should not perform the examination without a chaperone if you feel uncomfortable in doing so, and in this scenario, leaving the examination to the following day will not adversely affect your patient's health. Asking your patient to see a female GP (E) may be an appropriate response as both your female colleague and the patient may feel more comfortable for the examination to be carried out without a chaperone. In this case, the examination should be carried out to obtain further clinical information, and your patient has already consented to the examination, therefore basing your diagnosis and treatment on history

alone (D) is inappropriate. Performing the examination without a chaperone present (B) makes you vulnerable to complaints and should not be carried out if you feel uncomfortable doing so. You may, however, examine the patient without a chaperone if the patient did not want a chaperone and you felt comfortable with this, but this would require careful judgement and documentation. Asking her partner who is in the waiting room (A) is not appropriate as a chaperone should be impartial and familiar with the intimate examination procedure. There may also be reasons why your patient does not want her partner present during the examination.

Recommended reading

General Medical Council (2013), Explanatory guidance, in *Intimate Examinations and Chaperones*.

2.35 Chaperones

B E   A   D   C

This example deals with chaperones for intimate examinations. Chaperones are advisable for every intimate examination as their presence protects both the patient and the doctor. An intimate examination includes that of the breast, genitalia and rectum. Chaperones should always be offered, even if the doctor and patient are of the same sex. This scenario is complicated by the fact that the patient appears to be drunk. In situations where the patient's recall may be clouded, such as when intoxicated, under the influence of drugs or undergoing anaesthesia or sedation, it is even more important to protect yourself from accusations by ensuring a chaperone is present. The best responses in this case are those that do not offer to undertake the examination without a chaperone. Option B is the most appropriate as this placates the patient by explaining why chaperones are so important and that you do not feel like you can continue without. Option E is the next best response as you are asking for advice. Although, in option D, you don't perform the examination, you have not dealt with the matter in hand and could be missing potentially serious information; therefore, it ranks second to last. The decision about whether a chaperone is present is ultimately up to you and the patient, and as long as this is detailed accordingly, proceeding to do the examination without a chaperone (A) is not necessarily wrong, although it is potentially more risky for yourself. Option C similarly involves risk but also means you are lying to the patient because being rushed for time is absolutely not a reason to proceed without a chaperone; therefore, this option is the least appropriate.

Recommended reading

General Medical Council (2013), Explanatory guidance, in *Intimate Examinations and Chaperones*.

Medical Protection Society (2012), Morality and decency, section: Chaperones, in *MPS Guide to Ethics: A Map for the Moral Maze*, chapter 5.

The UK Foundation Programme Curriculum (2012), section 7.2: History and examination.

2.36 E-portfolio

A C B D E

Struggling to meet the objectives of both your educational and clinical duties as an FY1 is a common problem. You have to try and work together with senior colleagues to achieve your FY1 objectives, which may well involve a degree of compromise. The best person to talk to in this situation is your educational supervisor (A). If the only time your consultant is free to meet with you is during your annual leave, then you have to make allowances for this and attend the meeting, so option C is the next best response. Remember, you must complete your e-portfolio to pass FY1! Option B is ranked third; if you have persistently tried to meet with your supervisor and they refuse, this should be reported to the foundation programme director at your trust. Asking another consultant to bridge the gap (D) would be a proactive way of dealing with this problem, but you need to get this ratified with the foundation programme director as it is not usually permitted to choose your own supervisor. Option E would be the least appropriate course of action since writing a letter of complaint wouldn't deal with the problem in hand and is likely to cause friction between you and your supervisor.

Recommended reading

The Foundation Programme (2012), *Training Descriptor and Curriculum Matrix*.
The UK Foundation Programme Curriculum (2012).

2.37 Educational supervision

E A B D C

The most important thing here is to provide the medical care that is necessary to ensure patient safety while also remembering your own educational needs. You have arranged a meeting with your supervisor; therefore, it would be courteous to inform them that by seeing to a patient on the ward you will be late for this. Additionally, it would be advantageous to use this opportunity as a positive learning experience, so if your educational supervisor has already allocated this time for you, then it would be appropriate to ask them to complete a mini-CEX form with you (E). The next most appropriate responses are to move up the chain of on-call physicians as you have already finished your shift and should therefore utilise the on-call team. If the on-call SHO is not free (A), then the next person to contact would be the registrar (B). While it would mean that you are late for your meeting, if the nurses are concerned about a patient and the on-call team are busy, then you should go and see the patient yourself, but this should involve a full review (D) which is far better than simply glancing at the patient to alleviate the nurse's fears (C). Option D ranks higher than C as waiting for a proper review is better than you undertaking a poor review and then not having this followed up on.

Recommended reading

General Medical Council (2013), *Good Medical Practice,* paragraphs 44–45.

Medical Protection Society (2012), Professionalism and integrity, section: Professionalism, in *MPS Guide to Ethics: A Map for the Moral Maze,* chapter 3.

2.38 Clerking responsibilities

E   C   B   A   D

Medical clerking is a very common task for junior doctors, and it is a valuable learning opportunity as it allows you to see acutely unwell patients who require prompt investigations and management. The complexity and severity of cases varies from patient to patient, as does the ability of a doctor to complete their history and examination in a certain period of time. It is expected that more junior doctors will take longer to see a patient than more senior colleagues. In this scenario, your colleague may have a good reason for why they have taken a prolonged period of time to see one patient. It may be that they were seeing a particularly unwell patient or one with a complex case, or they may be struggling to make a diagnosis. In any event, approaching your colleague directly is always the best course of action (E). The medical registrar usually has general responsibility for newly admitted medical patients and contacting them about the current situation would be appropriate (options A and C). However, this would be better put in the context of voicing your concerns about your own workload (C) rather than the performance of your FY1 colleague (A), which would both be unproductive and could damage your professional relationship with your colleague. In fact, option A is less appropriate than option B, continuing to clerk. As a clerking doctor, it is your responsibility to see patients so continuing to clerk is important (B); however, this wouldn't provide any help or support for your colleague who could be having difficulty. Offering to take over your colleague's case is the least appropriate response (D) and could lead to confusion over the tasks to be completed.

Recommended reading

Medical Protection Society (2012), Professionalism and integrity, in *MPS Guide to Ethics: A Map for the Moral Maze,* chapter 3.

2.39 Emergency in the community

B   E   D   A   C

The General Medical Council (GMC) states that 'you must offer help if emergencies arise in clinical settings or in the community, taking account of your own safety, your competence and the availability of other options for care'. Therefore, in this scenario, the most appropriate course of action is option B, doing an assessment and providing care as best you can until emergency services arrive. The next best response is option E, to see if anyone has suitable training and then leave, although first-aid training is unlikely to be as good as your medical care since it could be outdated, or they could be inexperienced. Phoning for an ambulance (D) would alert the medical services, but the collapsed patient would have less chance of survival without CPR (if it was required) while waiting for the emergency services to arrive. Telling the crowd to call an ambulance (A) would be less appropriate as it could result in a delay in the emergency services being aware of the situation. Doing nothing (C) is the least appropriate response as a doctor does have a social and moral responsibility and a duty of care to patients in emergency situations in the community.

Recommended reading

General Medical Council (2013), *Good Medical Practice*, paragraph 26.

2.40 Unsafe on call

C   E   G

Part of your role as a doctor is to raise concerns when you believe that patient care or safety is being compromised by the practices of colleagues, systems, policies or procedures. To tackle this situation you first need to try and improve patient safety as best you can during your on-call, and secondly you should raise your concern through the appropriate levels after the weekend to improve a recurring situation. The most appropriate actions during your on-call are to inform the medical registrar (C), who is in a position to reallocate staff to where the clinical need is, and to prioritise your tasks (E) as best you can. After the weekend, you should highlight your concerns to your consultant (G), who should be able to give you advice and escalate the issue further, should you both deem it appropriate. Asking another colleague to come in on their day off (A) would be inappropriate as the on-call team should be able to reallocate staff without bringing in extra people. Option B, asking the nurses to contact you only when they are very worried about a patient, is inappropriate since it could result in unwell deteriorating patients being left until a critical point, when their further deterioration could have been prevented. However, informing nursing staff that you are extremely busy and making them aware that there may be a delay prior to your review would be sensible. Informing the SHO that you are not coping (D) is unlikely to be beneficial as he has already informed you that he is busy with the post-take ward round, and this may only serve to increase his own stress levels. Option F, seeing all of the unwell patients as quickly as possible and missing lunch, is both unprofessional and dangerous. By not being thorough you may miss important diagnoses, and breaks are vital to your working day and are known to improve productivity. Writing a letter to the medical director (H) may be useful if you feel your concerns are not being taken seriously, but in the first instance you should contact your consultant.

Recommended reading

General Medical Council (2012), *Raising and Acting on Concerns About Patient Safety*.

2.41 Complaint

D E B A C

Doctors find themselves in potentially compromising situations on a day-to-day basis, and it is important that you are mindful of how such situations may be perceived by the general public. You should adequately explain to patients what you intend to do prior to proceeding and should use chaperones for any procedure that involves close or intimate contact. In this scenario, your intentions were good, and there has been a simple misunderstanding. However, if handled badly, this complaint could become serious, so it is important to act with professionalism. The most appropriate response is to seek advice from your medical defence organisation (D) as this should always be your first action whenever any complaint is made against you. It is also prudent to allow the hospital to deal with the complaint (E). They will work on your behalf to resolve the situation and will notify you of any action necessary on your part. It is completely inappropriate to ask the patient to withdraw their complaint as this may be seen as coercion (C). Similarly, you should avoid approaching the patient (A), even if it is to explain that there has been a misunderstanding. This may worsen the situation or again be seen as an attempt to put pressure on the patient. While still unfavourable, it would be better for a colleague to approach the patient (B) rather than you since the patient may feel less uncomfortable talking to someone other than yourself. Option B therefore ranks higher than options A or C.

Recommended reading

General Medical Council (2013), *Good Medical Practice* paragraph 73.
Medical Protection Society (2012), Professionalism and integrity, in *MPS Guide to Ethics: A Map for the Moral Maze*, chapter 3.

2.42 Coroner statement

C E G

You are legally required to cooperate with all formal inquiries and should do so in a timely manner. Options D and F, which either ignore or delay this task, are therefore inappropriate. You are also legally obliged to take reasonable steps to ensure that the information you give is factually correct. The report should be based on the medical records, your recollection of the case and your usual practice. It would therefore be pertinent to re-familiarise yourself with the case using the patient's medical notes (E). To ask the nurses about their recollections (A) or to read what another doctor has written (B) may inadvertently lead you to write a false account of your personal involvement, so these are inappropriate courses of action. While giving a timely statement is important, to write the statement quickly and purely from memory (H) may again result in a factually incorrect statement. Writing a legal statement in the correct manner is clearly of paramount importance. It would therefore be advisable to seek advice both from your educational supervisor and a medical defence organisation (options C and G).

Recommended reading

General Medical Council (2013), *Good Medical Practice,* paragraphs 71–74.
Medical Protection Society (2013), *MPS Factsheet: A Guide to Writing Expert Reports.*
Medical Protection Society (2013), *MPS Factsheet: Report Writing.*

2.43 Angry registrar

D B E A C

As an FY1 you may feel like your job is right at the bottom of the ladder, but you are an important member of the team and a professional who should be treated as such. Shouting at a co-worker is not acceptable behaviour, so the best responses here both diffuse the situation immediately and take steps to stop it happening again. The most appropriate course of action is option D; it diffuses the situation but offers to discuss the matter in private when tempers have cooled. Option B ranks second as, again, apologising takes the heat out of this situation and by offering to go through the ways you can help better on the ward round in future could improve your own working day as well as that the rest of the team. An approach like this could result in a better working relationship. Option E ranks next: taking the matter to your consultant is a fair approach as shouting at you in front of staff and patients is highly unprofessional, and the team leader would want to be made aware. Option A is the fourth best option as it is confrontational and will not diffuse the situation, but it is potentially less dangerous than option C, where avoidance of your seniors could lead to a future failure in asking for help or escalating treatment because of your poor working relationship.

Recommended reading

General Medical Council (2013), *Good Medical Practice*, paragraphs 35–38.

2.44 EWTD breach

C B E A D

The European Working Time Directive (EWTD) was put in place to protect junior doctors from unhealthy working patterns and to protect patients from tired doctors. The best way to raise this issue of extra hours would be within your own team by speaking to your consultant (C). They are the head of the clinical team and will want to know if you are struggling with your workload and would be able to support you by delegating senior doctors to help with ward tasks or contacting medical staffing for a more permanent locum. Talking to your foundation programme director (B) is the next best response as they are there to ensure you are able to work safely and gain your foundation competencies. They would therefore be able to offer advice on this scenario. If this fails, then option E would be the next best course of action since contacting the CEO would ensure that the issue of working hours and pressures is seen by the management, although it would be prudent to try options C and B first. If you feel able to do so safely, continuing to work through this difficult rota would be the next best response (A). Rotations are four months long and, providing you are not exhausted and working safely, continuing to work extra hours is not unsafe in itself, although it may seem unfair. Option D is clearly inappropriate; not only is it dishonest, but taking sick days will put extra pressure on the already depleted team.

Recommended reading
British Medical Association, European Working time directive.
Government legislation: Statutory Instruments 1998 No. 1833: Terms and
    Conditions of Employment; The working time regulations 1998.

2.45 Responding to colleague's request

B A E D C
This question relies on your ability to maintain good communication and respect for your colleagues whilst under pressure as well as ensuring that you prioritise good patient care. Firstly, it is important to explain calmly and reassure the nurse that you are aware of the patient and are simply very busy (B). Creating an aggressive or hostile atmosphere is not professional and could impact good patient care. Whilst the nurse may be concerned that the patient is in pain, it would be irresponsible to prescribe analgesia before adequately assessing the patient and taking a full history (in particular drug history and allergy status). Option C is therefore the least appropriate, and morphine would also not be your first line drug of choice for pain. After explaining the situation to the nurse, it is courteous to maintain good communication with the patient (A) as this may help to prevent any resentment or ill feeling later on. Most patients are very understanding but appreciate knowing what is going on. Asking another doctor to see the patient may be appropriate, especially if you are worried about the patient, but remember that they probably have a heavy workload as well (E). Deliberately leaving the patient until last is petty, unprofessional and likely to simply cause more unnecessary hostility between you and your colleagues (D). More importantly, it could be detrimental to patient care, and you should prioritise patients based on clinical need rather than your own personal reasons.

Recommended reading
General Medical Council (2013), *Duties of a Doctor: Knowledge, Skills and
    Performance*.
General Medical Council (2013), *Good Medical Practice*, paragraphs 15, 16,
    32–34, 35–37, 46, 55, 56, 59.
Medical Protection Society (2012), *MPS Guide to Ethics: A Map for the Moral
    Maze*, chapters 7 and 11.
World Health Organisation, *Pain Ladder for Adults*. http://www.who.int/
    cancer/palliative/painladder/en/

Chapter 3

EFFECTIVE COMMUNICATION

QUESTIONS

3.1 Writing in the notes

You are reviewing a patient who has had an allergic reaction to penicillin. You treat the patient and document your history and examination in the notes. You mention the event to your senior house officer (SHO) when you next see them, which is at least three hours after the event. They ask you whether you examined their throat with a pen torch, which you did not. You return to the patient to re-examine them, and their throat looks normal. There have been several entries in the notes since your last one, and you are unsure how to enter this extra information in the notes.

Rank in order the following actions in response to this situation (1 = Most appropriate; 5 = Least appropriate).

A Do not record your further examination.
B Get an extra continuation sheet and file it out of order in the notes with your additional findings.
C Make a new entry detailing your additional examination.
D Remove that page from the notes and rewrite your entry.
E Write up your examination just underneath your last entry in the notes and make it clear that it is written in retrospect.

3.2 Requesting tests

You are trying to order a test for a patient, which your registrar asked you to do during the morning ward round. It is a complex radiological set of images, and when you submit the request to radiology reception, they inform you that you must discuss this in advance with the duty radiologist on call. You attempt to get in contact with the duty radiologist several times over the next few hours to discuss the request but cannot get through. If the request is not put in soon, the patient will not get the investigation until next week as it is a Friday.

Choose the **THREE most appropriate** actions to take in this situation.

A Contact your registrar explaining the difficulties and that the imaging may not happen today.
B Continue trying to get in contact and let the registrar know at the end of the day whether or not the imaging happened.
C Find out who and where the radiologist is and go and see them personally.

D   Get in touch with the consultant radiologist on call and inform them that their registrar is unobtainable.
E   Order a different set of tests for the patient, which is easier to organise.
F   Put the request card in the duty radiologist's office with a note asking them to approve it.
G   Return to radiology reception informing them that the duty radiologist has said yes to the request.
H   Speak to another radiologist with whom you get on well and ask them to approve the request.

3.3 Knowledge

A patient on your ward is due to have a colonoscopy later in the day. You are asked to go and talk to her as she has some concerns about the procedure. She asks you to explain the procedure and its associated risks since she has forgotten what has previously been said to her. You have seen a colonoscopy once before, but it was a long time ago, and you remember little about it. You cannot remember the risks.

Rank in order the following actions in response to this situation (1 = Most appropriate; 5 = Least appropriate).

A   Explain that you are not completely familiar with the procedure but that you will ask someone who is to speak with her as soon as possible.
B   Put off going to talk to her and hope that she finds someone else to speak to in the meantime.
C   So as not to damage her confidence in your abilities, give an explanation using your knowledge of other similar procedures.
D   Tell her as much as you can remember about the procedure.
E   Tell her that you do not know enough about the procedure to be able to discuss it with her.

3.4 Have I got cancer?

You are working as an FY1 doctor in a large hospital on a busy respiratory ward. You attend a multidisciplinary team meeting about a patient under your care. During the discussion, it is confirmed that this patient has a diagnosis of lung cancer. Your consultant informs you that she will talk with the patient that afternoon to give him the diagnosis. When you return to the ward, you are asked by the nurses to take some routine blood tests from the same patient. When you have finished taking the blood, the patient says. 'Have I got cancer doc?'

Rank in order the following actions in response to this situation (1 = Most appropriate; 5 = Least appropriate).

A   Ask the registrar who is currently on the ward for advice about what you should do.
B   Inform the patient that as far as you are aware, no diagnosis has yet been made and he should not worry.

C Inform the patient that your consultant wants to discuss the situation with him this afternoon and then find her to remind her of her promise.
D Take the patient with a senior nurse into a side room and inform him he has cancer.
E Tell the patient he has got cancer and tell him everything you know about lung cancer.

3.5 Drinking with friends

You are in a bar near the hospital that you work in, and one of your friends who is also a doctor has had a little bit too much to drink. A man enters the bar and sees the group of you sitting there and comes over to talk to your friend. While your friend does not say anything to jeopardise himself, he is slurring his words. The man says, 'It's good to see that doctors know how to wind down'. Your friend then hugs the man, and the man walks away. Your friend tells you that he is a relative of one of his patients.

Rank in order the following actions in response to this situation (1 = Most appropriate; 5 = Least appropriate).

A Excuse yourself and go to apologise to the relative about your friend.
B Don't do anything since the relative did not seem to be upset about the incident.
C Suggest to your friend that, the next time he sees him, he should apologise to the relative for being drunk.
D Suggest to your friend that he go and apologise to the relative now.
E Tell your friend that he should not return to the bar again.

3.6 Missing notes

You are reviewing an unwell patient on the ward who you suspect may have a chest infection. You have requested imaging and blood tests and started them on antibiotics. You want to record your history, examination, working diagnosis and treatment plan in the notes, but they have been taken off the ward for reviewing at a multidisciplinary team (MDT) meeting. You finish work in one hour, and they are unlikely to be back on the ward by then.

Rank in order the following actions in response to this situation (1 = Most appropriate; 5 = Least appropriate).

A Enter your notes a day late when the notes are back on the ward.
B Go to handover and explain what you've done to the evening team, so they are aware without needing the notes.
C Stay later than your finish time to enter your assessment when the notes are returned.
D Write your notes on a loose sheet of paper and pin it to the ward noticeboard.
E Write your notes on a loose sheet of paper and place it in a temporary ring binder in the notes rack.

3.7 Self-discharge

You are an FY1 working in general surgery. A nurse rings you from another ward informing you that a patient of yours, who has had major colorectal surgery earlier in the day, wishes to self-discharge.

Choose the **THREE most appropriate** actions to take in this situation.

A   Ask the on-call psychiatrist to assess his capacity.
B   Inform the patient that if he self-discharges, he won't be provided with any follow-up.
C   Inform your specialist registrar (SpR).
D   Recommend that he gets a friend/relative to stay with him overnight.
E   Refuse to prescribe analgesia if he self-discharges.
F   Ring his sister and tell her to persuade him not to leave hospital.
G   Talk to him, explore his reasons and let him go home if he has capacity.
H   Tell the nurses that it is not your responsibility to deal with the situation.

3.8 Patient requesting full-body scan

You are an FY2 working in a GP surgery seeing your own list of patients. The next patient on the list is a 52-year-old woman who has been to see you several times in the last few weeks. Each time you have seen her, she has complained of an array of symptoms but never has any clinical signs. You have carried out several investigations already and have not found a cause for her symptoms. The patient list indicates that she has asked to see you as she would like a 'whole-body scan', which you presume is because she would like to know what is causing her symptoms.

Choose the **THREE most appropriate** actions to take in this situation.

A   Discuss her symptoms with your supervisor before the appointment.
B   Explain the test results that you have so far and ask her if her symptoms have changed or developed.
C   Explore with the patient the reasons why she would like this scan.
D   Organise a full-body magnetic resonance imaging (MRI) scan.
E   Prescribe anxiolytic medications.
F   Reassure her that her symptoms are not caused by anything physical.
G   Refer her to the psychologist as you suspect that she has a functional disorder.
H   Refer the patient to one of your senior colleagues for a second opinion before you see her.

3.9 Foreign patient

You have just returned from a period of annual leave and have been asked to complete a discharge letter and make follow-up arrangements for a patient on the ward who speaks little English. The ward sister has asked you to discharge him as soon as possible since there is a bed shortage. The patient's family is keen to know what is going to happen to the patient when he leaves the hospital.

Choose the **THREE most appropriate** actions to take in this situation.

A   Ask for help from a doctor on another team who speaks the same language as the patient.
B   Ask your specialist registrar (SpR) to talk to the patient and his family about follow-up while you complete the discharge letter.
C   Book a translator so that you can tell the patient what follow-up plans are in place and which medications he needs to take and when.
D   Complete the discharge letters for the patients who are leaving tomorrow first so that you can then spend more time focusing on this patient.
E   Explain to the ward sister that you are making this case a priority but that you need to ensure the patient has understood the plan for his care following discharge.
F   Get the ward sister to talk to the family and let them know what the plans are for this patient following discharge.
G   Give the patient the discharge letter with the follow-up instructions written on it and discharge the patient with his medications.
H   Inform the family that you are making arrangements for a translator so that the patient fully understands what will happen when he leaves the hospital.

3.10 Suicidal patient wanting to talk

You are an FY1 doctor working on the medical assessment unit (MAU). A patient has been admitted after an intentional overdose. The patient calls you over and says that they want to discuss their overdose with you. The patient's family is present.

Rank in order the following actions in response to this situation (1 = Most appropriate; 5 = Least appropriate).

A   Tell them that you will ask your senior to talk to them about it.
B   Ask the family to leave.
C   Find a quiet place on the ward to discuss it.
D   Inform the patient that the psychiatric doctors will discuss it with them later.
E   Ask the patient if they would like a nurse present.

3.11 Cancer diagnosis

One of your patients asks to speak with you to discuss the results of their recent computed tomography (CT) scan. You know that there is a suspicious lesion in the lung, which has features of malignancy and that the patient will be discussed at the regional lung cancer multidisciplinary team (MDT) meeting. The patient has not been informed of their suspected diagnosis and is not aware that their chronic cough could be caused by cancer.

Rank in order the following actions in response to this situation (1 = Most appropriate; 5 = Least appropriate).

A Ask your registrar to come with you to discuss the results with the patient.

B Refuse to speak to the patient and ask the nurses to tell the patient that you are too junior to interpret the scans.

C Take the patient into the quiet room and discuss the probability of cancer with them.

D Tell the patient that the results of the scan are not back yet.

E Tell the patient that the scan has shown a mass, but you are not sure of the origin. Explain that it will be discussed at an MDT meeting and arrange a meeting with your registrar tomorrow.

3.12 Referral

You are at the beginning of your shift when your consultant approaches you. She asks you to refer a patient to cardiology immediately so that the patient will be seen by the cardiology team that day. You have never met the patient and know very little about them.

Rank in order the following actions in response to this situation (1 = Most appropriate; 5 = Least appropriate).

A Inform the patient of the plan to refer them to cardiology and gain consent for you to share their information.

B Make the referral immediately.

C Read the notes before making the referral.

D Take a history and examine the patient before making the referral.

E Tell your consultant that you don't feel able to make the referral.

3.13 X-ray reporting

You are an FY1 working on a care of the elderly ward. A patient is admitted to your ward with hip pain. She has had an X-ray on admission, which was reported as 'normal, no fracture'. However, her hip pain persists, so she is sent for another X-ray one week later, which reveals a fracture that was also present in the former X-ray, which was reported as normal.

Choose the **THREE most appropriate** actions to take in this situation.

A Inform the patient and her family that missing the fracture was the fault of the reporting radiologist.

B Inform the patient of the situation and apologise.

C Inform the patient that she has a fracture but omit the fact that the previous X-ray also showed a fracture.

D Make a complaint against the first reporting radiologist.

E Refer the patient to orthopaedic care.

F Speak to the reporting radiologist and ask him why he did not see it.

G Submit an incident form.

H Write a letter to the medical director about the incident.

3.14 Family wanting to know results

You are an FY1 on a care of the elderly ward. You are approached by the daughter of one of your patients, and she is angry. She wants to know why her mother has not been fully informed about her current management plan. The patient has experienced severe headaches and a computed tomography (CT) scan of her head has revealed a mass. Your senior specialist registrar (SpR) has specifically asked you not to inform the patient of the results as she are very anxious and he thinks these results would be better coming from either himself or your consultant.

Choose the **THREE most appropriate** actions to take in this situation.

A Admit to the daughter that the patient has been poorly managed.
B Apologise to the daughter about the current situation.
C Ask the daughter what she understands about the current situation and what her particular concerns are.
D Ask the patient if she would like to know the results of her scan.
E Explain that you are a junior doctor so are unable to help her with this query.
F Inform the daughter of the scan results but explain why you don't think the patient should be made aware of the results at this stage.
G Organise a consultant meeting with the family.
H Tell the patient and the daughter about the scan results.

3.15 Internet printouts

You are working as an FY2 doctor in a GP surgery, seeing a patient with type 2 diabetes. He has had poor control of his blood glucose levels for years and has tried many different medications. He is now being treated with insulin along with a few other medications. The patient has come to see you because he has heard of a new drug that can treat his disease. He says he heard about it on the television and has printed off information about the drug for you. He asks you to read the article and prescribe the drug for him. You read the article but have never heard of the drug before.

Rank in order the following actions in response to this situation (1 = Most appropriate; 5 = Least appropriate).

A Ask the patient to book an appointment with you in a week, allowing you time to research the topic and discuss it with your GP supervisor.
B Ask the patient to book another appointment with a different GP.
C Discuss the medication with your GP supervisor mid-surgery to ask for advice.
D Prescribe the medication based on the article and the information in the British National Formulary (BNF).
E Tell the patient that the drug isn't suitable for him and refuse to prescribe the drug.

3.16 Difficult questions about cancer

You are working as an FY1 doctor on an oncology ward in a large cancer unit, and you are seeing a patient who is suffering from oesophageal cancer. He has undergone surgery, radiotherapy and chemotherapy. You have attended a multidisciplinary team meeting during which the patient's case was discussed. During the meeting, you learnt that his cancer has metastasized, and he now has a very poor prognosis. Your consultant came to the ward especially to see the patient that morning to discuss the progression of the cancer. As you are about to leave the ward that evening, the patient asks to see you. He asks you several complicated questions surrounding his disease that you do not know the answers to.

Choose the **THREE most appropriate** actions to take in this situation.

A Answer the patient's questions to the best of your ability.
B Apologise and explain that you do not know the answers to his questions.
C Ask the patient to wait until the ward round on the following day when you know your consultant will be on the ward.
D Ask the senior nurse on the ward to help answer his questions.
E Bleep the on-call oncology registrar and ask them to see the patient and answer his questions.
F Offer to read out your consultant's entry in the notes from the morning.
G Read the latest journal article about the disease and attempt to answer the patient's questions.
H Telephone your consultant and inform him of the situation.

3.17 Breaking bad news

You are an FY1 working in the emergency department. A woman who has recently been diagnosed with lung cancer presents with left-sided facial weakness. A computed tomography (CT) scan of her head reveals a mass in the right frontal lobe of her brain. The radiologist has reported that this is likely to represent a metastasis, and you have referred the patient to the on-call medical team. Your consultant advises you not to tell the patient the results of the scan, but when you go to see the patient, she asks you whether her cancer has spread.

Rank in order the following actions in response to this situation (1 = Most appropriate; 5 = Least appropriate).

A Explain to the patient that the scan was normal.
B Say that you do not know what the scan showed.
C Tell her that an abnormality was detected, and while you can't be certain, it is likely to be cancer.
D Tell her that the scan has shown that the cancer has spread.
E Tell her that an abnormality was detected, but at this stage, you don't know what it is.

3.18 Explicit posters

The doctors' office is shared by a large group of doctors, the majority of whom are male. A couple of your male colleagues have put up posters of naked women on the walls. While your female colleagues have made no comments, you have noticed that they have been using the office less and are working elsewhere.

Rank in order the following actions in response to this situation (1 = Most appropriate; 5 = Least appropriate).

A Ask your male colleagues to remove the posters as you think that they are deterring female colleagues from using the office.
B Continue as before and enjoy the extra space in the office without your female colleagues.
C Explain to your male colleagues that you think the posters are inappropriate and remove the posters yourself.
D Raise the issue with the ward manager.
E Remove the posters when no one is looking.

3.19 Consent HIV test

You are caring for a patient with oesophagitis. Your senior house officer (SHO) asks you to take blood for a human immunodeficiency (HIV) test as this is a potential cause. You remember reading somewhere that counselling prior to performing an HIV test is no longer required.

Rank in order the following actions in response to this situation (1 = Most appropriate; 5 = Least appropriate).

A Ask one of the genito-urinary medicine (GUM) doctors to come and consent the patient for the test.
B Ask your SHO to show you how to consent for the test.
C Do not consent the patient for the test, take the blood for the test and communicate the results with them afterwards.
D Have a discussion about the test with the patient to gain their consent and record this in the notes.
E Obtain written consent from the patient.

3.20 Smoking

You are working as an FY1 on a respiratory ward. You have been spending a lot of time with a very unwell patient who is suffering from chronic obstructive pulmonary disease (COPD). His condition is deteriorating; despite this, the patient continues to go off the ward to smoke. You know that his continuing smoking is contributing to his considerable deterioration.

Rank in order the following actions in response to this situation (1 = Most appropriate; 5 = Least appropriate).

A   Do not discuss smoking with the patient since he should already be aware of the risks.
B   Explain to the patient that his smoking is contributing to his deteriorating condition and you think it would be beneficial if he stopped.
C   Give the patient some leaflets about stopping smoking.
D   Prescribe a nicotine patch for the patient.
E   Tell the patient that he must give up smoking or he will die.

3.21 Disclosure to relatives

You are looking after an elderly patient with pneumonia. Her daughter lives abroad but has flown over to visit, and she asks to speak to you. She tells you that she is aware of her mother's diagnosis of lung cancer and wants to know what treatment is available. You know that the patient does not have lung cancer. You tell the daughter that you need to get consent from the patient to discuss her care. When you ask the patient, she tells you that she has been lying to her daughter so that she will move back to the United Kingdom.

Choose the **THREE most appropriate** actions to take in this situation.

A   Document the event in the patient's notes.
B   Encourage the patient to be honest with her daughter.
C   Inform the daughter that her mother does not have cancer.
D   Reflect on the incident in your e-portfolio.
E   Talk to the patient's daughter as if the patient did have a diagnosis of cancer.
F   Tell the daughter that you are unable to discuss her mother's treatment with her.
G   Tell the patient that, if she does not tell her daughter that she does not have cancer, you will.
H   Tell the patient that you feel uncomfortable about what she is doing and therefore can no longer be involved with her care.

3.22 Uninformed consent

You are an FY1 working in general surgery. A surgical specialist registrar (SpR) offers you the opportunity to witness him obtaining consent for a laparoscopic appendicectomy. The patient signs the consent form, but you feel that the patient does not understand what he has been told as your SpR has been using a great deal of complex medical jargon.

Rank in order the following actions in response to this situation (1 = Most appropriate; 5 = Least appropriate).

A   Advise the patient to make a complaint about the SpR.
B   Ask another senior colleague to discuss the procedure with the patient afterwards.
C   Away from the patient's bedside, suggest to the SpR that you do not think that the patient understood his explanation.

D Do nothing as you do not want to upset the SpR.
E Read about the complications of the procedure and go back to discuss this with the patient.

3.23 Refusing medication

You are an FY2 working in a GP surgery. A patient comes to see you with her husband and tells you that she has had a major nosebleed two weeks after starting aspirin, which you had initiated to reduce her risk of cardiovascular disease. She wants to stop taking aspirin.

Choose the **THREE most appropriate** actions to take in this situation.

A Advise her to find another doctor as she has not listened to your previous advice.
B Ask a more senior GP colleague to discuss it further with her.
C Ask her husband to try and convince her to continue taking aspirin.
D Discuss the reasons why she does not want to take aspirin.
E Ensure that she knows the indication for commencing aspirin and the risks of not taking it.
F Respect her decision.
G Seek the advice of a medical indemnity society.
H Tell her that she has to follow your advice.

3.24 Confused patient refusing antibiotics

You are an FY1 working on a care of the elderly ward. A nurse approaches you and tells you that a patient is refusing her intravenous (IV) antibiotics. You go to assess the patient and find them to be febrile, very confused and disorientated due to sepsis from a lower respiratory tract infection (LRTI). The patient is still refusing IV antibiotics because 'it is poison' and tells you that she is in a lot of pain.

Rank in order the following actions in response to this situation (1 = Most appropriate; 5 = Least appropriate).

A Assess the patient's capacity to make this decision and give the antibiotics against her will if she lacks capacity.
B Contact the patient's husband and ask for his consent to give the antibiotic.
C Find an oral alternative for the antibiotic.
D Section the patient under the Mental Health Act.
E Tell her that you are giving her a painkiller but give her the intravenous antibiotic instead.

3.25 Language barriers

You are the FY1 on a busy surgical ward with many tasks to complete. You are required to insert a cannula and explain to an 87-year-old woman that she requires intravenous antibiotics for a severe chest infection. The woman is originally from Pakistan and doesn't speak any English. You know she has never been in hospital before and is unfamiliar with hospital procedures.

Choose the **THREE most appropriate** actions to take in this situation.

A   Ask her daughter to translate for you at the bedside.

B   Ask the in-hospital translator to help translate the decision.

C   Ask your FY1 colleague, who speaks the same language as the patient, to consent her.

D   Ignore the cannula and wait for someone else to do it.

E   Insert the cannula without talking to the patient.

F   Provide written information in her own language about what the procedure involves.

G   Switch to oral antibiotics instead of intravenous.

H   Use hand gestures to show what you are going to do and see if she understands.

3.26 Contraception and young people

You are an FY2 working in a GP surgery, and a 15-year-old girl has come to see you requesting contraception. She says she has been in a stable relationship with her boyfriend, who is 15, for two years and would like to start having sexual intercourse. She has investigated the different options and would like your help in deciding which contraceptive to choose. On questioning her, she appears to understand the situation well and is mature for her age. She says she doesn't want her parents to be informed because they wouldn't approve. When asked if she would have sexual intercourse without contraception, she shrugs her shoulders and says 'maybe'.

Choose the **THREE most appropriate** actions to take in this situation.

A   Ask the patient to book an appointment with her mother and come to see you together.

B   Ask your patient to book an appointment with a senior doctor, who will be able to provide more accurate advice.

C   Attempt to persuade her to inform her parents and provide the necessary support but still supply contraception if she refuses.

D   Document your conversation and seek advice from a senior doctor during the consultation.

E   Provide contraception only if she informs her parents.

F   Provide the girl with condoms for contraception and ask the patient to book an appointment in a week's time, then seek help from your educational supervisor about the correct course of action.

G   Provide the girl with contraception but inform her mother during her next appointment.

H   Suggest that the girl should refrain from sexual intercourse until she is of the legal age for consent and refuse to provide her with contraception.

3.27 Self-discharge

You are the FY1 on a general surgical ward. A patient who was admitted with diverticulitis is being treated with intravenous (IV) antibiotics. They tell you that they have had enough of being in hospital and are leaving today. You have no reason to believe that they lack the capacity to make this decision.

Rank in order the following actions in response to this situation (1 = Most appropriate; 5 = Least appropriate).

A Ask the patient to wait until your registrar can come to discuss their condition and the implications of going home at this stage.
B Discuss the risks of going home now, fill in a self-discharge form, and order medication for the patient to take home with them.
C Inform the patient that it would be unwise to go home at this stage and fill in a self-discharge form.
D Tell the patient that they cannot leave as their treatment hasn't been completed.
E Tell the patient that they have the right to walk out at any time.

3.28 Family translating

You are the FY1 working on a surgical ward. An elderly woman has been admitted with bowel obstruction. Your team go to discuss the options with her. Surgery could be life-saving, but there is also a high risk that she could die during or soon after the operation. The patient does not speak, any English. There is a group of family members with her for the consultation, and her daughter says that she will translate for you. You feel that she is saying relatively little to her mother compared with how much information your team is conveying. When your registrar asks whether the patient has any questions, the daughter says 'No', without any interaction with her mother, and tells you that she will have the surgery.

Rank in order the following actions in response to this situation (1 = Most appropriate; 5 = Least appropriate).

A Book the patient for surgery on tomorrow's emergency theatre list.
B Book the patient onto the theatre list, contact the hospital translator service and arrange for a translator to attend for the surgeon's and anaesthetist's pre-operative consultations.
C Tell the daughter that you do not believe that she is translating accurately.
D Tell your registrar that you are concerned about whether the patient is fully informed.
E Wait until the relatives have left, call Language Line™ and use it to discuss the situation with the patient.

3.29 Blood transfusion

You are the FY1 working on a general surgery ward and are looking after a patient with anaemia of chronic disease. After the ward round, your consultant asks you to consent the patient for a blood transfusion as her latest haemoglobin level was 4.5 g/dl, and she is scheduled for theatre in the next couple of days. As you explain the reasons for requiring a blood transfusion along with the risks and benefits, she tells you that her religion does not permit her to have the procedure and that, no matter what may happen to her, she will not agree to it. You know her to have mental capacity.

Choose the **THREE most appropriate** actions to take in this situation.

A Arrange for the patient to sign a proforma confirming that she does not want a blood transfusion under any circumstances.
B Ask the other FY1 on the ward to come with you and talk to the patient to try and persuade her to agree to the transfusion.
C Document your conversation in the notes, explaining that she does not want a transfusion despite the likely consequences of her severe anaemia.
D Explain the situation to your specialist registrar (SpR) and ask for their advice.
E Ignore the patient's wishes as she is likely to die without the transfusion, and it is in her best interests.
F Order the blood for the patient's operation anyway.
G Speak to the blood bank to get some advice.
H Tell the senior house officer (SHO) to come and talk to her to see if they can persuade the patient to change her mind.

3.30 Blind patient

You are the FY1 on a general surgical ward. Last night you clerked in a blind patient with right upper quadrant pain and jaundice. The following morning, after seeing the patient, your consultant asks you to discuss having a magnetic resonance cholangiopancreatogram (MRCP) and possible laparoscopic cholecystectomy with the patient and says that he will come and formally consent her for the procedure after his clinic. He tells you to look on the intranet for guidance on the procedures.

Rank in order the following actions in response to this situation (1 = Most appropriate; 5 = Least appropriate).

A Access the local guidance on consenting for these procedures so that you can talk to the patient.
B Ask your senior house officer (SHO) to speak to the patient about what these procedures involve and let her think about it.
C Print off the local guidance from the intranet and give it to the patient's husband to read to her.
D Speak to the ward sister to see if information in braille is available to give to the patient.
E Tell the patient about these procedures using the local guidance and give her husband an information leaflet to read before the consultant returns.

3.31 Refusing medication

You are the FY1 on a surgical ward. While reviewing a patient's drug chart, you notice that the nurses have been indicating that the patient is refusing to take their prescribed potassium supplement. Their potassium level remained slightly low on today's blood test. You have no concerns about the patient's capacity to make this sort of decision.

Rank in order the following actions in response to this situation (1 = Most appropriate; 5 = Least appropriate).

A Prescribe potassium as an additive to their IV fluids.
B On the consultant's ward round tomorrow, bring up the fact that the patient is refusing medications.
C Speak to the patient to find out why they are declining the medication and discuss the options.
D Do nothing as the patient has a right to refuse.
E Bleep your registrar to let them know that the patient has not been getting their potassium supplementation.

3.32 Seeking assistance to die

You are an FY2 working in a GP surgery. A patient with metastatic prostate cancer books an appointment with you. He would like advice from you about assisted suicide.

Choose the **THREE most appropriate** actions to take in this situation.

A Arrange to get the patient sectioned under the Mental Health Act.
B Ensure that the patient has no unmet palliative care needs.
C Explain that you are unable to help the patient with what he requests as it is illegal.
D Get another GP to talk to the patient.
E Listen to and discuss the patient's reasons for wanting to end his life.
F Refuse to engage in a conversation about this subject.
G Tell the patient that he are being selfish in wanting to die.
H Tell the patient that you are no longer able to provide care for him as he has voiced this wish.

3.33 Ward round

You and your consultant are doing a ward round. An elderly man has been newly admitted, and on his clerking sheet, you both notice that he is positive for the human immunodeficiency virus (HIV). Your consultant draws the curtains around the patient's bed and proceeds to talk loudly because the patient is hard of hearing. He goes on to ask the patient about his HIV diagnosis, but he is talking so loudly that you are sure the neighbouring patients will be able to hear the conversation.

Choose the **THREE most appropriate** actions to take in this situation.

A   Apologise to the patient on behalf of the consultant.
B   Ask the patients in the neighbouring beds whether they heard any of your conversation.
C   Ignore the situation.
D   Move the patient to a side room after the ward round to avoid a similar situation in the future.
E   Stop the consultant and suggest that he continues the conversation somewhere more private.
F   Suggest at the end of the ward round that the consultant offer the patient an apology.
G   Suggest to the patient that he make a complaint against the consultant.
H   Talk to the consultant about what happened at the end of the ward round.

3.34 Secret pregnancy

You are working on a general surgical ward. One of your patients needs a computed tomography (CT) scan; however, a pregnancy test has unexpectedly revealed that she is pregnant. She can no longer have the CT scan because of the pregnancy. The next day, the patient's husband asks you angrily why his wife is still waiting for her CT scan.

Choose the **THREE most appropriate** actions to take in this situation.

A   Ask the husband to calm down.
B   Ask the patient what she would like you to tell her husband.
C   Discuss with the patient why she has not told her husband that she is pregnant.
D   Encourage the patient to tell her husband that she is pregnant.
E   Explain to the husband that the patient no longer needs the CT scan.
F   Explain to the husband that you need to ask the patient's permission to discuss her treatment.
G   Suggest that the husband discusses the CT scan with his wife as you cannot discuss anything with him at this point.
H   Tell the husband that his wife can no longer have the CT scan because she is pregnant.

3.35 Discussion with relative

A patient was admitted to your ward with a chest infection. Two days after her admission, she becomes more unwell and suffers a seizure. Her husband approaches you and tells you that his wife is an alcoholic. He is worried that her alcohol withdrawal has caused her to become more unwell while in hospital. He asks you not to tell his wife about your discussion since she had not wanted the hospital staff to know about her alcohol dependence.

Rank in order the following actions in response to this situation (1 = Most appropriate; 5 = Least appropriate).

A Ask the patient about her alcohol use without mentioning your discussion with her husband.
B Ignore what the husband has told you since the patient has always denied alcohol use.
C Inform the husband that you will need to tell the patient about your discussion in order to investigate whether her deterioration is related to alcohol use.
D Tell the patient that her husband has told you that she is an alcoholic and ask her whether this is true.
E Treat the patient for alcohol withdrawal without asking her whether she is alcohol dependent.

3.36 Knife wound

You are an FY1 working in the emergency department. You clerk a young man who has been stabbed. He says that he was attacked but doesn't want the police to know.

Rank in order the following actions in response to this situation (1 = Most appropriate; 5 = Least appropriate).

A Inform the patient that you have a professional responsibility to tell the police.
B Inform the police without telling the patient that you are going to do so.
C Refuse to treat the patient unless he consents to you informing the police.
D Respect the patient's wishes and do not tell the police.
E Try to persuade the patient to consent to you informing the police during his time in hospital.

3.37 Telephone conversation with relative

While working as an FY1 on a care of the elderly ward, you are asked by a nurse to talk to a patient's son on the phone. He wants an update from a doctor on his father's condition as he is unable to come into the hospital to talk to you.

Choose the **THREE most appropriate** actions to take in this situation.

A Advise the son to speak to his father himself.
B Ask the nurse to speak to the relative.
C Ask the patient if he will allow the telephone conversation.
D Establish that you are talking to the son.
E Give the son a brief update on his father's condition.
F Refuse to speak to the son.
G Tell the son that you will only speak to him in person.
H Tell the son to phone the consultant's secretary to ask the consultant for information.

3.38 Contact tracing

You are currently working on a gynaecological ward. Results of a swab come back on one of your patients: she has tested positive for chlamydia. Your patient says she will take a course of antibiotics but does not want her boyfriend to know about it.

Rank in order the following actions in response to this situation (1 = Most appropriate; 5 = Least appropriate).

A   Ask a nurse to talk to the patient about it.
B   Discuss the options with your consultant.
C   Explore her concerns and discuss ways of informing her boyfriend.
D   Inform her that it is your duty to tell her boyfriend.
E   Respect her wishes and don't tell her boyfriend.

3.39 Prophylactic antibiotics

You are working as an FY2 doctor on the medical take in a busy admissions unit. You are treating a young man who has a headache. He has been diagnosed with meningitis and has already been given antibiotics and fluids. You inform your senior doctor, who tells you that anybody who has recently stayed in the same house as the patient overnight will need prophylactic antibiotics. He says that he stayed at a party last night with many of his friends and doesn't want you to contact them because he feels embarrassed.

Choose the **THREE most appropriate** actions to take in this situation.

A   Allow him to contact his friends to ask them if they are having similar symptoms.
B   Allow him to leave the department when he feels better, giving him several packs of antibiotics to give to his friends.
C   Explore the reasons for him not wanting to disclose the information and try to alleviate his concerns.
D   Inform the local public health consultant, who can help to trace and treat his friends at the party.
E   Inform your consultant immediately and ask for advice on the issue.
F   Refuse to treat him if he will not reveal the identity of his friends.
G   Respect his wishes and treat him without informing his friends.
H   Wait to see how severe his infection is before contacting relatives.

3.40 HIV and death certificates

You are an FY1 doctor working in a palliative care unit and are caring for a patient with end-stage human immunodeficiency virus (HIV). He has a malignancy associated with his HIV infection, and he is also suffering from tuberculosis. Your consultant informs you that the patient is unlikely to survive for more than a couple of days. The next day, on the ward round, he asks to discuss the possibility of him dying. He informs you that he doesn't want his HIV infection status to be written on his death certificate because he hasn't told his family of his condition. He asks you to promise that you will not write this on the certificate.

Choose the **THREE most appropriate** actions to take in this situation.

A   After his death, complete the certificate by mentioning a 'viral infection'.
B   Ask your consultant for advice before your patient passes away.
C   Inform his family of his condition before he dies so that you can complete the death certificate truthfully.
D   Inform the patient that you will have to complete the death certificate fully, including his diagnosis of HIV.
E   Promise to omit the infection and after his death, mention only the malignancy and the tuberculosis.
F   Promise to omit the infection from the certificate but after his death, complete the certificate with all the information disclosed.
G   Refuse to complete the certificate as you want to respect the patient's wishes.
H   Seek further information about his concerns and encourage him to tell his family before his death.

3.41 Drug overdose

While working in the emergency department, you treat a young female patient who has overdosed on an unknown substance. The patient claims she has not taken any illicit drugs, but she is unwell and requires treatment. She came in after a night of drinking alcohol at a party with her friends. Her friend asks to talk to you in private and says that she gave the patient a recreational drug without her knowing because she thought that she would have a 'better night out'. The friend asks you not to tell anyone because she might get into trouble. The overdose can easily be treated with an antidote, and the patient will likely make a full recovery.

Rank in order the following actions in response to this situation (1 = Most appropriate; 5 = Least appropriate).

A   Inform the friend that you will not be able to keep confidentiality and treat your patient for the overdose with senior support.
B   Inform the friend that you will not be able to keep confidentiality as it may put your patient at risk and phone the police after gaining the patient's permission.
C   Keep the information confidential and do not document where the information came from while treating the patient.
D   Phone the police and report a case of drugging.
E   Refuse to speak to the patient's friend again on the basis of confidentiality and dismiss her previous comments.

3.42 Safeguarding children

You are an FY1 working on a busy medical ward. A patient becomes tearful when you go to review her one afternoon, and she discloses to you that she is worried about going home because her partner has been very aggressive towards her recently. She does not answer your questions about whether there has been physical violence and strongly denies that there is any danger to her two young children but admits that they are in the house when they argue. She asks you not to share the information she has told you.

Rank in order the following actions in response to this situation (1 = Most appropriate; 5 = Least appropriate).

A Call your registrar and ask them to come and take over the situation.
B Explain to the patient that you are worried about this situation, that you have an obligation to record what she has told you in her medical notes, and ask for her consent to contact social services.
C Explain to the patient that you are worried about this situation, that you have an obligation to record what she has told you in her medical notes and then call the safeguarding children officer for the hospital.
D Listen and offer support to the patient, and record what she tells you in the notes.
E Make a full, formal referral to social services.

3.43 Lost notes

You are the FY1 on a general medical ward. The medical notes of a patient with a complex medical history have gone missing since his transfer from another ward. The nurses report that they have looked thoroughly for the notes. During the ward round, you are unable to locate them, and the matter is discussed in front of the patient at the beginning of their consultation. The patient is frustrated that their notes are missing and expresses a wish to make a formal complaint.

Choose the **THREE most appropriate** actions to take in this situation.

A Apologise to the patient.
B Ask the patient not to complain until you have had some more time to look for the notes.
C Ask the ward clerk to start a new set of temporary notes.
D Discuss the situation with your educational supervisor.
E Explain to the patient that the porter must have left the notes somewhere.
F Fill in an incident report form.
G Go to medical records to look for the notes.
H Wait to document the outcome of the ward round until the notes are found.

3.44 Employee disclosure

You are the FY1 working on orthopaedics and are looking after a 50-year-old man who is scheduled for an operation this afternoon to mend a fractured tibia and fibula. Just before lunchtime, you receive a phone call from a man who reports to be your patient's new employer. He wants to know how long the patient will be in hospital and off work so that he can offer his job to someone else. He says he doesn't have the luxury of time or money to be 'waiting around for a disabled employee to get fit for work again'.

Choose the **THREE most appropriate** actions to take in this situation.

A Ask the staff nurse to talk to the employer for you as you are about to go for your lunch.
B Do not give the caller any information but speak to the patient and find out whether he wants you to talk to his employer.
C Do not mention what the patient's condition or treatment is but say that they will not be able to work for a long time and that they should find an alternative employee.
D Inform the caller that he is having surgery that afternoon and will be out of work for at least six weeks.
E Politely tell the employer that you cannot give any information over the phone without the patient's permission.
F Pretend that you don't know anything about the patient and ask them to call back at a time when you will not be on the ward.
G Seek advice from the sister in charge and ask her to come and talk to the patient with you.
H Tell the caller that it is illegal to terminate employment on the basis of a disability and that you are going to report him to the relevant authorities.

3.45 Child confidentiality

You are working in paediatrics, and you are caring for a five-year-old patient named Chloe who has leukaemia. You are completing the day's jobs when a man who says that he is Chloe's father approaches you and asks for an update on Chloe's clinical condition. You are aware that the girl's parents are divorced and that her mother attends the ward every day, but you have never met her father.

Rank in order the following actions in response to this situation (1 = Most appropriate; 5 = Least appropriate).

A Ask Chloe's mother's permission to discuss Chloe's health with her father.
B Invite both parents together for a meeting to discuss Chloe's condition.
C Explain that you cannot give the man any information without proof that he is Chloe's father.
D Ask the man to get an update from Chloe's mother rather than yourself.
E Ask him to wait while you get a senior doctor to speak with him.

3.46 Handover sheet

You leave work in a hurry to get to the supermarket before it closes. In your haste, you decide to leave shredding your handover sheet until the morning and put it safely in your bag instead. When you get home, you realise that it is no longer in your bag and must have fallen out at the supermarket checkout. The sheet contains a great deal of confidential information.

Choose the **THREE most appropriate** actions to take in this situation.

A Ask your registrar for advice.
B Call the police to assist you with looking for your list.
C Call your clinical supervisor to explain what has happened.
D Ensure you never leave the hospital with confidential patient information again.
E Forget about the loss of the handover sheet.
F Go and speak to the patients on the ward explaining your mistake.
G Offer to do a teaching session on confidentiality to your FY1 colleagues.
H Phone the supermarket to see if someone has handed the sheet in to customer services.

3.47 Consultant names

You are working with a consultant on a surgical firm consisting of ten FY1s. Your consultant has not learnt any of your names and simply refers to you as 'boy' or 'girl' depending on the gender.

Rank in order the following actions in response to this situation (1 = Most appropriate; 5 = Least appropriate).

A Gather all the FY1s together and go to discuss the matter with the consultant as a group.
B Let your educational supervisor know that your consultant is referring to you in this way.
C Request your consultant to call you by your name as you find it demeaning to be only distinguished by your gender.
D Report your consultant to the General Medical Council (GMC) for improper conduct.
E Tell your consultant that unless he learns your name, you will not do any of the jobs he asks of you.

3.48 Degrading nursing staff

You are about to enter the doctors' office on your ward when you hear the senior house officer (SHO) and registrar comparing the nursing staff's physical attributes. They are speaking loud enough that you can hear them outside the office, which many of the nursing staff regularly walk past.

Rank in order the following actions in response to this situation (1 = Most appropriate; 5 = Least appropriate).

A Enter the office and tell the SHO and registrar that you are disgusted with their conversation and that you will report this to your consultant.
B Enter the office loudly to make it seem as if you did not hear their conversation.

C Close the door so that no one passing by will hear the conversation.
D Remind your colleagues that the nursing staff demand more respect than to be reduced to their physical attributes.
E Walk on by and return to the office later.

3.49 FY1 vs SpR

One evening you enter the doctors' office to find a fellow FY1 colleague in tears. He says that his registrar had just left having told him that he was a 'useless doctor and the hospital would run more smoothly without him'.
He tells you that this is because he declined to request a computed tomography pulmonary angiogram (CTPA) for a patient as the radiologist had not thought it was indicated.

Choose the **THREE most appropriate** actions to take in this situation.

A Ask your colleague's educational supervisor to talk to the registrar.
B Comfort your fellow FY1 and explain that it is not a reflection on them if the radiologist does not think a scan is indicated.
C Find the registrar later in the shift to let them know that what they said to your colleague was inappropriate and upset them.
D Go with your colleague to find the registrar and discuss what was said.
E Phone the consultant responsible for the team and tell them about the registrar's comments.
F Say nothing: the registrar probably just needed to vent frustration at someone and therefore it is probably best to let it go.
G Suggest to the FY1 that he discusses how upset he was with the registrar tomorrow when they have both had time to reflect on the situation.
H Volunteer to carry your colleague's bleep for the rest of the day so that they can have some time to recover.

3.50 Patient concerns about GP

You are the FY1 working on a medical ward. When you go to take a blood sample, one of your patients tells you that they are worried about how their care was handled by their GP. The patient had visited their GP multiple times over several months before any investigations were performed. They ask you about whether you think it would have made a difference if their GP had picked up earlier that there was a serious underlying cause for their symptoms.

Choose the **THREE most appropriate** actions to take in this situation.

A Agree with the patient that there was a delay in their diagnosis.
B Contact the General Medical Council (GMC) about the delay.
C Contact the GP to let them know that the patient is complaining about them.
D Explain that it isn't possible for you to comment on the decisions the GP made at the time of their consultation.

E   Inform your registrar and consultant that the patient has these concerns.
F   Listen to the patient's concerns.
G   Reassure the patient that the GP did everything correctly.
H   Refuse to be involved in a conversation about another doctor's decisions.

3.51 Registrars conflicting plans

You are the FY1 working on a surgical team. The radiology report from an investigation for a patient has suggested further imaging. However, when you checked this earlier in the day with one of your registrars, he decided it was not clinically indicated. Later in the day, a different registrar does a ward round and declares, in front of the patient, that they need further imaging.

Rank in order the following actions in response to this situation (1 = Most appropriate; 5 = Least appropriate).

A   Say nothing but don't organise the imaging.
B   Say nothing and organise the imaging.
C   Tell the second registrar and the patient that the first registrar thought imaging was unnecessary.
D   Explain to the second registrar and the patient about the first registrar's decision, and ask the second registrar to call them and discuss the matter between themselves.
E   Call the first registrar yourself to let them know that their decision is being altered.

3.52 Complaints

You go to perform venepuncture on a patient on the ward. While you are there, the patient tells you that he is upset about the way he was spoken to by the consultant on the ward round that morning. You were not on the ward round, but the patient explains what was said and asks if you agree that the consultant was rude.

Choose the **THREE most appropriate** actions to take in this situation.

A   Advise the patient to speak to the consultant about these concerns.
B   Agree that it sounds as if the consultant was rude.
C   Apologise to the patient on behalf of the consultant.
D   Decide to avoid the patient as they may complain about you too.
E   Explain that you cannot comment since you were not present on the ward round.
F   Recommend that the patient contacts the Patient Advice and Liaison Service (PALS) to make a complaint against the consultant.
G   Speak to the consultant yourself about the patient's concerns.
H   Tell the patient that you do not think that the consultant was rude.

3.53 Consensual Dr–Dr relationship

You are an FY1, and the sister on your ward approaches you after the ward round and asks you to have a word with the other FY1 on your ward. She says that he is behaving inappropriately with your SHO while at work. You are aware that they are in a relationship but have never witnessed this type of behaviour yourself.

Choose the **THREE most appropriate** actions to take in this situation.

A Ask other members of the ward staff if they have witnessed similar behaviour.
B Ask the nurse whether she thinks that patient care is being compromised as a result of their behaviour.
C Explain that you think their behaviour is fine and that if they are happy, it doesn't matter.
D Explain to the nurse that you have never witnessed this kind of behaviour.
E Say that if she has real concerns, she should speak to a more senior member of the medical team.
F Tell the nurse that she should speak to the doctors in question.
G Tell the nurse to document her concerns formally.
H Tell your educational supervisor about the sister's concerns.

3.54 Putting arm around relative

You are the FY1 on a busy colorectal firm, and the sister in charge asks for a private talk as she says that someone has made a complaint about you. The son-in-law of one of your patients, a woman who has just been diagnosed with colon cancer, says that you put your arm around his wife while talking to her yesterday, and he thought that this was inappropriate behaviour.

Rank in order the following actions in response to this situation (1 = Most appropriate; 5 = Least appropriate).

A Explain to the nurse that you were simply comforting the woman after she learned of her mother's diagnosis.
B Talk to your educational supervisor about the complaint.
C Apologise to the son-in-law and explain the reasons for your behaviour and assure him that it won't happen again.
D Tell the son-in-law that you were comforting his wife and that your behaviour was not inappropriate.
E Tell the nurse to explain to the son-in-law the reasons for your behaviour.

3.55 Interrupting the SpR

You are working in the genito-urinary medicine clinic and need to talk to one of your senior colleagues. One of the nurses tells you that she thinks the registrar is in one of the clinic rooms. You knock, and the registrar shouts for you to come in, but on opening the door, you discover that the registrar is doing cervical swabs on a lady who is in the lithotomy position. She is covered with a sheet over her legs.

Rank in order the following actions in response to this situation (1 = Most appropriate; 5 = Least appropriate).

A   Apologise and say that you'll come back later.
B   Enter the room and wait for the registrar to be free.
C   Enter the room and ask the registrar for their advice.
D   Shut the door immediately and come back later.
E   Let the nurse know that she put you in an awkward situation and that you are not happy.

3.56 Upset patient

You are an FY1 working in oncology. One of the patients under your care has been found to have metastases in the lungs. You walk into the bay after the consultant has broken the news. You see that the patient is still clearly upset by the news, and you go over to comfort them. To offer comfort and support, you take their hand. However, after leaving the bay, one of the nurses comes to find you and tells you that the patient found it very inappropriate that you touched them without their permission and would like to make a formal complaint.

Rank in order the following actions in response to this situation (1 = Most appropriate; 5 = Least appropriate).

A   Apologise to the patient immediately.
B   Ask the nurse to go and explain that they were mistaken.
C   Await the complaint as you feel you did nothing wrong.
D   Confront the patient and tell them that you think it is unfair they are complaining about you when they are clearly just upset about the progression of their disease.
E   Take the nurse back in with you, apologise to the patient and explain that you were trying to be comforting.

3.57 Assisted suicide

You are working as an FY2 doctor in a GP surgery when you see a patient who has recently been diagnosed with motor neurone disease. Both you and the patient know that this condition is terminal and that she has a poor life-expectancy. She has begun to experience debilitating symptoms that she feels are humiliating and uncomfortable. She breaks down in tears during the consultation and asks for your help to commit suicide. She says she has been thinking about it since she received her diagnosis and would like further information about how she might achieve this.

Rank in order the following actions in response to this situation (1 = Most appropriate; 5 = Least appropriate).

A Suggest she books an appointment with a senior GP to discuss the issues around assisted suicide and offer instead to focus on treating her symptoms.

B Offer to listen to her concerns and treat her symptoms with appropriate medications but explain that assisted suicide is a criminal offence.

C Offer to listen to her concerns but explain that assisted suicide is a criminal offence and that you cannot help her.

D Prescribe the patient large doses of opiate medications and suggest that she can make her own decisions regarding further management.

E Refer her directly to the psychiatric and palliative care teams because she has voiced suicidal intent.

3.58 Comments on abortion

You are working as an FY2 doctor with a specialist registrar (SpR) in obstetrics and gynaecology. You are undertaking a joint clinic and are seeing a patient together. The SpR is leading the consultation with a 17-year-old pregnant woman who wishes to have a termination. She has discussed the situation with the specialist nurse and now wishes to discuss this with her doctor. As you are discussing this, the SpR informs the patient that 'abortion is wrong' and shouldn't be done under any circumstances. The patient immediately starts to cry and leaves the room.

Choose the **THREE most appropriate** actions to take in this situation.

A Ask for the patient to return to the room and tell the SpR to apologise.

B Ask the nurse to see the patient and arrange for her to see another doctor.

C Ask the SpR to discuss the case immediately with the consultant responsible for the clinic.

D Discuss the situation with the consultant responsible for the clinic after the clinic has finished.

E Discuss the situation with your educational supervisor following the clinic.

F Discuss your concerns about the situation with your SpR asking her to explain why she made the comments.

G Document your concerns in the notes about the consultation.

H Remain silent as the consultation was led by the SpR.

3.59 Racism

You are an FY1 working on a gastroenterology ward when a nurse approaches you visibly upset. She reports that a patient in her bay has just refused to let her take his observations because she is black. You approach the patient to enquire about this matter, and he repeats to you 'I will not be treated by a black nurse, I have told her this already'.

Choose the **THREE most appropriate** actions to take in this situation.

A Advise the nurse that she should fill in an incident form and report the matter to her ward manager.

B Comfort the nurse, explain that the patient's behaviour will not be tolerated but that for patient safety he must have care from nursing staff and arrange for another nurse to care for him.

C Discharge the patient immediately from hospital but write a letter to his GP for follow-up care.

D Explore the patient's concerns more fully, and then approach your registrar for advice on how to care for this patient.

E Refuse to see the patient because of his unacceptable behaviour.

F Reprimand the patient for his behaviour and write a paragraph in the notes warning other staff members of his racism.

G Tell the patient that he is behaving disrespectfully and that this matter will be reported to senior doctors, nurses and ward managers. Then move the patient into another bay to be cared for by another nurse.

H Tell the patient that, if he will not accept care from this nurse, he will get no nursing care at all, and direct the nurses to ignore the patient all day.

3.60 Refusing treatment for children

You are working as an FY1 in a paediatric emergency department. A mother brings her one-year-old baby in for you to examine a rash on her daughter's leg. When you inspect the rash you, recognise severe eczema with infected areas from scratching. You plan to prescribe an antibiotic cream alongside emollients and mild steroid cream, but the mother refuses saying that she doesn't believe antibiotics work, and it is better for her child's immune system to beat the infection herself. She takes the prescription for the other creams and leaves the surgery.

A Call the patient's mother at home to try and explain the importance of this treatment and urge her to return.

B Call the police to recover the child and initiate antibiotic treatment.

C Discuss this matter with a senior doctor in the practice.

D Call social services to report the neglect of this child.

E Discuss the matter with another FY1 who has recently completed a paediatric rotation.

3.61 Inappropriate dress at work

You are the FY1 on a busy medical ward, and one morning the sister approaches you to voice some concerns about your fellow FY1 colleague. She has noticed that the FY1 often has a bare midriff, wears bracelets and long earrings and her knickers are often visible riding up above her skirt when she bends over. You admit to yourself that you have also noticed that her standard of dress is not always appropriate.

Rank in order the following actions in response to this situation (1 = Most appropriate; 5 = Least appropriate).

A Speak directly to the FY1 in question when there is the opportunity to speak in private.
B Keep an eye on her clothing over the next few days and keep a record of her dress.
C Mention your observations and the sister's concerns to your specialist registrar (SpR) and ask for advice.
D Speak to your housemate, another FY1 working on a different ward at the hospital.
E Report her dress to her educational supervisor.

3.62 Late colleague

You are working the early shift on a busy medical admissions unit (MAU), and you are due to finish in five minutes. You have chased all the investigation results for your patients and finished your job list, but it is another half an hour before the FY1 who is due to take over from you turns up for work. You have noticed that he has been late for work on repeated occasions over the past few months.

Choose the **THREE most appropriate** actions to take in this situation.

A Ask the sister in charge to mention something to your colleague.
B Ask your colleague if he realises that he is late for work and if there is a reason for it.
C Ask your other colleagues in the medical team whether they have noticed lateness in your FY1 colleague.
D Explain to the FY1 that it isn't professional to repeatedly turn up late for work without an explanation.
E Mention your colleague's behaviour to your consultant and ask for him to be moved into another team.
F Speak to your educational supervisor about your observations.
G Take your colleague into the doctors' office when he arrives and speak to him sternly about always being late.
H Write an anonymous note detailing in bold what time the shifts start and finishes and pin it up in the doctors' office.

3.63 Registrar responsibility

While working on a medical ward, you have noticed that when you ask one of the junior registrars to review patients you are concerned about, they often just give advice and don't follow this up by seeing the patient themselves. You are concerned that this means that the advice they give is not always in the patient's best interests.

Rank in order the following actions in response to this situation (1 = Most appropriate; 5 = Least appropriate).

A Ask the registrar to come and see patients with you rather than simply asking them to do it alone.
B Raise the matter with your consultant.
C Ask other members of the team if they have had the same problem.
D Ignore the registrar's advice: you have seen the patient; therefore, your plan is superior to theirs.
E Take the registrar's advice, write the plan in the notes and state that the registrar gave this advice.

3.64 Gift from patient

You are the FY1 working on an elderly care ward. In making conversation with one of your patients, you make an admiring comment about their watch. When they are discharged home, they approach you and give you the watch, saying that it is a gift to show their thanks for all that you have done for them.

Rank in order the following actions in response to this situation (1 = Most appropriate; 5 = Least appropriate).

A Accept the watch, thanking the patient.
B Thank them for their kindness, but refuse the watch saying that it is important to them and that you want them to keep it.
C Ensure that the patient understands that your previous comment was not intended as a request and did not bear any significance to how you treated them; ask them to reconsider but accept the watch with thanks if they insist.
D Refuse saying that it is inappropriate for them to offer you a gift.
E Accept the watch but ask the patient to keep this a secret.

3.65 Promise to family

You are an FY1 working on a surgical team. One of your patients is on the high dependency unit following major surgery. Your team is concerned that she may be suffering from a major complication which would require returning to theatre for further surgery, including formation of a stoma. The patient's family ask to speak to you about her condition and what is going to happen next. The patient is very tired and unwell but nods when you ask if she is happy for the situation to be discussed with her family. You have several urgent jobs to do but agree to come back and speak to them later that morning.

Rank in order the following actions in response to this situation (1 = Most appropriate; 5 = Least appropriate).

A Call your registrar and ask them to come to the ward now to speak to the family.
B Leave the conversation for your registrar to have during the afternoon ward round.

C Return later in the morning and explain that you cannot discuss the details as you are not a surgeon.

D Return later in the morning, take the family to a private room and explain the nature of the suspected complication, what the surgery will involve, the risks and the likely outcomes.

E Return later in the morning, take the family to a private room and explain that there is still some uncertainty but there is a chance further surgery will be necessary and that one of your seniors will discuss this in detail with them later on.

3.66 Interpreter

You are an FY2 in a GP surgery, and a patient who speaks very little English attends with his friend who says that he will translate. You take a history about his headache, but you are worried that what you're saying is not being fully translated, and you feel like you cannot rule out a serious cause for his headache.

Rank in order the following actions in response to this situation (1 = Most appropriate; 5 = Least appropriate).

A Advise his friend to bring him back to the GP or to emergency services if he develops any 'red flag' symptoms.

B Book a consultation with a professional interpreter present.

C Use a telephone interpreter service in your consultation.

D Record that you tried to ask him about 'red flag' symptoms but weren't able to.

E Send the patient to the emergency department.

3.67 Breaking bad news

You are the FY1 working on hepatobiliary surgery. One of your patients who has previously had surgery for a cholangiocarcinoma is discussed in the multidisciplinary team (MDT) meeting in the morning, and it is confirmed that the cancer has already spread to the liver and peritoneum. That afternoon, the patient pulls you to one side and asks, 'Did you get all the cancer out in my operation?' You are the only doctor on the ward.

Rank in order the following actions in response to this situation (1 = Most appropriate; 5 = Least appropriate).

A Tell the patient that the MDT hasn't happened yet and that you don't know the answer to their question.

B Ask one of your senior colleagues when they anticipate they will be able to come and discuss the results with the patient.

C Explain that the more experienced doctors are not on the ward at the moment but as soon as they have arrived, they will come and discuss the results.

D   Take the patient into a private room and ask a nurse to come with you so that you can discuss any concerns that the patient may have.

E   Take the patient into a private room and ask a nurse to come with you whilst you explain that the results from the surgery have suggested that the cancer had already spread.

3.68 Refusing antibiotics

You are the FY1 working on a respiratory ward. One of your patients, Mr Splutter, who has a history of COPD has developed an atypical pneumonia. You have contacted microbiology who have recommended a rare combination of unusual antibiotics, but as you are explaining this to the patient, he says he doesn't want any as his 'wife was in hospital with pneumonia and the drugs didn't work, she just got more sick'.

Rank in order the following actions in response to this situation (1 = Most appropriate; 5 = Least appropriate).

A   Explain to the patient both the risks and benefits of his treatment options, ensuring he understands why you think this regime is the best choice.

B   Speak to your specialist registrar (SpR) about the situation and potential alternative treatment options.

C   Tell the nurses to administer the antibiotics anyway and don't tell the patient.

D   Document the patient's decision to refuse treatment.

E   Call your consultant and ask them to come and speak to the patient.

ANSWERS

3.1 Writing in the notes

C B E A D

A patient's notes are a legal document and should state the date and time when written, be legible and signed off fully with signature, name, General Medical Council (GMC) number and contact details. The best way of recording any new information is to make a new entry. Even if it consists of a minor additional examination, it should be recorded chronologically, which therefore makes option C the best response. Writing your additional examination on another sheet and filing it can cause some confusion about the order of the notes but will ensure that your entry is recorded accurately and fully, so option B ranks second. Option E is potentially a risky way of making an addendum; it is often not very obvious when notes have been added at a later date, and it may be construed as dishonest, especially if the notes are needed at a tribunal or an investigation. You should be very careful of this, and it is important that you write that your comment was written in retrospect. Option A is one of the least appropriate options: you should record all significant interactions with patients, and if it was important enough for you to return and re-examine a patient, the outcome should be recorded clearly. Removing pages from patient's notes (D) is illegal. The notes are a legal document and should not intentionally be tampered with, removed or destroyed.

Recommended reading

Medical Protection Society (January 2012), Writing good medical records, in
    GP Registrar, vol. 13, Issue 1.
Medical Protection Society (April 2013), *Medical Records Factsheet*.

3.2 Requesting tests

A C D

Safeguards against unneccesary tests exist to protect patient safety. It can be difficult to get tests and investigations quickly in a busy hospital, but the safeguards (such as approval by a specialist) should not be circumvented. The most appropriate answers include option A, which informs a senior member of your team that the test they were expecting may not occur and gives them the option to request another test if appropriate. Option C is also an appropriate response as it can be much easier to reach someone if you go to see them face to face rather than trying to call them repeatedly on the phone when they are busy, a visit in person is harder to ignore. Although it is generally better to contact the on-call registrar first, going directly to the consultant (D) is a valid option if the appropriate person is unavailable and the test is urgent. Option B demonstrates a lack of ingenuity in attempting to contact the radiologist, and option F means the request card could potentially be lost if left on an unattended desk. The remaining options are not appropriate due to their dishonesty (G) and avoidance of patient safeguards (H), while deciding to order another set of imaging that is easier to obtain (E) is outside the competence of an FY1 and should only be done if ratified by a senior.

Recommended reading

Student BMJ (2013), Junior doctor survival guide: How to cope with on-calls, night shifts, and everything else, *BMJ*, 21, f4014.

3.3 Knowledge

A E D B C

You must make every effort to ensure that the information you provide to patients is accurate. You must always be honest in your communications and work within the limits of your knowledge. In addition, if you do not have the appropriate knowledge or skills, it is your responsibility to find someone who does; option A is therefore the most appropriate response. Declining to discuss the procedure with her (E) is the next best option since it avoids being untruthful; however, it does not fulfil your responsibility to provide the information. While option D gives the patient some of the information, you may not remember important aspects of the procedure; however, the patient will wrongly assume that you have provided all the relevant information. Ignoring the situation (B) does not aid the patient in any way and neglects your duty of care. Improvising based on your other medical experiences (C) is wholly inappropriate since you may provide false information, and it is dishonest with regard to your level of knowledge.

Recommended reading

General Medical Council (2013), *Good Medical Practice*, paragraph 32, 34, 68.
Medical Protection Society (2012), Honesty, in *MPS Guide to Ethics: A Map for the Moral Maze*, chapter 6.

3.4 Have I got cancer?

C A D E B

As the doctor on the 'front line' on the wards, you are often faced with difficult questions from patients and relatives, which you may not necessarily have the competence or knowledge to answer. In this scenario, while you may know the diagnosis, you will not have the necessary information on hand to answer the inevitable further questions your patient may have. Honesty and integrity is always of the utmost importance, and this makes option B the worst response as you should not lie or mislead your patient. Lying to the patient is not acceptable, and in doing so you may be offering him false hope, which could be very damaging. The best course of action would be to ask your consultant to discuss the situation with the patient as planned (C). Failing this, your registrar is likely to have the experience and knowledge required to speak to the patient in the meantime (A). Informing the patient yourself, in this scenario, is completely inappropriate. However, it should be noted that all personal and potentially distressing conversations should be performed in private with a colleague present, which makes option D preferable to E.

Recommended reading

British Medical Association, *Real Life Advice: Breaking Bad News,* http:// bma.org.uk/developing-your-career/foundation-training/real-life-advice/ breaking-bad-news.

3.5 Drinking with friends

C   B   A   D   E

As a doctor you are, of course, allowed to enjoy a private life, but you must remember that as a professional you are always in the public eye. You must therefore try to remain professional in public, otherwise the medical profession risks losing the trust of the public. While embracing a relative in an amicable manner outside the clinical situation, as in this scenario, is not entirely improper, it does cross the boundaries of professional conduct. The best option here is to suggest that your friend apologises to the relative when sober and in a professional situation (C). The next best option, however, would be to not do anything about the situation as the relative did not seem upset (B). This is better than risking worsening the situation. If you feel that you need to say something, then it would be better for you to apologise to the relative (A) as you are not drunk, than for your friend to go and do this (D). Telling your friend not to return to the bar would be the wrong response here (E) as this would be imposing social barriers, and this is unfair on your friend.

Recommended reading

General Medical Council (2013), *Good Medical Practice,* paragraphs 55b and 65.

Medical Protection Society (2012), Personal conduct, in *MPS Guide to Ethics: A Map for the Moral Maze,* chapter 12.

3.6 Missing notes

B   E   D   C   A

All medical professionals have a duty of care to record important patient information clearly and legibly in the notes to facilitate good handover and informed care of patients. Notes are often taken from the wards into meetings, so sometimes it is not possible for you to make entries as they happen. In this situation, you need to make sure that the information is safely handed over, otherwise there is no way the doctors or nurses later in the evening will know that you have formally reviewed this patient. The best answer is option B: informing the evening team of your plan for this patient directly means that they won't repeat what you have already done and that they will understand the background if they are called to see this patient again. Writing on loose sheets of paper is not a safe way to keep information as it can easily get lost but keeping them in a ring binder removes some of this risk, so option E is the second-best option. Pinning notes to the ward staff noticeboard (D) is not ideal as it is not usually a place staff would think to check, so the notes could easily be missed. However, this response is better than having to stay on the ward for an indeterminate time until the notes are returned (C) or failing to make any documentation at all that day (A).

Recommended reading
Medical Protection Society (April 2013), *Medical Records Factsheet.*

3.7 Self-discharge

C   G   D

It is important that you respect a patient's wishes, even if you deem them foolish. In this scenario, you should first speak to the patient and assess his capacity. If you judge that he has capacity to make this decision, he must not be held in hospital against his will, and he should be allowed to self-discharge, provided he is aware that this is against medical advice (G). You should recommend that he has someone to monitor and care for him at home overnight (D). Your SpR should be informed about the situation as they may also want to speak to the patient (C). Asking the on-call psychiatrist (A) to assess his capacity would be inappropriate as this should be something you should be able to do; however, if you find it difficult to make an assessment, it would be appropriate to involve your seniors. Not allowing him follow-up (B) or analgesia (E) if he self-discharges would be unacceptable in this case as he has had major surgery and should have both to avoid complications. Ringing his sister to ask her to persuade him not to self-discharge (F) is something that you could suggest to the patient, but she should not be involved without the patient agreeing to it first as this would be breaking patient confidentiality. Option H is unprofessional as you are part of a team responsible for the patient's care.

Recommended reading
General Medical Council (2013), *Good Medical Practice,* paragraph 59.
Medical Protection Society (2012), Duty of care, in *MPS Guide to Ethics: A Map for the Moral Maze,* chapter 4.

3.8 Patient requesting full-body scan

A   B   C

Working in general practice throws up challenges that are often very different to those that you will encounter while working within a hospital. In this scenario, your investigations and actions would very much depend upon what symptoms she is complaining of. However, situational judgement test questions often don't include all the information you would like. In this scenario, you must think what the most sensible course of action would be. Discussing with the patient her symptoms and requests would be the most appropriate first action to take (options B and C). This would allow you to explore her concerns and narrow down your own differential diagnosis. You must also seek advice from your educational supervisor when you are unsure, particularly in complicated cases such as this (A). They may be able to suggest relevant further investigations, or they may suggest seeing the patient themselves to come up with a suitable management plan. Directly referring the patient to another colleague (H) before even seeing her would be inappropriate as you may be able to deal with the situation yourself. Organising full-body scans of any kind are rarely indicated, and you would not be expected to do this as an FY2 (D). Making a diagnosis of a functional disorder may be correct; however, you do not have enough information to do this yet (G). Reassurance can be very valuable (F); however, it is more appropriate to rediscuss her symptoms and get the opinion of your supervisor before making this decision to ensure you have not missed any pathology. Prescribing anxiolytics (E) would be inappropriate without exploring her concerns and making a formal diagnosis.

Recommended reading
General Medical Council (2013), *Good Medical Practice,* paragraph 16.

3.9 Foreign patient

C E H

This question is assessing your ability to communicate effectively with patients, their families and also other colleagues. It is important that when patients cannot speak English, you make every effort to provide information to them in a way that they can understand, for example via the use of a translator (C). Another effective way to do this would be using patient information leaflets written in the relevant language. You also have a duty to communicate effectively with those who are close to the patient (H), especially if they are going to have a role in caring for the patient outside of the hospital. When delivering and making arrangements for patient care, it is also courteous to keep your colleagues informed of your plans; this helps to maintain good professional relationships and will have a positive impact on the service that your patient receives overall. Option E is therefore also appropriate. While option A may be a suitable action to take if you cannot get hold of a translator, your colleague is likely to be busy with their own patients; therefore, you should explore alternative options first. Similarly, B is less appropriate, since part of your role as an FY1 is to complete discharge letters and ensure that your senior's plans are implemented when patients are discharged. Option F may be suitable, in part, when dealing with English-speaking patients; however, this case requires additional support to ensure the patient and his family understand the plans, and you should always be working in conjunction with the nursing staff to discharge patients. Option D does not demonstrate good prioritisation; while your reason for completing the other discharge letters first may have merit, this patient's needs are more urgent (especially considering the need to involve translators). Finally, ignoring the language barrier (G) is certainly not appropriate as patients have the right to have information presented to them in a way that they can understand. Failure to do so could negatively impact patient safety.

Recommended reading
General Medical Council (2009), *The New Doctor,* paragraph 9.
General Medical Council (2009), *Tomorrow's Doctors,* paragraph 15.
General Medical Council (2013), *Good Medical Practice,* paragraphs 32, 33.
Medical Protection Society (2012), Duty of care, in *MPS Guide to Ethics: A Map for the Moral Maze,* chapter 4.

3.10 Suicidal patient wanting to talk

C E B A D
As a junior doctor you will sometimes need to have sensitive conversations that you may not feel particularly comfortable with. In this case you do not know what the patient wants to discuss: for example, they may want to be discharged, or they may be concerned about their medical health. The most appropriate response would be option C, finding a quiet place on the ward to talk to the patient, as the information that they disclose is likely to be sensitive and warrants privacy. Asking the patient if they would like a nurse present (E) is also appropriate as the nurse looking after the patient may have built up more rapport with them and may be able to give more information. Asking the family to leave (B) may be useful, but it would be better if you asked the patient if they wanted to talk in private or if they would prefer their family to be present. Simply telling them that you will ask your senior to talk to them (A) is not appropriate at this stage as you do not know what their concerns are; however, you could offer this after having had a conversation with the patient. Option D, informing the patient that the psychiatric doctors will discuss it with them later, is the least appropriate option as it would close the conversation and could leave the patient upset or angry, especially given the stigma that surrounds psychiatry as perceived by many members of the public.

Recommended reading
General Medical Council (2013), *Good Medical Practice,* paragraphs 31–34, 46–48.

3.11 Cancer diagnosis

A E D B C
In this situation, the bad news should be broken by a senior doctor who can explain the suspected diagnosis and treatment options fully and accurately answer any questions that the patient may have. A registrar is best placed to do this, and so option A is the best response. Option E is the next best as you are being honest with the patient yet only giving basic information and a basic plan. The patient may be worried after this conversation; however, by

providing some information you have stayed within your competence, and your senior can have a follow-up conversation, if needed, to explain things in more detail. Option D is the next best answer: if you cannot break the news well, it is best not to break it at all. Telling the patient that the results are not back yet buys some time to ensure you can get a senior to speak with them and will hurt them a lot less than if you gave incomplete and incorrect information; however, it is dishonest so should be avoided if at all possible. Avoiding speaking to the patient and placing nursing staff between you (B) is unprofessional, and if a patient wants to speak with you, you should not refuse. An important conversation such as breaking bad news should always be between the patient and a senior registrar or consultant. It is beyond your competency as an FY1 as you cannot answer all the questions that the patient might have, which makes option C wholly inappropriate.

Recommended reading
Patient.co.uk (2010), *Breaking Bad News.*

3.12 Referral

A   D   C   E   B

The process of referral involves the arrangement for another practitioner to provide a service that is beyond your professional competence. It is important to inform patients of any plans for referral to other departments as well as to gain consent to share their information with the appropriate people (A). It is also important, when making a referral, that you provide enough information. This enables the healthcare professional in receipt of the referral to assess whether it is appropriate for them to become involved in the patient's care. In this scenario, you need to gather the relevant information before making the referral. While the information may be available in the notes, it is best not to rely on the assessments made by others. It is preferable to take a history and examine the patient yourself: option D is therefore preferable to C. If you have no knowledge of the patient, it may be appropriate to tell your consultant that you are not able to make the referral (E). This would be more appropriate than making the referral without any information about the patient (B).

Recommended reading
General Medical Council (2013), Explanatory guidance, in *Delegation and Referral,* paragraphs 6, 9.

3.13 X-ray reporting

B   E   G

Learning from our mistakes is an integral part of the educational process and thus improves competence. Errors should be analysed to ascertain how they happened to prevent reoccurrence. In this situation, you should submit an incident form (G) to allow root cause analysis to take place. The other most appropriate responses are to inform the patient of the situation and

apologise (B) and refer the patient to orthopaedic care (E). The General
Medical Council (GMC) states that, in the event of a mistake relating to
patient management, you should do three things: put matters right if possible,
apologise and explain the situation, including the likely short-term and long-
term effects. Informing the patient and her family that missing the fracture is
the radiologist's fault (A) would be unprofessional and could undermine public
confidence in the profession. Option C, informing the patient but omitting
the fact that the fracture was visible in the previous X-ray, does not involve
being completely honest and open with the patient. If the patient discovered
this at a later stage, this could also affect their trust in the medical profession.
Making a complaint about the first reporting radiologist (D) is one way of
raising concerns, but in this situation, it would be more appropriate to submit
an incident form as you cannot be absolutely sure that any blame lies with
the radiologist. Speaking to the first reporting radiologist and asking why he
did not see the fracture (F) may be perceived as confrontational, especially
if you are not already familiar with the radiologist. Writing a letter to the
medical director (H) would raise concerns around the incident, but the most
appropriate channel would be to submit an incident form.

Recommended reading
General Medical Council (2013), *Good Medical Practice,* paragraph 55.
Medical Protection Society (2012), Competence, in *MPS Guide to Ethics: A
Map for the Moral Maze,* chapter 10.

3.14 Family wanting to know results

B   C   G
This is a tricky scenario. As an FY1, you should not be expected to break
bad news of this nature, especially when you have been asked not to discuss
it by a senior colleague. In this situation, you should think about the patient's
autonomy and her right to know any scan results if she wishes and also confidentiality as the patient may not want her daughter to know the scan results.
Therefore, you should do three things: apologise to the daughter about the
current situation (B), empathise with the daughter and discuss both what she
already knows and what she is particularly concerned about (C) and organise a
consultant meeting with the patient and her family as soon as possible (G). The
latter option would depend on whether the patient wishes to attend and, if the
patient gives consent, to let her daughter know about the situation. Admitting
to the daughter that her mother has been poorly managed (A) would be unprofessional even if you thought it was true and could damage her opinion of your
colleagues and even the medical profession. Asking the patient if she would like
to know the results of the scan (D) would be imperative for breaking the bad
news; however, as already established, this should be done by a more senior
colleague. Explaining that you are a junior doctor and that you cannot help
(E) would not be useful; you should instead explain that it would be better to
speak to senior colleagues and make arrangements for this to happen. Speaking
to the daughter but not informing the patient (F) is unethical, unless you

have spoken to the patient first and received her permission to do so. Telling the patient and her family the results of the scan (H) should not be done by a junior doctor, as discussed earlier.

Recommended reading
Medical Protection Society (2012), Patient autonomy and consent; Competence, in *MPS Guide to Ethics: A Map for the Moral Maze,* chapters 8; 10.

3.15 Internet printouts

A   C   B   E   D

The internet has changed access to medical information forever. Information that used to be only available to doctors and research scientists is now accessible at the click of a button. However, not all the information is genuine and not all of it has an evidence-based rationale. Often it can be frustrating for patients to hear that the miracle cure they have found online is no more than an old wives' tale or a preliminary small-scale trial abroad. As a doctor, you must be understanding of this and not dismiss your patient's concerns. In this scenario, it is possible that the patient has found a drug that may be a treatment option. As a junior doctor, you may lack the knowledge required to answer all of your patient's questions. It is not a sign of incompetence or weakness to admit that you do not know the answer and to refer to a colleague for help. Here, discussing the case with your GP supervisor (C) could provide a quick answer that could help to satisfy your patient. However, as this is not an urgent issue, the preferred option would be to give yourself the opportunity to research the topic and discuss it with your supervisor at a more convenient time (A). Prescribing a drug you do not know anything about (D) would be potentially very dangerous and should be avoided. Refusing to prescribe the drug (E) would be an unhelpful response without researching and explaining your reasoning; however, it is preferable to a blind prescription. Booking your patient in with another GP (B) may solve your patient's problems; however, this would not address your own learning needs around the topic.

Recommended reading
Medical Protection Society (2012), Competence, section: Referrals, in *MPS Guide to Ethics: A Map for the Moral Maze,* chapter 10.

3.16 Difficult questions about cancer

B   E   H

As an FY1, you are often the medical 'point of contact' for the patients on the ward. You spend the majority of your time on the ward and see the patients every day. This can often lead to a situation where you are asked questions that you do not know the answers to. This is not a sign of incompetence as you could not be expected to possess the same depth of knowledge as a consultant at this early stage in your training. In these scenarios, the best course of action is honesty. The majority of patients will respect your honesty if you admit that you cannot answer their questions, apologise and offer to help find them the answers. Therefore, option B would be the best course of initial action. You must then assess how you can help to answer his questions and who would be the most appropriate source of information. Technical questions about metastatic cancer should be addressed by registrars and consultants. In this scenario, most consultants would appreciate a courtesy phone call (H) and may suggest that you discuss the case with the specialist registrar or even come to see the patient themselves. If the questions were to do with his nursing care, a senior nurse may be an appropriate source of help (D); however, this is not the case in this scenario. In attempting to answer his questions (options A and G), you may inadvertently communicate some incorrect information and possibly false hope, even if your intentions were good. Offering to read your consultant's entry in the notes (F) is likely to cause more harm than good as the entry hasn't been designed as a patient explanation. Finally, if these were questions that the patient was not necessarily worried about, it could be appropriate to delay them until the consultant ward round on the following day (C); however, given the change in the patient's diagnosis, on balance, it would be better to address his issues immediately.

Recommended reading
Medical Protection Society (2012), Competence, section: Referrals, in *MPS Guide to Ethics: A Map for the Moral Maze,* chapter 10.

3.17 Breaking bad news

C   E   B   D   A

Breaking bad news is a difficult but important skill that is usually left to more senior members of the team. However, there are situations where you are left with no choice but to discuss important results with patients. In this instance, although you do not know for certain that the brain lesion is a metastasis of your patient's lung cancer, this is the most likely explanation. While you could choose not to discuss the scan results with the patient yourself, in this instance, she has asked you outright. It would therefore be wrong to withhold the information you have. Explaining that the scan is normal (A) is completely inappropriate since this is untrue. Similarly, telling her that the cancer has definitely spread (D) is also potentially untrue and would cause her undue distress in the unlikely event that the lesion were found to be non-cancerous. To tell the patient that you do not know what the scan shows (B) is also dishonest but does not pose future repercussions, as options A and D. Option E is a suitable response as it is true to say that there is an abnormality but that you don't know exactly what it is. Option C, however, is the most appropriate option: although you can emphasise that you have no definite answers, it is indeed likely that this is a metastasis. A useful tool in breaking bad news involves 'warning shots', where ideas can be introduced before definite answers are given. This prepares the patient in advance of them receiving a definitive diagnosis once more investigations have been performed.

Recommended reading

General Medical Council (2013), *Good Medical Practice,* paragraphs 31–33.
Patient, Breaking Bad News, http://www.patient.co.uk/doctor/
  breaking-bad-news.

3.18 Explicit posters

C A E D B

The doctors' office is part of the workplace and should be treated as such. It is therefore inappropriate to display sexually explicit posters on the walls. In this scenario, it is even more important to tackle the issue since the posters are also making colleagues feel uncomfortable. A good first response is option C: both explaining to your male colleagues that the posters are inappropriate and removing them yourself. This is preferable to asking your colleagues to remove the posters themselves (A) since by removing them yourself you are ensuring that they are indeed removed. Taking down the posters when no one is looking (E) does not alert your colleagues to the reason why they have been removed, although it does still ensure that they are removed. While the ward manager may be able to help (D), you should at least be able to attempt to solve the situation yourself. Doing nothing (B) when the posters are obviously having a negative impact on female colleagues is unacceptable as it shows a lack of respect and a poor professional attitude.

Recommended reading

General Medical Council (2013), *Good Medical Practice,* paragraphs 36
  and 59.

3.19 Consent HIV test

D B E A C

A few years ago, it used to be routine to formally counsel patients before testing them for HIV. This was because it held implications for people's health care insurance if they had the test as, even if it was negative, it was seen as an admission of risky behaviour. Currently there is a big push to routinely test people more widely and part of achieving that is to try and reduce the stigmatisation of the testing. Option D is the best response: you should still consent the patient for the test as you would for any other test, and you should record your conversation in brief in the notes. An FY1 should be able to do this, but if you do not feel confident in doing so, learning from a senior can help (B). Option E comes third; it is not necessary to obtain written consent for an HIV test, and it defeats the new movement to make it more routine; however, you are getting valid consent in this way, and it is not entirely inappropriate. You can always ask the advice and support of other medical professionals when dealing with something outside of your comfort zone; however, consenting for an HIV test is something within the remit of an FY1 and asking for the attendance of another doctor outside of the department might not be appreciated (A). The worst response here is option C, to not consent for the test and 'surprise' them with the result; it doesn't show respect for the patient and their right to provide consent, not to mention that this is also deeply unprofessional.

Recommended reading
British HIV Association (2008), *UK National Guidelines for HIV Testing.*

3.20 Smoking

B C D A E

As a doctor, it is your responsibility to promote healthy lifestyle choices and to encourage patients to take responsibility for improving and maintaining their own health. However, you should also respect a patient's autonomy even if their decisions result in a risk to their health. The most appropriate response is to discuss your concerns with the patient and encourage him to give up smoking (B). Providing information leaflets is also appropriate (C), although less favourable than option B since there is no opportunity for discussion or questions. Prescribing a nicotine patch (D) is inappropriate without prior discussion with the patient about whether they wish to give up smoking. However, this is a more favourable response than option A, which does not attempt to address the patient's smoking. Option E is wholly inappropriate. You should not attempt to 'tell' a patient what to do and neither should you try to scare a patient in order to manipulate their decisions.

Recommended reading
General Medical Council (2013), *Good Medical Practice*, paragraphs 46–49, 51.

Medical Protection Society (2012), Patient autonomy and consent, in *MPS Guide to Ethics: A Map for the Moral Maze,* chapter 8.

3.21 Disclosure to relatives

A B F

While you can listen to a patient's family's concerns without the patient's consent, you cannot disclose any information without consent. You therefore cannot tell the patient's daughter that she doesn't have cancer (C), unless the patient gives her consent. You should tell the daughter that you cannot discuss her mother's case with her (F). You should never lie on behalf of a patient (E). You can encourage the patient to be honest with her daughter (B), but you should not coerce the patient into telling the truth (G). Similarly, your opinion of a patient's actions should not influence the care you give (H). It is good practice to document all conversations you have with patient's relatives (A). This may be particularly important in this case since the daughter may become upset that you did not disclose the truth if she were to later discover her mother's true diagnosis. While it is important to reflect on incidents such as this (D), it is not the most appropriate response in this scenario.

Recommended reading
General Medical Council (2009), Explanatory guidance, in *Confidentiality,* paragraphs 64, 66.
Medical Protection Society (2012), Confidentiality, in *MPS Guide to Ethics: A Map for the Moral Maze,* chapter 9.

3.22 Uninformed consent

C B E D A
When obtaining consent, it is imperative to check a patient's understanding. If a patient does not fully understand the risk of complications, then they are not making an informed decision and could seek legal compensation should such a complication occur. In this scenario, you should suggest to your colleague that you do not think that the patient fully understood (C); this may upset your colleague, but ultimately they should know this, and it gives them a chance to change their practice and avoid complaints and litigation. Another good option would be to ask a senior colleague to discuss the procedure with the patient (B) as this would enable the patient to get the information required from an experienced colleague; however, this would not help your SpR to change his practice, so it is less suitable than option C. Option E would improve the patient's understanding; however, as a junior doctor, you are likely to lack the necessary experience and knowledge needed to provide this information. Doing nothing (D) would be negligent; however, advising the patient to make a complaint about your colleague (A) would be unprofessional. As a doctor, you should provide the correct channels for a patient if they wish to make a complaint, but you should not suggest that a patient makes a complaint about a colleague.

Recommended reading
General Medical Council (2008), Explanatory guidance, in *Consent: Patients and Doctors Making Decisions Together,* paragraphs 7–11.

3.23 Refusing medication

D E F
As a doctor you should respect a patient's autonomy and their right to refuse treatment or medication; however, you should also make sure that they have made an informed decision. The most appropriate actions in this case are therefore to discuss it further with the patient and empathise with her reasons for not wanting to take aspirin (D), to ensure that she understands the benefits and the risks of aspirin (e.g. bleeding) and also the risks associated with not taking it (E) and to respect her decision (F). Options A and H, advising

her to find another doctor or telling her that she must take your advice, are outdated and unprofessional as you should not force a patient into treatments or withdraw treatment, even if you disagree with their beliefs. Asking a senior GP colleague to speak to your patient (B) could be helpful if you felt out of your depth or wanted reassurance; however, this should be a situation that a junior doctor can deal with. Asking her husband to convince her to take it (C) would be disrespectful towards your patient and their right to make a decision. Seeking advice from a medical indemnity society (G) would be unnecessary in this situation.

Recommended reading
Medical Protection Society (2012), Patient autonomy and consent, in *MPS Guide to Ethics: A Map for the Moral Maze*, chapter 8.

3.24 Confused patient refusing antibiotics

A   C   B   D   E

In this scenario, it is obvious that at this point in time that the patient does not have capacity to make this decision. When a patient lacks capacity, you can give treatment against their wish if it is in their best interests. Sepsis is potentially life-threatening, and here the patient should be given the antibiotic against their will, although you should remain respectful (A). Finding an oral alternative for the antibiotic (C) may be appropriate in some cases, but IV antibiotics are more effective in sepsis, especially when a patient is still febrile. Asking the patient's husband for consent (B) is not necessary but may be useful to glean the patient's views and beliefs to decide whether you would be acting in the patient's best interests. Getting the patient sectioned (D) is inappropriate as the confusion is likely to resolve with treatment of the sepsis. Telling the patient that you are giving her a painkiller but instead giving her the antibiotic (E) is deceitful and dishonest.

Recommended reading
General Medical Council (2008), Explanatory guidance, in *Consent: Patients and Doctors Making Decisions Together,* paragraphs 75, 76.

3.25 Language barriers

B   C   F

Despite this being a relatively minor procedure, you are still required to obtain verbal consent from the patient, so options E and H are inappropriate. Either ignoring the situation (D) or changing the management plan (G) could result in the patient receiving sub-optimal care and could potentially be dangerous. You will need to communicate with the patient in her own language, and therefore, options B and C would be the most appropriate as they ensure impartial communication of consent. Option F is also appropriate, although less so, but it is preferable to A because it ensures that the information relayed to the patient is the information you wish to communicate.

Recommended reading
General Medical Council (2013), *Good Medical Practice*, paragraph 32.

3.26 Contraception and young people

C D F

This question focuses on a famous case concerning consent and young people. It is appropriate for a doctor to provide contraception for a child under the age of 16 without parental consent and knowledge if:

- She is mature enough to understand the nature and implications of the contraception.
- She cannot be persuaded to discuss the situation with her parents or allow the doctor to do so.
- She is likely to have sexual intercourse with or without contraception.
- Her physical or mental health may suffer unless she receives contraception.
- The contraception is given in her best interests.

If a young person under the age of 16 fits these criteria, they are said to be Gillick competent. Option C would be the best course of action to ensure she has competence. Option D is a possibility as FY2 doctors should feel they can approach an educational supervisor for support, and it would immediately tackle the issue. It is also important to ensure that you have fully documented the conversation you have had with your patient should any difficulties subsequently arise with her parents. Option F, though not ideal, would provide contraception while allowing you time to gain support and advice. Options A and G are inappropriate as the patient clearly does not want to inform her parents and in so doing you would break confidentiality. Option H would harm your doctor–patient relationship and not solve the issue as she intends to have sexual intercourse regardless. Option E is inappropriate as she does not have to inform her parents if she does not wish to and should not be pressured into doing so. Finally, asking the patient to book an appointment with a senior doctor (B) might eventually solve the problem, but she may have unprotected sexual intercourse in the meantime.

Recommended reading
General Medical Council (2008), Explanatory guidance, in *Consent: Patients and Doctors Making Decisions Together*, paragraphs 54–56.

3.27 Self-discharge

A B C E D

If you can convince the patient to wait, it is best for a senior to be involved in situations of self-discharge (A). This will ensure that the risks have been explained fully and all efforts have been made to help the patient understand the importance of staying in hospital. However, you can manage the situation yourself as an FY1 and indeed you may have to if a senior is not available at the time. You would need to have a discussion with the patient and complete the appropriate paperwork (B). Option C ranks lower than B because it describes a one-way communication of the risks rather than a two-way discussion and makes no mention of ensuring the patient gets their medications to take home with them, which is important for patient safety. You cannot take a passive role in this context: telling the patient that they are free to leave the ward is true but you must follow the necessary processes (E). Telling the patient that they must stay (D) is the worst response as it is both untrue and would be a complete violation of the patient's autonomy.

Recommended reading
Medical Protection Society (2012), Patient autonomy and consent, section: Free will, in *MPS Guide to Ethics: A Map for the Moral Maze*, chapter 8.
Raine T, McGinn K, Dawson J, Sanders S, Eccles S, Being a doctor: Self-discharge, in *Oxford Handbook for the Foundation Programme* (3rd edn.), chapter 1.

3.28 Family translating

E   B   D   C   A

This situation implies that you have major concerns over whether the patient can give informed consent, so the worst response here is to ignore the issue and just book her for theatre (A). The other four options involve different methods of approaching the problem. Using Language Line™ promptly but without the family present (E) is the best response because it gives the patient an opportunity to have the situation explained independently, without the influence of her family, which could potentially be persuasive. Although translation is more effective in person than via the telephone, option B is not as good as E because it delays the discussion until immediately before the operation. This has service planning implications and may make the patient feel pressurised to continue with the plan. Asking your registrar to deal with the situation (D) is a way to raise your concerns but is passive, and you can be more proactive with the higher ranking options. Challenging the daughter (C) is provoking confrontation, and this may not do much to help solve the problem. However, this is still better than ignoring your concerns, as in option A, which is entirely inappropriate.

Recommended reading
Communication in difficult circumstances (2012), in *Foundation Programme Curriculum*, Section 2.3.
General Medical Council (2013), *Good Medical Practice*, paragraph 32.

3.29 Blood transfusion

A   C   D

This question focuses on respecting patient autonomy in situations where, as a doctor, you may not agree with the decision the patient makes. It is also important to remember to maintain good communication with the patient and your colleagues. If the patient has capacity, you must act according to their wishes and remember to document accurately and clearly any conversations you have with them, while ensuring that the patient completes any necessary paperwork. Options A and C are therefore wise actions to take initially, while ignoring the patient's wishes by proceeding to arrange the transfusion would be inappropriate (E and F). As a less experienced doctor, it is also sensible to talk to a senior about your conversation (D) and to see whether there is anything else that needs to be done. This would be preferable to discussing the case with another FY1 colleague (B), who is likely not to have any more experience in these types of situations than you. You must be satisfied that the patient is aware of the risks of refusing treatment, but your aim should not be to coerce them into agreeing with you (H); instead, simply make sure that they are provided with all of the information they need so that they can make a fully informed decision. The blood bank may be able to give you some advice about the paperwork that needs to be completed (G), but your team should be the first port of call for help in dealing with these situations. You should always involve a senior colleague.

Recommended reading

General Medical Council (2008), Explanatory guidance, in *Consent: Patients and Doctors Making Decisions Together.*

General Medical Council (2013), Duties of a doctor, in *Good Medical Practice.*

General Medical Council (2013), *Good Medical Practice,* paragraphs 11, 14, 17, 19, 21, 31, 46–49, 54, 68, 71.

Medical Protection Society (2012), Patient autonomy and consent, in *MPS Guide to Ethics: A Map for the Moral Maze,* chapter 8.

3.30 Blind patient

D E A B C

This question concerns one of the duties of a doctor: that of making sure you give patients information in a way they can understand. This is always important, especially when the situation involves obtaining informed consent. Option D is the most appropriate initial response in this case as, in doing this, you are showing regard for the patient's disability as well as ensuring that she still receives the information she needs. Option E would also be suitable (discussing the procedures with the patient and supplying the patient's husband with an information leaflet); however, it would be courteous to the patient to provide her with the written information as well as her husband, if possible. This would be better than simply talking things through, as in option A, so that the patient can consolidate the verbal conversation with written information and helps to ensure that she doesn't forget anything important. Similarly, option B is less appropriate, but it is worse than option A because, in addition, you are asking one of your colleagues, who may be very busy, to do one of your jobs without good reason. You may wish to ask for advice regarding giving the information, but you should attempt to complete the task before referring to a senior to complete it. Option C would be the least courteous as the patient would probably not be able to read the information herself, and you would be directly ignoring your consultant's request by failing to discuss the procedure with the patient and her immediate family.

Recommended reading
General Medical Council (2013), Duties of a doctor, in *Good Medical Practice*.
General Medical Council (2013), *Good Medical Practice,* paragraphs 18, 31, 32, 33, 46, 49, 51, 60.
Medical Protection Society (2012), Patient autonomy and consent, in *MPS Guide to Ethics: A Map for the Moral Maze*, chapter 8.

3.31 Refusing medication

C   E   B   A   D
In reality, the only correct answer here is to go and speak to the patient (C). You need to understand their perspective and discuss the situation with them. You do not need senior input at this stage (E); you should be able to attempt to resolve the issue yourself, which is why option E is less preferable to option C. Option B is a poorer choice because it involves delaying resolving the problem until the next day. In addition, the patient may feel embarrassed that you have brought up the issue in front of the whole team, and this could undermine your relationship with them. These first three options have all involved some attempt to respond to the problem so that a solution can be found that will hopefully lead to a mutually acceptable, effective treatment. However, options D and A do not lead to this outcome and are therefore ranked lowest. Prescribing potassium by an alternative route (A) does ensure that the low potassium doesn't go untreated because, in extreme cases, this could have potentially fatal effects. However, it fails to deal with the underlying issues or to involve the patient in communication. The worst answer is to do nothing (D) as this could lead to harm to the patient. While patients do have a right to refuse any treatments, that doesn't mean that doctors should accept this with no further action. The doctor and the patient should be working together to find a management plan that is acceptable to both parties.

Recommended reading
General Medical Council (2013), *Good Medical Practice,* paragraph 2.
The UK Foundation Programme Curriculum (2012), *Relationship and Communication with Patients*, chapter 2.

3.32 Seeking assistance to die

B   C   E
This is a difficult situation; the General Medical Council (GMC) has produced guidance for this issue. You should try to remain compassionate while ensuring that you do not contravene the law by encouraging or assisting the patient to

commit suicide. Therefore, you should address a number of issues during your consultation. Discussing your patient's reasons for wanting to end his life, while explaining that you are unable to provide him with advice about suicide is the best course of action (options C and E). You should also ensure that he has no unmet palliative care needs, referring to the appropriate services that he may require (B). Arranging to section the patient under the Mental Health Act (A) would be inappropriate at this stage as the patient may not have a psychiatric disorder. Getting another GP to speak with your patient (D) could be useful as you are likely to need support dealing with this situation; however, options B, C and E are more important at this point in time. Telling the patient that they are being selfish (G) would be very unsympathetic and unprofessional. Informing the patient that you can no longer provide care (H) is incorrect; the patient has confided in and asked you for advice, not to help them physically end their life. Once you have established that you cannot provide the patient with this information, you should seek other ways of improving his condition, for example with symptom control or psychological and social support. You should listen to and respect your patient's decisions, and for this reason, option F, refusing to engage in a conversation about this subject, would be unsuitable.

Recommended reading
General Medical Council (2013), *When a Patient Seeks Advice or Information About Assistance to Die.*

3.33 Ward round

A E F

Patients have a right to confidentiality, which is central to the trust held between doctors and their patients. While it is inevitable that patients on a ward will unintentionally learn information about each other, this should be avoided wherever possible. This is particularly important when discussing sensitive information, such as an HIV diagnosis. You should therefore stop the consultant and suggest that he takes the patient somewhere more private (E). This may prevent any further information from being disclosed and enable a more open discussion between your consultant and the patient. You should also suggest that the consultant apologises to the patient (F). It is appropriate for you too to apologise on behalf of the consultant (A). While talking to the consultant at the end of the ward round (H) may alert him to his mistake and prevent a further breach of confidentiality, it does nothing to rectify the current situation. Similarly, asking other patients whether they heard the conversation (B) does nothing to help. Moving the patient to a side room (D) is unnecessary and may make them feel stigmatised. Indeed, if you act appropriately at this stage, there should be no similar situations in the future. Although your consultant has acted poorly, this was undoubtedly unintentional. An apology to the patient may be all that is needed to resolve the issue, so suggesting that the patient make a complaint (G) may cause unnecessary upset. Ignoring a breach in confidentiality (C) is inappropriate and fails your duty as a doctor.

Recommended reading

General Medical Council (2009), Explanatory guidance, in *Confidentiality*, paragraphs 6, 13.
General Medical Council (2013), *Good Medical Practice*, paragraph 55.

3.34 Secret pregnancy

C   F   G

While, in most cases, a patient is happy for their family to be fully informed about their treatment, there are instances where this is not the case. You should therefore be mindful when talking to relatives about what you can and can't discuss. In this scenario, your patient has clearly felt unable at this point to tell her husband that she is pregnant, and it is not your place to tell him. You should therefore explain to the husband that you cannot discuss his wife's treatment without her permission (F). It is also appropriate to ask the husband to discuss the CT scan with his wife in the meantime (G). This gives the patient the opportunity to tell her husband what she would like him to know. You could discuss with the patient why she has not told her husband (C) so that you have a better understanding of her situation and are able to offer some support if necessary. In this scenario, you should not encourage the patient to be honest with her husband about the pregnancy (D) as it is entirely her decision whether to inform him or not. You should not normally lie on behalf of a patient, so telling the husband that his wife no longer needs the scan is inappropriate (E). Similarly, asking the patient what she wants you to tell her husband (B) is not ideal as she may want you to lie on her behalf. Telling the husband about the pregnancy (H) is a breach of confidentiality, so it is clearly unsuitable. Asking the husband to calm down (A) is also inappropriate since this may further anger him and offers no solution to the problem.

Recommended reading

General Medical Council (2009), Explanatory guidance, *Confidentiality*, paragraphs 6, 64, 66.
Medical Protection Society (2012), Confidentiality, in *MPS Guide to Ethics: A Map for the Moral Maze*, chapter 9.

3.35 Discussion with relative

A   C   D   E   B

While you should maintain patient confidentiality when speaking to relatives, you can and should listen to any concerns that a relative wishes to discuss with you. You should, however, make it clear that you may need to inform the patient of your conversation. In this scenario, you need to speak to the patient about her alcohol use in order to establish whether her symptoms are attributable to alcohol withdrawal. You do not necessarily have to disclose your conversation with her husband in order to do that (A). It would not be inappropriate, however, to tell her about your conversation with her husband, although you should warn him that this is your intention (C). To tell the patient about your conversation without forewarning her husband (D) is less favourable as this may risk damaging both their relationship and the trust that the husband has in you. You should not treat the patient for alcohol withdrawal without establishing whether she is alcohol dependent nor should you provide treatment without informing the patient of what it is for (E). Having said that, ignoring the husband would fail to investigate a potentially serious condition, which is why option B ranks last.

Recommended reading
General Medical Council (2009), Explanatory guidance, in *Confidentiality*, paragraph 66.

3.36 Knife wound

A   B   E   D   C

In cases of knife or gunshot wounds, it is important to inform the police so that they can ensure the safety of the patient, hospital staff and the public. The police should be informed, even if the patient does not consent to disclosure. However, wherever practicable, the patient should be informed before the information is disclosed; therefore, option A is preferable to B. The police should be informed as quickly as possible so that any further harm can be prevented. Waiting for the patient to change his mind (E), although it seems courteous, is therefore unsuitable. A decision not to report knife or gunshot wounds is rare and should be made by the consultant in charge (D). Coercing the patient into giving consent is completely inappropriate (C).

Recommended reading
General Medical Council (2009), Explanatory guidance, in *Confidentiality*, paragraphs 36–39.
General Medical Council (2009), Explanatory guidance, in *Confidentiality: Reporting Gunshot and Knife Wounds.*

3.37 Telephone conversation with relative

C   D   E

This is a common scenario in hospital medicine. It is important, before discussing with relatives, to confirm with the patient that they are happy for you to speak to certain relatives (C). Without this consent, you may be breaching confidentiality. During telephone conversations, you should try to confirm that you are speaking to the correct person (D). You could do this by ringing the relative on a number given to you by the patient. On occasions when you are disclosing personal information about a patient, you should give only the minimum necessary information (E). Options B and H are both inappropriate as the son has requested to talk with a doctor, and as an FY1, you should be able to deal with this situation. Option A is unlikely to suffice as the son would like information from a doctor, and option F would be both rude and unprofessional. Having a face-to-face conversation would be preferable in this situation; however, the son has already specified that he is unable come into hospital (G).

Recommended reading
General Medical Council (2009), Explanatory guidance, in *Confidentiality*,
        paragraphs 9, 64–66.

3.38 Contact tracing

C   B   D   A   E

This question assesses your ability to communicate effectively with the patient and to know in what circumstances personal information can be disclosed against the wishes of the patient. In this situation, you should explore your patient's concerns and inform her of the importance of her boyfriend's treatment and discuss ways of implementing it (C). This should enable your patient to make an informed decision. Option B is the next step if the patient is still refusing to tell her partner. This is now an issue of public safety as her boyfriend may unknowingly infect others. It is important to make the consultant aware and to implement the contact tracing protocol of the genito-urinary medicine (GUM) clinic. Option D is the next best response; the patient should be informed that you may have to break confidentiality in the interest of public safety. Option A is not appropriate as this is shirking responsibility. Option E is the least appropriate course of action as the boyfriend may never find out and unknowingly carry a chlamydial infection, which, among other things, may seriously damage his future health.

Recommended reading
General Medical Council (2009), Explanatory guidance, in *Confidentiality*,
        paragraph 64.
General Medical Council (2013), *Good Medical Practice*, paragraphs 31, 50.

3.39 Prophylactic antibiotics

C   D   E

This is a difficult situation and one that is not commonly faced. In the majority of situations, most patients will be happy to disclose information if it will protect family and friends. Meningitis is a potentially fatal infection and should be taken very seriously. The General Medical Council advises that a balance must be sought between your duty of care to the patient and your duty to protect others from serious harm. In this situation, you must inform the potential contacts at the party that they are at risk. The best way to do this would be with the help and support of the patient, so option C would be most appropriate. The local public health department or your consultant could also help and offer advice in this scenario, which also makes options D and E appropriate, especially if the patient is refusing to cooperate with your request. Allowing him to contact his friends himself (A) could potentially identify at-risk individuals; however, some of his friends may not show symptoms in the early stages of the infection. Additionally, you may run the risk of him failing to contact all of the necessary people. Relying on the patient to distribute antibiotics to his friends (B) is not a reliable method of providing appropriate prophylaxis to potential contacts. Refusing to treat him (F) is a breach in your duty of care to the patient, while respecting his wishes (G) would breach your duty of care to the public.

Recommended reading

General Medical Council (2009), Explanatory guidance, in *Confidentiality*, paragraphs 68, 69.

3.40 HIV and death certificates

B   D   H

The completion of death certificates is a common task for an FY1 doctor. General Medical Council (GMC) guidelines set out several situations where you should disclose relevant information about a patient who has died. One of those situations is on death certificates, which must be completed honestly and fully. While this patient is dying from a malignancy and tuberculosis, his HIV infection is also a key contributor to his death, and therefore, it must be mentioned on his certificate. Option E is therefore inappropriate. Documenting a 'viral infection' (A) would not be completing the certificate fully so is also inappropriate. You should be open and honest with your patient about your duty (D), while also trying to allay his fears (H). In a difficult situation, you should always contact a senior for help if you are unsure about what to do (B). Informing his family of the condition before he dies (C) would involve breaking patient confidentiality and is therefore inappropriate. Of the responses left, lying to your patient is bad practice (F) and refusing to complete the certificate (G) would ignore the issue and leave this task to a fellow colleague to deal with, which is inappropriate.

Recommended reading

General Medical Council (2009), Explanatory guidance, in *Confidentiality*, paragraph 71.

3.41 Drug overdose

A   B   C   D   E

In this type of situation, it is important not to guarantee to a friend/relative/partner that you will keep a conversation confidential. This is because the information they give you may prove to be important in the treatment of your patient (as in this case). Good communication with all parties from the outset is key to ensuring that there is no confusion and will prevent difficult situations from arising. Considering these points, the two most appropriate responses are options A and B. Of the two, A is more appropriate as it deals with the patient who currently requires treatment and involves senior support in a difficult situation. Refusing to speak to the patient's friend (E) could potentially lead to sub-optimal care and the incorrect treatment, so this ranks last. Phoning the police to report a case of drugging (D) would be inappropriate before liaising with seniors, the patient and the friend of the patient; however, this is technically a criminal matter, so this could be considered. Keeping the source of the information confidential and treating the patient (C) ensures immediate patient safety; however, it may put the patient at risk in the future of a similar episode.

Recommended reading
General Medical Council (2009), Explanatory guidance, in *Confidentiality*, paragraph 66.

3.42 Safeguarding children

C A B E D

As a healthcare professional, you have an ethical and legal responsibility to take action if you become aware of children who could be at risk. You should explain each step of what is happening to the patient, and the best person to contact is the safeguarding officer in your hospital (C). You could defer responsibility to your senior (A), but this is not the best response as the patient has disclosed to you, and you should be able to respond to this yourself. Referring to social services (options B and E), an external agency, is a decision that should only be taken after seeking support from within your organisation. Asking for consent is a problematic issue because you may need to disclose this information to social services even if the person involved refuses their consent for this. Nevertheless, option B is better than E because it explains to the patient and attempts to involve them in the decision, which is polite. The worst response in this scenario is to take no action, even if you do document your findings (D). These children are living in a house with the potential for domestic abuse, and this must be investigated by the appropriate services.

Recommended reading
General Medical Council (2007), Explanatory guidance, in *0–18 Years: Guidance for All Doctors*, paragraphs 56–63.

3.43 Lost notes

A C F

The first action you should take in this situation is to apologise to the patient (A). However, you should not seek to pin the blame on any particular member of staff (E), especially when it is not clear how the notes were lost. You should never try to discourage a patient from making a complaint if they wish to (B). After speaking to the patient, you should take action to address the problem. It is likely to take up a lot of time to search for the notes yourself in the medical records department and is unlikely to be successful (G). Involving the ward clerk so that they can start a new temporary file (C) is appropriate, and they will also be a valuable aid in trying to locate the originals. Using a temporary file is better than waiting to document (H) as you should be recording what is happening to the patient in a thorough and timely manner to protect patient safety. This would also minimise the risk of human error in forgetting what has been said about the patient's management. It is important to raise this to a higher management level as this ensures that any underlying system issues are investigated to try to prevent future occurrence of the problem. The best way to do this in this situation is to fill in an incident form (F). This is a better response than talking to your educational supervisor (D) as it relates to a ward management issue.

Recommended reading
Foundation Programme Curriculum (2012), section 2.4: Complaints.
General Medical Council (2013), *Good Medical Practice*, paragraph 55.

3.44 Employee disclosure

B E G
This question tests your ability to maintain patient confidentiality, specifically for the purposes of protecting against discrimination. You should not disclose information to third parties, as in options C and D, without the patient's permission. In this scenario, it would therefore be wise to have a conversation with the patient about his wishes (B), and if you are unsure as to how to approach the situation, a more experienced member of staff on the ward may be able to help you with this (G). It would also be polite to explain to the caller in a professional manner about your obligation to protect the patient's confidentiality (E), which would show good communication skills and respect for the caller in addition to the patient. Threatening or aggressive behaviour towards the caller (H) would simply inflame the situation and would not demonstrate good professional behaviour. Shirking your responsibility onto another member of the team (options A and F) is unprofessional and would show a disregard for your professional responsibilities.

Recommended reading
Disability Discrimination Act (2005), chapter 13.
General Medical Council (2009), Explanatory guidance, in *Confidentiality*.
General Medical Council (2013), Duties of a doctor, in *Good Medical Practice*.
General Medical Council (2013), *Good Medical Practice,* paragraphs 31, 34, 46, 47, 50, 68.
Medical Protection Society (2012), Confidentiality, in *MPS Guide to Ethics: A Map for the Moral Maze*, chapter 9.

3.45 Child confidentiality

B C D A E
According to the General Medical Council (GMC), divorce does not affect parental responsibility, and both parents should be allowed equal access to information about their child. The best responses establish that this man is

definitely Chloe's father. It is difficult when you have never met family members before to ensure that they are who they claim to be. Option B would ensure both parents had fair access to updates about Chloe and also seamlessly allows you to discover if this man is Chloe's father, since his ex-partner will surely recognise him. Option C is the next best response as validating whether this man is Chloe's father is reasonable before discussing confidential information. If you explain sympathetically that you need proof of his identity and that it is in the interest of Chloe's confidentiality, most people will gladly oblige. Asking the man to ask Chloe's mother (D) is not a very helpful response on your part, but at least you are avoiding a potential breach in confidentiality. However, you cannot be sure how amicable their relationship is, so deflecting the man to Chloe's mother may land you in the middle of a family feud. Option A is ranked fourth because asking Chloe's mother's permission to speak to her father would ensure that both parties know that they are each involved (avoiding an argument), but it comes after option D because you do not actually need the mother's permission to discuss Chloe with her father. The least appropriate response is Option E: asking help from seniors in complicated situations is always advised, but an FY1 is capable of giving simple updates to family members and shouldn't need senior support, unless things become more complicated.

Recommended reading
General Medical Council (2007), Explanatory guidance, *0–18 Years: Guidance for All Doctors*, paragraph 55.

3.46 Handover sheet

A F H
Handover sheets are a necessity on the wards to ensure essential patient information is always at hand. Unfortunately, they are therefore one of the most concise summaries of an entire patient history, simply written and easily understood by the public. You should never take sensitive patient information home where members of the public could see it and where appropriate disposal might not be available. In this scenario, one of the best responses is to attempt to retrieve the lost handover sheet (H). This could recover the information without too many people seeing it. The second best option is to ask for the advice of someone senior, and your registrar who knows the patients in question and the details on the handover sheet is the best person to ask for help (A). Finally, to apologise to the patients is going to be difficult, but it is important that you do so as it is their information that could potentially have been made public (F). Simply ignoring the potential loss of confidential patient information (E) is inappropriate; this is not the behaviour of an honest and trustworthy doctor. To call the police (B) is not appropriate for the loss of one handover sheet. The rest of the options involve you trying to prevent this happening again, which is important but doesn't retrieve the lost handover sheet. Informing your clinical supervisor (C) could be productive as you could both sit down and come up with ways of preventing it happening again. Option D is

a good personal learning point, although does little for the situation at hand. Teaching other FY1s about confidentiality (G) would also be a valuable learning experience, although again it does little to remedy the immediate situation.

Recommended reading
General Medical Council (2013), Protecting information, in *Confidentiality*, paragraphs 12–14.

3.47 Consultant names

C A B D E

The best response here is to go straight to the source and tell your consultant how you feel (C). Some older, more traditional consultants may refer to you in the same way that their seniors did them, and they simply need reminding that this is not an appropriate way to address colleagues. The next best response is to discuss the matter as a team (A), followed by going to your supervisor (B). Your consultant is not in breach of the GMC's guidelines, so reporting him (D) is unlikely to be of any benefit to you. However, this is more appropriate than refusing to perform any of the jobs for the consultant (E), which is both unprofessional and would put patient safety at risk; therefore, this option has to rank last.

Recommended reading
General Medical Council (2013), *Duties of a doctor*, paragraph 1.
General Medical Council (2013), *Good Medical Practice*, paragraph 36.
Medical Protection Society (2012), Relating to colleagues, in *MPS Guide to Ethics: A Map for the Moral Maze*, chapter 11.

3.48 Degrading nursing staff

D A B C E

Option D is the best response by far since politely reminding your colleagues that a) they should be more respectful towards the nursing staff and b) they are in a place where anyone could overhear their conversation are important actions here. Option A ranks next as it involves making your colleagues aware that their discussion should not be taking place, but it is preferable not to be confrontational in your approach to this, which would likely make your working situation very difficult with them and is unprofessional. Option B is perhaps the next best response as making it seem like you did not overhear the conversation is likely to put an end to it, while reminding your colleagues that others can overhear. Option C is preferable to E as, by closing the door, at least you are attempting to make their conversation private, whereas doing nothing (E) could result in one of the nursing staff overhearing their conversation.

Recommended reading
Medical Protection Society (2012), Respect, in *MPS Guide to Ethics: A Map for the Moral Maze*, chapter 7.

3.49 FY1 vs SpR

B   D   G

Your colleague is upset so therefore the first thing you should do is comfort him (B). It is important that the registrar learns how your colleague feels and that what he said was inappropriate, but this is best coming from the person involved (options D and G) rather than their educational supervisor (A) or yourself (C). However, while it is better to discuss the matter directly with the registrar, if they do not listen, then you should escalate the matter to their consultant. Ignoring the situation (F) is never appropriate; all doctors have bad days, but this should not be taken out on more junior colleagues. Offering to take on your colleague's duties (H), while chivalrous of you, is not going to help the situation and will only result in further problems as you try and cover too many patients.

Recommended reading

Medical Protection Society (2012), Relating to colleagues, in *MPS Guide to Ethics: A Map for the Moral Maze*, chapter 11.

3.50 Patient concerns about GP

D   E   F

You should always take the time to listen to patients' concerns (F). It would be rude and uncaring to refuse any discussion (H). However, you must be objective when making any comment on the work of another practitioner, and in this situation, you are not in a position to either confirm the patient's concerns (A) or refute them (G). If you make disparaging comments about the care of the GP, this could be seen as defamation (A). It is best to remain neutral and explain to the patient that you do not have enough evidence to give your own professional opinion (D). You certainly do not have enough evidence to be concerned enough to contact the GMC at this point (B). However, you should let your seniors know, both so that they can look into the matter further if necessary and so that they are aware that the patient is likely to ask their opinions too (E). If you were to involve the GP in discussions about what had taken place (C), this should be done carefully so that the patient does not feel you had abused their trust when they confided their concerns. It should not be done in an inflammatory or confrontational manner.

Recommended reading

Medical Protection Society (2012), Relating to colleagues, section: Commenting upon the work of others, in *MPS Guide to Ethics: A Guide to the Moral Maze*, chapter 11.

3.51 Registrars conflicting plans

D   E   C   B   A

You are in a difficult position here in the midst of poor team communication. Nevertheless, it is important that you address the conflicting decisions (options D and E) rather than avoiding this. Option D is preferable to option E because the patient is expecting to go for the investigation, and the last entry in the patient's medical notes will specify that this is the plan, so there needs to be an open discussion about it, initiated by the second registrar. By calling the first registrar (E), you are avoiding them feeling undermined in future when they discover that the imaging was performed, and this will hopefully lead to a discussion between the two registrars. Option C is the next best response, and is preferable to A or B because it raises the opposing view; however, it involves challenging the second registrar in front of the patient, which they are likely to find embarrassing. This conversation would be better left until away from the patient's bedside to maintain professionalism. To ignore the situation (options A and B) is unprofessional and shows a lack of respect and appropriate responsibility on your part; in particular, to let the investigation remain unperformed (A) could potentially be damaging to patient care if the procedure was required, so this is the worst response.

Recommended reading
Medical Protection Society (2012), Relating to colleagues, section: Differences in opinion, in *MPS Guide to Ethics: A Map for the Moral Maze*, chapter 11.

3.52 Complaints

A C E

The NHS Litigation Authority confirms that providing an apology does not admit liability. Doctors should be prepared to apologise to a patient or relative regardless of whether they themselves were responsible for the incident (C). You cannot, however, comment on what may or may not have happened when you were not present, and this should be explained to the patient (E). It would also be highly inappropriate to either agree or disagree with the patient's view of the incident (options B and H). The doctor involved is best placed to comment and you should advise the patient to raise their concerns with the consultant directly (A). You are not in possession of all the facts, and it would be inappropriate for you to discuss the complaint with the consultant yourself (G). This incident may well be resolved simply by an apology from the consultant without the need for a formal complaint (F). Patients should be free to make complaints about their treatment without fear that their care will be compromised, so avoiding the patient (D) is inappropriate. In addition, personal views should not affect your relationship with the patient.

Recommended reading
General Medical Council (2013), *Good Medical Practice*, paragraphs 59, 61.

3.53 Consensual Dr–Dr relationship

D E F

In this situation, you have a duty both to protect patients against any behaviour that may potentially compromise care and to maintain good professional relationships with your colleagues and not to judge based on hearsay. It would therefore be sensible to clarify to the nurse that you had not observed this behaviour yourself (D). The sister should speak to the doctors in question (F) as you are not involved. If she determines that it is necessary, a more senior member of the medical team should be involved (E). It would be unlikely that there was a direct impact on patient safety (B); however, their behaviour may cause discomfort to other staff and therefore impact the team's functioning. Escalating the concerns of others when you have none yourself (H) or suggesting that a formal complaint should be made (G) are inappropriate responses. While remaining impartial, it is important to support your colleague in doing the right thing, and therefore, option C would be inappropriate.

Recommended reading

General Medical Council (2013), Duties of a doctor, in *Good Medical Practice*.
General Medical Council (2013), *Good Medical Practice*, paragraphs 16, 22, 23, 24, 25, 35–37, 56, 59, 65, 68.
Medical Protection Society (2012), Morality and decency, in *MPS Guide to Ethics: A Map for the Moral Maze*, chapter 5.

3.54 Putting arm around relative

C A B E D

This question concerns good communication and the necessity to apologise to patients and their relatives when they are dissatisfied with your behaviour. As a doctor, a position with social and public responsibility, putting a comforting arm around someone may not seem to you to be inappropriate, but you need to respect the fact that different cultures or religions may think differently. It is therefore imperative that you apologise in the first instance and reassure them that this will not happen again (C). Failing to apologise (D) would be unprofessional and could lead to further action if the person in question wished to make a formal complaint. It would also be inappropriate to ask the nurse to speak to the relative for you (E) because it is your professional duty to speak to the complainant in person; however, since they would still be receiving an apology, it is therefore not as inappropriate as option D. Explaining your behaviour to the nurse (A) is also courteous and wise so that they can support you in any further conversations; and informing your educational supervisor (B) would also be wise from an educational and reflective perspective. However, these courses of action should occur after apologising to the family.

Recommended reading

General Medical Council (2013), Explanatory guidance, in *Maintaining a Professional Boundary Between You and Your Patient*.
General Medical Council (2013), Duties of a doctor, in *Good Medical Practice*.
General Medical Council (2013), *Good Medical Practice*, paragraphs 31, 33–36, 46–48, 53, 55, 61, 65, 73.
Medical Protection Society (2012), Morality and decency, *MPS Guide to Ethics: A Map for the Moral Maze*, chapter 5.

3.55 Interrupting the SpR

A D B C E

This scenario raises a few different issues, most of which suggest that the registrar was not acting professionally, which puts you in a difficult position. First, the door should be locked during intimate examinations; second, the registrar should have had a chaperone present who could have answered the door for them and third, you should have been asked to remain outside. The most important thing is to make these points clear to the registrar, but you must also apologise to the patient (A). The next best response would be to close the door immediately and leave the patient alone (D); hopefully, the registrar would then apologise for the interruption. Following this, the preferable response of those remaining is to enter the room and wait (B) rather than to proceed to discuss another patient with the registrar while the patient remains on the table (C). The least appropriate response here is to blame the nurse incorrectly (E) as this ill only make your working relationship difficult.

Recommended reading

Medical Protection Society (2012), Morality and decency, in *MPS Guide to Ethics: A Map for the Moral Maze*, chapter 5.

3.56 Upset patient

E A B C D

This is obviously a difficult situation for the patient, and the most likely reason for the complaint is a product of their grief reaction. However, the first thing you must do in this scenario is apologise to the patient for any misunderstanding (options E and A), although this is best done with someone else present as a witness (E). Of the remaining options, B is the next best as having a third party explain the situation, while not ideal, ensures that an apology is made. Waiting for the situation to run its course (C) is not practical but is far superior to antagonising the patient (D).

Recommended reading

Medical Protection Society (2012), Morality and decency, in *MPS Guide to Ethics: A Map for the Moral Maze*, chapter 5.

3.57 Assisted suicide

B A E C D

This is a very difficult scenario, with equally difficult responses to choose from. Thankfully, for practitioners, there is helpful guidance available to answer these kinds of questions. Assisted suicide is a criminal offence in the United Kingdom, and any doctors found to be taking part in such activities would be liable to prosecution. In this scenario, however, your patient is clearly making a plea for help. She is experiencing severe symptoms, which are likely having a strong effect on her mood. The General Medical Council (GMC) advises that doctors should be open to discuss requests from patients but should also reiterate that this request in particular is illegal in the UK. The most important factor in this scenario, however, is to ensure that you offer your patient help and support for her symptoms as well as discuss her comments about suicide. For this reason, option B is the most appropriate response. Asking a senior colleague to discuss the issues (A) could be appropriate, but as an FY2 doctor, you would be expected to at least briefly discuss the issues and assist her with her symptoms. Referring her to the psychiatric and palliative care teams (E) may be appropriate; however, you should be attempting to manage aspects of the situation that are within your realm of competence (i.e. symptom control) initially before making a referral. Not offering to support your patient (C) would be inappropriate and could lead to unnecessary suffering. The most dangerous (and potentially illegal) option would be to prescribe large doses of opiate medication (D) as this could be seen as being compliant with suicide. Opiate-based medication may have a place in this patient's care but should be used according to appropriate guidance from experts such as the specialist palliative care team.

Recommended reading
General Medical Practice (2013), *When a Patient Seeks Advice or Information About Assistance to Die.*

3.58 Comments on abortion

B   C   F
This scenario deals with a number of issues that a foundation doctor may face. First, the doctor–patient relationship portrayed in this situation is clearly poor, and this must be addressed. Furthermore, there are also issues about relating to colleagues as well as the moral issues surrounding abortion. The SpR in this scenario is entitled to conscientiously object to providing a termination service for the patient, but the situation should have been handled very differently. The General Medical Council (GMC) offers good advice about how to tackle such a situation. While a doctor may object to a particular procedure, they must provide the patient with the opportunity to see a medical practitioner who could offer assistance. The most appropriate response here would be to discuss the situation with your SpR (F) as this would allow her to analyse the consultation and would hopefully lead to her addressing the obvious issues. Arranging for the patient to see another doctor (B) would ensure that the patient's needs are met. Asking the SpR to discuss the situation with a senior doctor immediately (C) would ensure that you have included senior support and that the patient's needs would be addressed before leaving the department. Discussing the situation after the clinic (options D and E) may well be appropriate, but this does not leave the patient with the support and advice she requires at this instance. Returning the patient to the room without discussing the situation (A) could potentially cause further distress and is therefore inappropriate. Documenting your concerns would also be appropriate (G), but the priority here is to ensure that

the patient's needs are met first. Remaining silent despite having concerns (H) is unacceptable in this scenario as this neglects the patient and would lead to ongoing poor practice by the SpR.

Recommended reading
General Medical Council (2013), *Personal Beliefs and Medical Practice.*

3.59 Racism

B   D   G
This question deals with the issue of racism at work. Racism is not tolerated within the NHS and faces severe disciplinary action if detected among staff. It is more complicated when patients are racist towards staff members as despite their behaviour, there remains a duty of care for that patient. This is a scenario that is likely to stir strong emotions, but it is important to remain civil and professional. There is a duty of care for any admitted patient; therefore, any option that involves ignoring the patient or discharging them without further assessment (options C, E and H) is inappropriate. Although it seems like avoidance of the situation, options B and G, which involve placing the patient under the care of another nurse, are the safest courses of action for a junior doctor to take. Although the scenario seems to make the patient's views quite clear, it is always a good idea to explore the true roots of patients' concerns, and when unsure of how to take matters forward, to seek senior advice; therefore, option D is also one of the best responses. Incident reporting would be inappropriate in this case, so option A is not one of the most appropriate responses, although it would be sensible to advise the nurse to report this higher through nursing channels. Reprimanding patients (F) is not the place of a junior doctor and should be avoided in all situations.

Recommended reading
General Medical Council (2013), *Good Medical Practice*, paragraphs 36, 59.
Medical Protection Society (2012), Morality and decency, in *MPS Guide to Ethics: A Map for the Moral Maze*, chapter 5.

3.60 Refusing treatment for children

A   C   E   D   B
This question tackles issues surrounding the protection of children. Although this example of a skin infection may seem trivial, the implications of receiving improper treatment may lead to serious morbidity. The best response in this question is option A. Calling the mother to properly explain the intended treatment may calm her concerns once she is properly informed. This is within the scope of your role as an FY1 and would be both proactive and helpful. Option C is the next best response: getting advice on the situation and how to proceed from a senior doctor is useful in complicated scenarios, particularly those involving child safety. Discussing the issue with another FY1 (E) would rank third because, although your colleague may not be able to give you the best advice directly, they are perhaps more likely to be familiar with the

issues surrounding child protection than you are. Option D ranks fourth: it is difficult to understand when people make different choices for themselves and their children to the ones the medical profession would advise, but this does not necessarily amount to neglect. Raising such a concern with social services without concrete evidence would cause distress for the family and generate distrust of healthcare professionals in future. Calling the police (B) would result in similar mistrust and distress. However, in cases of life and death, and where other routes have been exhausted, the police should be called to rescue a child who needs to be admitted for life-saving treatment.

Recommended reading

General Medical Council (2007), *0–18 Years: Guidance for All Doctors*, paragraphs 42–52.

3.61 Inappropriate dress at work

A C D B E

This question requires you to demonstrate good communication with staff, while remembering the duty of a doctor to maintain a professional appearance. It is possible that your colleague is not aware that she is dressing inappropriately; therefore, your first action should be to speak directly to her at a suitable time (A). Speaking to a senior colleague may be helpful if you need guidance in this (C) and is probably more appropriate than your friend who has no supervisory role in this situation (D). Monitoring the situation is less appropriate (B) as you have admitted that her dress is a problem, and this would therefore delay addressing the issue. However, this is slightly more suitable than reporting her to her educational supervisor (E), which would only serve to jeopardise your professional relationship and does not give your colleague a chance to either explain herself or rectify the situation.

Recommended reading

General Medical Council (2007), *Medical Students: Professional Behaviour and Fitness to Practice*.
General Medical Council (2012), *Continuing Professional Development: Guidance for All Doctors*.
General Medical Council (2013), Duties of a doctor, in *Good Medical Practice*.
General Medical Council (2013), *Good Medical Practice*, paragraphs 24, 25, 35–37, 43, 59, 65.
Medical Protection Society (2012), Professionalism and integrity, in *MPS Guide to Ethics: A Map for the Moral Maze*, chapter 3.

3.62 Late colleague

B D F

This question relies on your ability to balance maintaining a good professional relationship with colleagues with the requirement that doctors should be reliable and punctual. You have a duty to explore and try to rectify this issue as you have observed on multiple occasions a lack of punctuality in your colleague. Option A, to ask the sister to talk to him, and option H, to write an anonymous note, are therefore not appropriate responses as this does not involve you personally communicating the issue to your colleague. Gathering information from other colleagues (C) is not necessary before you take action, although you may wish to discuss the matter with someone else in the team. You do not know, however, whether there has been a good reason for the lateness, and therefore your first response should be to enquire as to why he is often late (B). As a colleague you should try to help out if you can. It would be unprofessional to exhibit aggressive behaviour (G) in any situation. Explaining to your colleague why his behaviour isn't professional (D) would be appropriate and may help him to understand why it is important that he turns up on time for work in the future. As mentioned earlier, you may want to get advice from a senior, and your educational supervisor is a useful point of contact, as in option F. However, asking your consultant to move the FY1 from your team (E) is not your right and nor does it help to find the reason behind why he is often late.

Recommended reading

General Medical Council (2013), Duties of a doctor, in *Good Medical Practice.*

General Medical Council (2013), *Good Medical Practice*, paragraphs 22, 24, 25, 36–38, 43, 44, 59, 68.

Medical Protection Society (2012), Professionalism and integrity, in *MPS Guide to Ethics: A Map for the Moral Maze*, chapter 3.

3.63 Registrar responsibility

A C B E D

If you ask your registrar to review patients you are concerned about, then they should always review them themselves and should not simply rely on your assessment as an FY1. This is a tricky situation since you do not want to damage your professional relationship or be seen to be undermining their authority. The best way to get the registrar to review the patients directly is by going with them to see the patient so that you can demonstrate the areas causing your concern (A). Discussing the matter with colleagues to see if others have had a similar experience would be useful (C), prior to discussing with your consultant (B), as it would add weight to your concerns. Taking the registrar's advice may be the right thing to do, but ensure that it is documented in the notes that this advice came from a senior (E). It is important to remember though that, if you are really concerned about patient safety, you must escalate the situation as quickly as possible to the appropriate seniors. Option D is obviously the worst choice; you are an FY1, and thinking that your plans are preferable to that of a registrar is both dangerous and unprofessional as you do not have their level of experience.

Recommended reading

General Medical Council (2013), *Good Medical Practice*, paragraphs 39–42.
Medical Protection Society (2012), *Medical Records: An MPS Guide*, pp. 8–10.
Medical Protection Society (2012), Professionalism and integrity, in *MPS Guide to Ethics: A Map for the Moral Maze*, chapter 3.

3.64 Gift from patient

C B D A E

It is appropriate to accept small gifts from patients as long as this cannot be seen to have affected the way you have treated them, which needs to be clarified in this situation (C). If you have not clarified this, it would be best to decline the watch in order to protect yourself from any accusations of manipulating the patient or being induced to treat them differently (B). Option B is also a kind and compassionate way of declining, which shouldn't have a detrimental effect on the patient's opinion of you, as opposed to implying that the patient is being improper (D). Option D could come across as rude but still ranks higher than options A or E. This is because you should refuse the gift, unless you have ensured that the patient does not consider it a deal you made for the treatment you gave them or have any other misconceptions. Option A fails to address these questions, while option E is immoral as it suggests that you do feel the gift is inappropriate but want to accept it anyway. You should always be prepared to be open and honest about all of your interactions with patients.

Recommended reading

General Medical Council (2013), *Good Medical Practice*, paragraph 68 and 80.
Medical Protection Society (2012), Professionalism and integrity, section: Conflicts of interest, in *MPS Guide to Ethics: A Map for the Moral Maze*, chapter 3.

3.65 Promise to family

E C A D B

One of your duties of a doctor is to provide patients and relatives with the information that they require in a way that they can understand; however, as a junior doctor, it is often difficult to give them adequate details due to both time pressures on the ward and a lack of clinical experience. You have made an agreement to go back and speak to the family, so the worst option here is to avoid the conversation altogether and leave it to the registrar who won't be there until the afternoon (B). The family may no longer be on the ward when the afternoon ward round takes place, leaving them feeling completely let down by you. However, you do not have the knowledge to fully discuss the complexities of the situation (D), so that is also an inappropriate response. Asking the registrar to come (A) is preferable, because the family will get an explanation from somebody more qualified, and this will take place before the time agreed. Your registrar does not need to attend the ward immediately, however, as this is not an emergency, and you should be able to manage an interim conversation. Meeting with the family as agreed but explaining that you are unable to discuss things further (C) meets your agreement to speak to them but is likely to come across as cold, and the family may feel that you are intentionally withholding information from them. It is best to explain what you can to the family, with an acknowledgement of the limitation of your experience (E).

Recommended reading

General Medical Council (2013), *Good Medical Practice*, paragraph 14.
Medical Protection Society (2012), Professionalism and Integrity, section:
    Professionalism, in *MPS Guide to Ethics: A Map for the Moral Maze*,
    chapter 3.

3.66 Interpreter

C E A B D

The General Medical Council (GMC) states that 'you should make sure that arrangements are made, wherever possible, to meet patients' language and communication needs'. In this scenario, these needs are not being met. In the first instance, you should do everything you can to rule out a life-threatening cause of headache. This would be best carried out by using a professional interpreter. This needs to be accessed immediately using a telephone interpreter (C). Sending the patient to the emergency department (E) is the next most appropriate response; however, they will most likely come across the same barriers of communication and need the services of an interpreter. Advising the friend to take him to emergency services or reattend the GP if any worrying symptoms occur (A), which is otherwise known as 'safety-netting', would normally be a good course of action, but in this scenario, you cannot be sure that this information would be translated effectively to the patient through his friend. Booking a consultation with a professional interpreter present (B) would be a good approach with a non-urgent consultation, but the delay could be potentially life-threatening in this scenario. Option D, recording that you were unable to rule out a sinister cause of headache, is the least appropriate option as this would be recording the fact that you neglected your duty to your patient.

Recommended reading

General Medical Council (2013), *Good Medical Practice*, paragraph 32.

3.67 Breaking bad news

C B D E A

This is a challenging situation as it is important to remain open and honest with your patients whist ensuring that you are not working beyond the limits of your competence. As an FY1, it is not your responsibility to break bad news such as this as it is unlikely that you will know enough to answer further questions and provide reliable information about the future course of action (E). However, this is slightly more preferable than lying to a patient about the MDT (A), which is never acceptable. You should explain that the senior doctors will come and discuss the results (C) as they are better placed to do this, and it would then be sensible to speak to one of your colleagues about when they anticipate that they will be able to attend the ward (B). In the meantime, it may be beneficial for the patient to voice any concerns to you in private (D), and a chaperone is often useful in these situations. You can then ensure that the senior doctor addresses these concerns later.

Recommended reading

General Medical Council (2013), *Duties of a Doctor: Communication, Partnership and Teamwork*.

General Medical Council (2013), *Good Medical Practice*, paragraphs 14, 16, 31–34, 46, 49, 68.

Medical Protection Society (2012), *MPS Guide to Ethics: A Map for the Moral Maze*, chapter 7.

National Council for Hospice and Specialist Palliative Care Services (2003), *Breaking Bad News Regional Guidelines*.

3.68 Refusing antibiotics

B A D E C

This question highlights a situation where you may need to respect a patient's autonomy and their right to refuse treatment, even if you disagree with it. Asking for advice from your registrar (B) is the most appropriate option in the first instance as it is important to ensure you have all the information ready to present to the patient before giving them the opportunity to make an informed decision. Asking for a senior's advice would be a sensible action to take before speaking to the patient yourself (A). It is probably unnecessary to bother your consultant at this point if the SpR is available; therefore, option B is more appropriate than E, however it is important to keep them informed. As always, accurate documentation is important, and after speaking to the patient and receiving their decision, this should be your next step (D). Administering medication that a competent adult has refused is not allowed. Despite the fact that you may think it in their best interests, you should always maintain an open and honest relationship with patients, and therefore option C is not appropriate.

Recommended reading

General Medical Council (2010), *Treatment and Care Towards the End of Life Good Practice in Decision Making*.

General Medical Council (2013), *Duties of a Doctor: Communication, Partnership and Teamwork*.

General Medical Council (2013), *Good Medical Practice*, paragraphs 14–17, 19, 21, 31, 46–49, 68.

Medical Protection Society (2012), *MPS Guide to Ethics: A Map for the Moral Maze*, chapter 7.

Chapter 4

PATIENT FOCUS

QUESTIONS

4.1 Ordering wrong test

You are working on a busy ward and accidentally request a chest x-ray for the incorrect patient. You notice them returning from the radiology department before you realise your error; therefore, the wrong patient has had the scan.

Choose the **THREE most appropriate** actions to take in this situation.

A   Apologise to the patient and arrange a meeting with your clinical supervisor to find a way to prevent this from happening again.

B   Apologise to the patient and explain your error but do not inform your seniors of your mistake.

C   Apologise to the patient for your error, look at the x-ray and inform your seniors of your mistake.

D   Fill in an incident form due to the unnecessary radiation that the patient has been exposed to.

E   Look at the x-ray to ensure that nothing is wrong and then forget all about the event.

F   Make a comment to the nurses about how this further proves that your registrar requests too many tests.

G   Pretend that the x-ray in question has never happened and order one for the correct patient.

H   Write a false entry in the notes about the patient reporting a cough that justified the x-ray.

4.2 Signing sick note

You are one of the FY1 doctors on urology. It is the end of a busy shift, but you still have some jobs to complete from the morning's ward round. A patient, who has been admitted under a different team with suspected pyelonephritis, approaches you for a sick note as he says his doctor said he would be allowed to go home that evening and that this is the only obstacle delaying his discharge.

Rank in order the following actions in response to this situation (1 = Most appropriate; 5 = Least appropriate).

A   After looking through the patient's notes to find out what his doctor advised regarding fitness to work, provide the patient with a note in line with these recommendations.

B   Explain to the patient that, because you are not familiar with his case, you would need to look in his notes and speak to the doctor who has been looking after him before you would be able to sign a sick note.
C   Quickly write out and sign a sick note for the patient, asking him how long he needs it for and the details of his admission.
D   Say that you will look into it to keep the patient quiet, but hurry off to cannulate one of your patients who has been waiting an hour already.
E   Say to the patient that you are very busy at the moment with more pressing jobs for your own patients and that you do not have time to be dealing with sick notes.

4.3 End of life care

You are an FY1 working in oncology. It is Friday afternoon and the computed tomography (CT) scan results for one of your patients show multilevel bowel obstruction from metastatic cancer. Your consultant tells you that the prognosis is now very poor; the patient is palliative, and she needs a nasogastric (NG) tube as she is to be nil by mouth for the foreseeable future. When you go to insert the NG tube, the patient asks you what this means for her future. You are aware that your consultant is planning a meeting with the patient and her family the following morning to discuss the progression of her disease with them.

Rank in order the following actions in response to this situation (1 = Most appropriate; 5 = Least appropriate).

A   Ask the senior house officer (SHO) to go and talk to the patient instead of yourself.
B   Decline to comment and tell the patient that she must wait for the consultant to talk to her.
C   Explain to the patient that you don't fully understand the situation but that you know that her prognosis is now much worse than previously thought.
D   Tell her that she will be fine once the NG tube is in.
E   Tell the patient that she only has days to weeks to live.

4.4 Discussing options with patient

You are an FY1 working on a surgical ward. Your consultant calls you in the afternoon and says that he has seen test results for one of his patients. The results indicate that they need imaging of their abdomen. Your consultant tells you to request a computed tomography (CT) scan because this will be available sooner than other imaging modalities, even though this involves a significant radiation exposure.

Rank in order the following actions in response to this situation (1 = Most appropriate; 5 = Least appropriate).

A   Put in a request for the CT scan as your consultant has asked.
B   Call your registrar and ask them to come out of theatre to discuss the scan with the patient.

C Tell the consultant that you cannot organise the scan because they have not discussed it with the patient.

D Discuss the benefits and risks of the scan with the patient, in addition to the benefits and risks of doing nothing.

E Inform the patient that the consultant has asked you to organise a scan, and put in a request for it.

4.5 Imminent cardiac arrest

You are working as an FY1 and have already stayed an hour longer than your shift finish time, in order to complete some jobs, when a nurse asks you to see a patient urgently. This patient is well known to you because you and your team have been looking after her for several weeks. She is a 54-year-old woman who was initially admitted with severe pneumonia. The nurse tells you that she thinks this patient may be about to have a cardiac arrest. She says the patient still has a pulse and is breathing.

Rank in order the following actions in response to this situation (1 = Most appropriate; 5 = Least appropriate).

A Ask the nurse to assess the patient and call the crash team if appropriate; then leave the ward.

B Ask the nurse to call the on-call FY1 to assess the patient; then leave the ward.

C Ask the nurse to perform a full assessment of the patient including a set of observations, while you phone a member of the on-call medical team for help.

D Immediately assess the patient with the nurse using the ABCDE approach and call the crash team if required.

E Start CPR (cardio-pulmonary resuscitation) at a rate of 30 compressions to 2 breaths.

4.6 Chest drain at nighttime

You are an FY1 on a quiet medical night shift. A senior house officer (SHO) that you are working with offers to assist you in performing a chest drain in a patient with a pleural effusion. You have never inserted a chest drain before. The patient is currently comfortable and stable; they are not likely to deteriorate during the night.

Rank in order the following actions in response to this situation (1 = Most appropriate; 5 = Least appropriate).

A Seek learning opportunities in the daytime instead.

B Suggest that the SHO speaks to the registrar about it.

C Do the procedure as learning opportunities don't arise very often.

D Ask the SHO to do it so you can observe.

E Say that you think it should be left to the daytime staff.

4.7 Poor equipment

You are in the urology day case centre and are asked by your senior house officer (SHO) to catheterise a woman before she goes for urological investigations.
There is one private room in the day case centre, but it does not have a curtain
that can pull across the window, and there isn't a nurse available to chaperone.
The patient is due to go down to the urodynamics department in 15 minutes.

Rank in order the following actions in response to this situation (1 = Most
appropriate; 5 = Least appropriate).

A Ask your SHO to come and help you catheterise and chaperone the patient
in the private room.
B Call the urodynamics department to see if you can delay the study for an
hour to allow you to safely catheterise the patient.
C Catheterise the patient in the treatment room without a chaperone, using a
towel to protect her dignity.
D Send the patient down for the tests uncatheterised.
E Take the patient across onto another ward to catheterise her, thereby
making her late for her test.

4.8 Nurse prescribing

You are the FY1 working in vascular surgery, and one of the nurses on your
ward asks you to prescribe a heparin infusion for a patient who has just
returned from theatre. When you arrive, the patient has already been started
on the infusion without a prescription, and when you review the operation
notes, you realise that they don't, in fact, need it at all. The nurse in question
often decides to give patients medication without checking with the medical
team first and then asks you to prescribe it later.

Choose the **THREE most appropriate** actions to take in this situation.

A Assess the patient, stop the infusion and apologise. Ask your registrar for
advice regarding taking the incident further the next time you see them.
B Continue with the infusion to save the nurse's embarrassment.
C Stop the infusion and bring up safe prescribing of heparin at your next
team meeting.
D Stop the infusion and fill out an incident form.
E Stop the infusion and inform the nurse of their error.
F Stop the infusion and tell your colleagues to avoid working with this nurse.
G Stop the infusion, apologise to the patient and detail the incident in the notes.
H Stop the infusion, inform the nurse of their error and speak to the ward
matron as well as your consultant about this incident.

4.9 Staying late

You are working on a busy surgical ward. Over the last week, you have
been struggling to get all of your work done and have been going home late.

Your shift has now finished, and you are ready to leave when a nurse asks you to prescribe some analgesia for a patient who is in severe pain.

Rank in order the following actions in response to this situation (1 = Most appropriate; 5 = Least appropriate).

A Bleep the on-call team to hand over the patient.
B Ignore the request.
C Leave a note in the doctor's office asking the on-call team to prescribe the analgesia.
D Review the patient and prescribe the analgesia.
E Tell the nurse to ask another doctor since your shift has finished.

4.10 Faulty equipment

You are working on a cardiology ward. A patient needs an urgent electrocardiogram (ECG), but when you go to use the machine, you find that it is broken.

Choose the **THREE most appropriate** actions to take in this situation.

A Complete an incident form.
B Find another machine on a neighbouring ward and perform the ECG.
C Put a note on the machine to indicate that it is broken.
D Put the machine back and hope that the next person to use it will sort it out.
E Report the fault to the medical equipment department.
F Report the fault to the ward manager.
G See if you can replace the machine with one from a neighbouring ward.
H Try to fix the machine yourself.

4.11 Child protection

You are an FY1 working in the accident and emergency department. You see an eight-month-old baby who has been brought in by her parents. They are concerned that she has been having difficulty breathing. You take a history and begin to examine the baby when you notice a large bruise across her back. You are worried that this could be a non-accidental injury.

Rank in order the following actions in response to this situation (1 = Most appropriate; 5 = Least appropriate).

A Ask the parents to explain how the baby sustained the bruise.
B Ask the parents to leave the room while you continue your examination.
C Continue to examine the baby.
D Discuss your concerns with the emergency consultant.
E Take a picture of the bruise using your phone.

4.12 Abortion

A patient who has recently undergone an abortion is admitted to your ward. She has developed complications following the abortion and requires in-patient care. You are the FY1 responsible for her ward care. However, you have a religious objection regarding abortion.

Rank in order the following actions in response to this situation (1 = Most appropriate; 5 = Least appropriate).

A Ask your FY1 colleague on a neighbouring ward to take over the care of the patient.
B Avoid the patient and provide only essential care.
C Inform the patient that you are unable to care for her because you do not agree with abortion.
D Inform the ward manager that you are unable to care for the patient and ask them to find another doctor to care for the patient on the ward.
E Treat the patient as you would any other patient on your ward.

4.13 Sleeping tablets dementia

You are an FY1 working on a care of the elderly ward. The daughter of an elderly patient with advanced dementia asks you to prescribe a sleeping tablet for her mother for when she is discharged. She is the sole carer for her mother and says that her mother keeps her up all night by frequently waking up and disturbing her sleep. She is worn out and feels that she can't cope.

Rank in order the following actions in response to this situation (1 = Most appropriate; 5 = Least appropriate).

A Advise the daughter to put her mother in a residential home.
B Prescribe the sleeping tablet and ask the patient's GP to review the medication.
C Refuse and advise the daughter to speak to the patient's GP about increasing the patient's package of care on discharge.
D Refuse but organise a multidisciplinary team (MDT) assessment of the patient during her time in hospital to assess her nighttime activity and whether she needs any more care.
E Suggest that the daughter sees her own GP to discuss her mood and anxiety.

4.14 Group and save

You are an FY1 in general surgery. You are asked to prepare a patient for major abdominal surgery; part of this task is ensuring that the patient has had a blood test (group and save) to ensure that the blood bank can readily provide blood of the patient's blood group either during or after surgery. The patient goes into theatre, and you realise that you forgot to send a group and save blood test.

Rank in order the following actions in response to this situation (1 = Most appropriate; 5 = Least appropriate).

A Complete an incident form.
B Do nothing.

C Inform your specialist registrar (SpR).
D Ring the operating theatre and let them know.
E Take the blood test from the patient as soon as they leave the operating theatre.

4.15 Disruptive intravenous drug user patient

You are an FY1 in general surgery. The nurses contact you and tell you that a patient on the ward, who is a known intravenous drug user, is disruptive, is not engaging with treatment and keeps leaving the ward and returning seemingly under the influence of recreational drugs. They would like you to discharge the patient.

Rank in order the following actions in response to this situation (1 = Most appropriate; 5 = Least appropriate).

A Contact your registrar or consultant for advice.
B Discharge the patient from hospital care.
C Signpost the patient to drug misuse and addiction services.
D Speak to the patient about their behaviour and inform them that if it continues then they will be discharged.
E Tell the nurses that they must continue to care for the patient.

4.16 Waiter with diarrhoea

You are an FY2 in a GP surgery, and a patient comes to see you with his uncle. The patient works for his uncle in a fast-food restaurant and has been experiencing some diarrhoea. His uncle explains that his nephew needs a medication called loperamide to reduce diarrhoea symptoms so that he can work in the restaurant. You are concerned that he may have an infectious cause of diarrhoea.

Choose the **THREE most appropriate** actions to take in this situation.

A Advise him not to take loperamide at this time.
B Advise him to keep excellent hand hygiene at work.
C Ask the patient to provide a stool sample.
D Notify the Health Protection Agency (HPA).
E Prescribe the loperamide.
F Report the restaurant to the local newspaper.
G Tell him that he must not work until the diarrhoea has stopped for 48 hours.
H Tell him that he needs to get in touch with the occupational health department.

4.17 Hyperkalaemia and chasing blood tests

You are working as an FY2 in a GP surgery and are completing your paperwork at the end of the day. You are reading through your documentation of a consultation with a 54-year-old male patient with diabetes, hypertension and chronic kidney disease. He came to see you today for an annual review and the results of his routine blood tests. As you are completing your writing, you notice that you missed his serum potassium result. You check the result, and it is 6.2 mmol/L (normal range 3.5–5.0). You know that high levels of potassium can have serious consequences. The patient seemed well during the consultation and had no complaints.

Rank in order the following actions in response to this situation (1 = Most appropriate; 5 = Least appropriate).

A   Ask your clinical supervisor for advice.
B   Assume that the sample was haemolysed as the patient was well and didn't have any chest pain or palpitations.
C   Book urgent repeat blood tests for the patient tomorrow with an appointment to see you afterwards to explain the situation.
D   Check all of your other consultations for the day to see if you missed any other important results.
E   Telephone the patient and ask him to attend hospital for repeat blood tests urgently.

4.18 Responsibility between teams

You are an FY1 working on a surgical ward. One of your patients, in addition to their acute surgical problem, has been reviewed by the neurology team as they have started a new anti-epileptic drug. You know that this drug can have serious side effects. When you look the drug up in the British National Formulary (BNF), you find that regular blood tests should be performed to monitor for these side effects, starting from the second day of treatment.

Choose the **THREE most appropriate** actions to take in this situation.

A   Add instructions for drug level monitoring to your team's daily handover sheet.
B   Call the neurology registrar to discuss the situation and get advice from them regarding monitoring.
C   Call your registrar and ask for their advice regarding appropriate monitoring.
D   Complete a request for the blood levels to be taken the next morning.
E   Cross the drug off the drug chart.
F   Perform the monitoring blood test now.
G   Write an entry in the notes describing the monitoring required.
H   Write an entry in the notes explaining that neurology are responsible for monitoring.

4.19 Ensuring follow up

You are an FY1 working on a medical team. One of your patients has been discharged with a plan for follow-up tests in six weeks, which are to be organised by their GP. You realise that you have forgotten to mention this in the discharge letter, which has been fully authorised on the computer system and cannot be retrieved for additions.

Rank in order the following actions in response to this situation (1 = Most appropriate; 5 = Least appropriate).

A Arrange the follow-up tests yourself.
B Explain to the patient which tests they need, and ask them to make an appointment with their GP in a few weeks' time.
C Make an out-patient appointment for the patient with your consultant to ensure that they receive the tests.
D Telephone the GP surgery, and leave a message with the receptionist regarding the follow-up tests.
E Write an additional letter to the GP detailing the follow-up tests required, and explain to the patient that they should make an appointment with their GP in a few weeks' time.

4.20 Negligence 1

You are the FY1 in colorectal surgery, and one of the patients your team is managing has developed an abscess. As part of the treatment, microbiology recommended that they should be commenced on gentamicin. They are now on day three of their treatment. At the end of the working day, you realise that you have forgotten to check their pre-dose level, and the next dose has already been given. You also remember that yesterday the dose had been increased. What should you do?

Rank in order the following actions in response to this situation (1 = Most appropriate; 5 = Least appropriate).

A Ask the nurse why she gave the dose before you had checked the gentamicin level.
B Call the senior house officer (SHO) on call and ask their advice.
C Explain what has happened to the patient, apologise and ensure that you check their levels tomorrow.
D Ring the microbiology department and ask for their advice.
E Tell your registrar that you had forgotten to check the levels and ask their advice.

4.21 Negligence 2

You are the FY1 working in general medicine, and you are called in the evening to see a patient with suspected diabetic ketoacidosis (DKA). You have never treated a patient with DKA on your own before, but you need to initiate treatment while awaiting help as your specialist registrar (SpR) is currently attending an emergency in A&E resus. You think you can remember the management steps.

Choose the **THREE most appropriate** actions to take in this situation.

A   Ask for help from your fellow FY1 on call.
B   Ask the advice of the ward matron who is present at the time.
C   Assess the patient using an ABCDE approach while awaiting help.
D   Call your senior house officer (SHO) for help.
E   Find the trust protocol online and follow it.
F   Manage the patient according to your memory of the required treatment.
G   Tell the nurses you cannot manage this patient alone and therefore will wait for the SpR to be free.
H   Use the section in a clinical medicine handbook on treating DKA, which you have with you, to manage the patient appropriately.

4.22 Challenging decisions

You are an FY1 working on a renal team. You receive a phone call from your consultant who is in the out-patient clinic and has just reviewed a patient with chronic kidney disease, who has been feeling unwell for a number of weeks. He would like the patient to be admitted to the ward following the consultation, so he has dispatched the patient to the phlebotomy department for some routine blood tests. Half an hour later, you receive another phone call from the clinic nurse informing you that the patient and consultant have now decided against the admission and opted instead for a follow-up clinic appointment in one week's time. The patient has gone home. You later review the results of the blood tests and notice that the patient's potassium level is raised at 6.4 mmol/L.

Rank in order the following actions in response to this situation (1 = Most appropriate; 5 = Least appropriate).

A   Ask the on-call registrar for advice.
B   Ask your educational supervisor to talk to the consultant as consultant-to-consultant communication may be more appropriate in situations like this.
C   Call the patient at home and tell them to come in, as their blood test results are abnormal.
D   Do nothing; the consultant has seen the blood results, and since he is their patient, you shouldn't change their management plan.
E   Ring the consultant yourself and ask them to clarify why the patient went home.

4.23 Breaking bad news

You are the FY1 in oncology and are seeing a patient with advanced loco-regional breast cancer. Her most recent computed tomography (CT) of chest, abdomen and pelvis shows that she has extensive liver metastases, which has not yet been communicated to her. Her consultant rings the ward and says that he is caught up in clinic at another hospital and therefore will not be able to come and see the patient today. He asks you to discuss with her the results of her scan.

Rank in order the following actions in response to this situation (1 = Most appropriate, 5 = Least appropriate).

A   Ask the FY2 to discuss the results with the patient as you do not feel comfortable doing so.

B   Ask the oncology registrar on call to discuss the results with the patient as they will have a better understanding of what the findings mean.

C   Inform the patient of the results but tell her you might not be able to answer her questions about what this means regarding further prognosis.

D   Research the prognosis and treatments of metastatic breast cancer on the internet and use this to discuss the scan with the patient.

E   Tell the consultant that this is outside of your competencies, and you do not feel comfortable having this discussion with the patient.

4.24 Analgesia

When you are seeing one of your outlying patients on the surgical ward, one of the nurses comes to ask you to prescribe some analgesia for a patient. The patient is not under the care of your consultant, but the nurse insists that this patient has been without analgesia all night and is in a lot of pain.

Choose the **THREE most appropriate** actions to take in this situation.

A   Ask the nurse to bleep the team's FY1 as you don't know the patient.

B   Bleep the FY1 for that team and let them know that their patient needs analgesia.

C   Perform a thorough check of the patient's notes to see what would be the most appropriate analgesia to prescribe.

D   Prescribe a variety of analgesics as required and ask the nurse to pick the most appropriate.

E   Prescribe paracetamol as required medicine (PRN) and ask the nurse to get a more comprehensive plan for the patient from their team later.

F   Refuse to prescribe the analgesia as this is not your patient and you know nothing about them.

G   Review the patient and take a history about the pain to prescribe the most appropriate analgesia.

H   Suggest that if the patient needs acute pain relief, then the nurse should refer them to the acute pain team.

4.25 MRSA patient

You are the FY1 working on a busy surgical ward. Yesterday you admitted a 63-year-old woman into an all-female bay; she was complaining of upper abdominal pain and vomiting. As part of her clerking, you took some bloods, and the nurses took swabs from her nose and groin as per local protocol. You are now chasing her blood results and notice that, as well as having slightly deranged liver function, her swabs have come back as methicillin-resistant Staphylococcus aureus (MRSA) positive. You do not think that the nurses are aware of this.

Rank in order the following actions in response to this situation (1 = Most appropriate; 5 = Least appropriate).

A   Ask one of the other nurses to inform the ward sister about the MRSA results as you need to contact your senior about the abnormal blood results.
B   Contact your registrar to let them know that the patient is MRSA positive and find out what steps you should take next.
C   Explain to the patient the results of the MRSA screen and let them know that they will have to be moved into a side room.
D   Immediately inform the sister on the ward of the results so that the patient can be barrier-nursed in a side room.
E   Put a plan in place regarding the deranged liver function tests (LFTs) and let the nurses deal with the MRSA screen as this is part of their job.

4.26 Arranging follow up

You are the FY1 working on breast surgery. One of your patients is about to be discharged after a wide local excision for a ductal carcinoma in situ. You think that you remember your consultant mentioning on the ward round that the patient will need a follow-up appointment in his clinic. Your colleague completed the discharge letter for this patient, but you notice that no follow-up arrangements have been documented.

Choose the **THREE most appropriate** actions to take in this situation.

A   Ask the patient what follow-up arrangements she needs and document this instead.
B   Change the discharge letter yourself so that a clinic appointment is arranged for the patient.
C   Discuss the matter with your colleague and make sure that the details for follow-up on the discharge letter reflect their understanding of the situation.
D   Discuss with your colleague your concerns about the follow-up arrangements.
E   Don't voice your concerns as arrangements for this patient's discharge were not your responsibility.
F   Look in the patient's notes to double-check what the consultant said on the ward round.
G   Speak to the consultant to reiterate what follow-up arrangements the patient needs.
H   Tell your colleague to change the discharge letter as you think the consultant said that the patient needed a follow-up appointment.

4.27 Antibiotic guidelines

You are the FY1 on a general surgical ward and are called to see a patient who is spiking a temperature of 37.9 degrees Celsius. After assessing the patient using an ABCDE approach, you find that she is also tachypnoeic and tachy-cardic, has oxygen saturations of 92% on air and crackles localised to the right lung base. You suspect a hospital-acquired pneumonia and want to start anti-biotics alongside further tests. However, the local treatment policy has recently changed, and you can't remember the recommended empirical treatment.

Rank in order the following actions in response to this situation (1 = Most appropriate; 5 = Least appropriate).

A Access the local clinical guidelines on the intranet and start empirical treat-ment as recommended.

B Ask your specialist registrar (SpR) what the empirical treatment is and prescribe according to their advice.

C Look in the *Oxford Handbook of Clinical Medicine* for the treatment of pneumonia and prescribe what it suggests.

D Prescribe treatment as per the old guidelines and inform the nursing staff to increase their frequency of observations as you will check later.

E Withhold treatment and ask the nurse to speak to microbiology for their advice.

4.28 ABG competence

You are watching your FY2 colleague take an arterial blood gas (ABG) sample. After a sample is collected, they leave immediately to process the sample with-out putting pressure over the artery as per standard procedure.

Choose the **THREE most appropriate** actions to take in this situation.

A Ask one of the nurses to put pressure on the area.

B Ask the patient to put pressure on the area.

C Ask your FY2 colleague to come back to put pressure on the area.

D Follow the FY2 to learn how to use the ABG analyser.

E Put pressure on the area yourself.

F Reflect on this scenario in your e-portfolio.

G Speak to the FY2's educational supervisor regarding retraining on ABG sampling for them.

H Write in the patient's notes the incorrect way the FY2 took the sample.

4.29 Keeping up to date

You are the FY1 working for a consultant in cardiology. You have started to notice that, on the ward rounds, your consultant is not using the most recent guidelines while making decisions about the management of heart failure or hypertension. As a consequence of this, you are worried that their patients are not receiving the best quality of care.

Rank in order the following actions in response to this situation (1 = Most appropriate; 5 = Least appropriate).

A Ask your consultant to explain the management of these conditions to you and use this teaching session to ask questions about the new guidelines.

B   Discuss the matter with your senior house officer (SHO) as they are more experienced than you.
C   Do nothing as you are the FY1 and your consultant probably has good reasons for managing their patients in the way they are.
D   Raise the matter with your educational supervisor at your next meeting.
E   Using your knowledge of the guidelines, prescribe medications as recommended instead of following your consultant's management plan.

4.30 Clinical skills

While working as an FY1 on the admissions unit, you see a male patient in acute urinary retention. After performing your baseline examination and investigations, your management plan includes catheterising the patient. You have only performed this procedure once before as a medical student, over a year ago, and do not feel fully confident performing the procedure; however, none of the nurses on the ward are trained in male catheterisation.

Rank in order the following actions in response to this situation (1 = Most appropriate; 5 = Least appropriate).

A   Ask a member of the nursing staff to come with you to chaperone and ask her to let you know if you start to do anything she thinks is wrong.
B   Ask your senior house officer (SHO) to catheterise the patient but go along to chaperone and watch closely to revise the procedure.
C   Ask your SHO to supervise you performing the procedure so that you feel confident in the future.
D   Call the continence nurse specialist and ask them to catheterise the patient.
E   Contact the clinical skills department and arrange a revision course on male catheterisation.

4.31 Incident reporting

During a medical on-call shift, you are called to see an elderly man who has become increasingly unwell. When you assess him, you realise that he was seen yesterday and started on antibiotics for pneumonia. However, when looking at the drug chart, you see that he has not yet received any doses of this. The doses are charted as 'drug not available'. When you ask the nurse responsible for the patient, she tells you that the antibiotic was not available on the ward, and the staff have been too busy to order it from the pharmacy. You know that the patient is deteriorating because he needs the antibiotics.

Choose the **THREE most appropriate** actions to take in this situation.

A   Ask the nurse to source a dose of antibiotic from another ward.
B   Ask the senior house officer (SHO) to review the patient.
C   Call the on-call pharmacist and ask them to provide a dose of antibiotics immediately.
D   Complete an incident form.

E Prescribe the second line antibiotic for pneumonia, which is readily available on the ward.
F Report the incident to the consultant responsible for the patient.
G Report the incident to the ward manager.
H Tell the nurse that she has endangered the patient by not ensuring that the patient received the antibiotics.

4.32 Patient handover

You are the FY1 doctor working on a busy general surgery ward, and you have started to address your tasks following the morning ward round. You are working quickly because you want to leave on time that evening to attend a friend's birthday party. Ten minutes before you are due to leave, one of the nurses asks you to assess a patient who has just fallen out of bed. She says that they didn't hit their head, but they are complaining of new pain in their right hip.

Rank in order the following actions in response to this situation (1 = Most appropriate; 5 = Least appropriate).

A Assess the patient using an ABCDE approach and ask the evening team to arrange any further investigations so that you can get to your social function on time.
B Assess the patient using an ABCDE approach, arrange any necessary investigations and ensure that the evening team are aware of the need to chase the results.
C Ask the nurse to put it on the handover board for the evening team to be aware of.
D Ask the nurse to arrange an x-ray of the right hip and put it on the handover board for the evening team to chase.
E Assess the patient using an ABCDE approach, arrange x-rays and an ECG and wait for the results to come back before leaving the hospital.

4.33 Non-accidental injury

You are working as an FY2 doctor in the emergency department of a children's hospital. You see Maisie, a six-month-old girl who has severe burns to her feet and ankles. You ask her mother how Maisie sustained her burns. She says she was giving her a bath and didn't realise that the water was so hot. Maisie has three sisters at home all under the age of ten. You are concerned this could be a non-accidental injury.

Choose the **THREE most appropriate** actions to take in this situation.

A Ask your senior registrar to take over the case.
B Document that you are concerned about non-accidental injury but don't inform Maisie's mum because it may have been a genuine accident.
C Inform Maisie's mum that, because of the nature of Maisie's injuries, you will need to discuss the case with the child protection team.

D   Inform Maisie's mum that she is likely to lose access to her children.
E   Inform the consultant in charge of the emergency department of your concerns.
F   Take a full history, perform a full examination of Maisie and start relevant treatment.
G   Telephone the police and ask them to check the temperature of the hot water in Maisie's house.
H   Telephone the police and inform them that several children are at risk of child abuse.

4.34 GP treatment final

On an FY1 GP taster day, you are sitting in with a GP whom you have not met before. Throughout the clinic you notice that they don't fully discuss treatment options with any of their patients, and most patients seem to leave quite dissatisfied. You ask the GP whether he thinks that his patients are compliant with their medications, to which he replies that all of his patients are compliant since they trust his judgement as a clinician. You find this a little unsettling.

Rank in order the following actions in response to this situation (1 = Most appropriate; 5 = Least appropriate).

A   Bring up the topic at lunchtime in the staff room so that you can discuss it with other members of the practice staff in a non-threatening environment.
B   Find one of the other GPs and sit in with them for the rest of the week as you feel that this way you will learn more.
C   Ignore the situation – at the end of the week you will no longer be working at the practice.
D   Suggest to the GP that he further discusses treatment options with his patients and make a comment about how this could lead to increased compliance.
E   When you finish for the day find the practice manager and suggest to them that this should be raised in their next practice meeting.

4.35 Consent for blood test

You are an FY1 working on a care of the elderly firm. Mrs Jones, a frail, elderly lady with known Alzheimer's disease, hypertension and atrial fibrillation, is admitted to your ward following routine monitoring by her GP of her international normalised ratio (INR), which was shown to be dramatically raised. On admission she is disorientated, agitated and is wandering around the ward. She is very unsteady on her feet, and therapy services have been unable to find a zimmer frame for her at present. You need to take a repeat INR, but she is refusing to let you take the blood sample.

Rank in order the following actions in response to this situation (1 = Most appropriate; 5 = Least appropriate).

A   Ask one of the nursing staff to help you return her to her bed and calm her down so that you can take the sample.

B   Explain to Mrs Jones the reasons why you need to repeat the sample, including the potential consequences of not doing so before proceeding to take the blood even if she still declines.
C   Ask your registrar for advice and to help you assess her capacity to refuse the blood sample.
D   Leave it: you have yesterday's result from the GP so you can try to repeat the sample tomorrow when she is more settled.
E   Wait for a couple of hours for Mrs Jones to become more orientated to the ward before talking to her again about taking the sample.

4.36 Jehovah's Witness

A patient you are caring for is a Jehovah's Witness. They inform you in advance of their abdominal aortic aneurysm repair that they do not want to receive blood products during the operation and that, if they bleed, they would prefer to die naturally.

Choose the **THREE most appropriate** actions to take in this situation.

A   Advise the patient against surgery due to the high risk of bleeding.
B   Ask the patient to contact their lawyer to draft an advanced directive.
C   Ask the patient to fill out a refusal of blood products form.
D   Ask the patient to make a donation towards the use of intraoperative blood-saving machines.
E   Ensure the theatre staff and the anaesthetic team are aware of this.
F   Ignore the patient's statement: they might never know they've been administered blood products.
G   Inform the patient's consultant of their wishes.
H   Write a message in the patient's medical notes detailing their wishes.

4.37 Advanced directive

A patient on your ward has advanced motor neurone disease and develops aspiration pneumonia. He has an advanced directive signed by himself, his lawyer and his wife stating that if he becomes too unwell to swallow and aspirate, he does not want to be treated with antibiotics. His wife tells you that she has changed her mind and wants you to actively treat him with antibiotics.

Rank in order the following actions in response to this situation (1 = Most appropriate; 5 = Least appropriate).

A   Ask your registrar to come and speak with the patient's wife about the advanced directive.
B   Call the patient's lawyer to check the status and legality of the advanced directive.
C   Console the patient's wife, explaining that you cannot go against his advanced wishes.
D   Get medico-legal advice from your medical malpractice insurer.
E   Treat your patient with antibiotics.

4.38 Refusal of treatment

An elderly patient on your ward has been recovering well following abdominal surgery. However, she subsequently goes on to develop a severe hospital-acquired pneumonia. While she appears to be improving with antibiotics, she still requires oxygen via a face mask in order to maintain her saturations. You are called to see her because she is now refusing to keep the mask on her face, and her saturations have become dangerously low. You explain that without the oxygen she may die but she continues to refuse, telling you that she wants to die.

Choose the **THREE most appropriate** actions to take in this situation.

A Ask your registrar to come and review the patient.
B Ask your registrar to complete a 'do not attempt cardiopulmonary resuscitation' (DNACPR) form urgently.
C Assess the patient's capacity to make a decision about receiving the oxygen.
D Call the crash team.
E Call your consultant to discuss the situation.
F Contact the on-call psychiatrist for advice.
G Respect the patient's wishes and leave the oxygen off.
H Sedate the patient and replace the face mask.

4.39 Capacity

You are working on a care of the elderly ward. One of your patients needs a colonoscopy to investigate anaemia. On the ward round earlier, your consultant had explained the procedure to the patient and asked her to sign a consent form. Later, you are talking to the patient, and she begins to ask you questions about the colonoscopy. She has clearly not understood or remembered what was explained to her earlier.

Rank in order the following actions in response to this situation (1 = Most appropriate; 5 = Least appropriate).

A Ask the nursing staff whether the patient is more forgetful or confused than she has been previously.
B Assess the patient's capacity to make the decision about whether or not to have the colonoscopy.
C Call endoscopy and cancel the colonoscopy.
D Explain the procedure again to the patient and continue planning for the colonoscopy.
E Inform your consultant that the patient has not understood or remembered his explanation.

4.40 Patient unsafe at home

You are an FY1 working on a diabetes and endocrine ward. One of your patients has been admitted several times due to recurrent falls at home. He is medically fit for discharge, but occupational therapists and physiotherapists

have completed assessments which conclude that he is unsafe at home.
The patient, however, is adamant that he wants to return home.

Rank in order the following actions in response to this situation (1 = Most appropriate; 5 = Least appropriate).

A Ask a psychiatrist to assess the patient's capacity.
B Ask the patient's family their opinion about how he will function at home.
C Assess the patient's capacity to make the decision.
D Reduce the patient's risks of falls at home by introducing home aids and implementing home care.
E Tell the patient that he is unable to return home as he is unsafe.

4.41 Family disagreement

You are an FY1 on a care of the elderly ward. A patient wishes to be discharged to her home after recovering from a urinary tract infection (UTI) that required hospital admission. She has been seen by occupational therapists and physiotherapists, who have found her to be safe to be discharged home. Her son and daughter, however, want her to go into a nursing home as they believe she cannot cope at home.

Rank in order the following actions in response to this situation (1 = Most appropriate; 5 = Least appropriate).

A Advise the family that it is not their decision.
B Advise the family that they should discuss this with your consultant.
C Inform the patient that it is best if they go into nursing care.
D Inform the therapy team of the family's concerns and ask them if they wish to carry out further assessments.
E Organise a family meeting with the multidisciplinary team (MDT), with the permission of the patient, to discuss her discharge destination.

4.42 Dementia and capacity

You are an FY1 on a care of the elderly ward looking after a number of sick patients. During a ward round, your team decides that a patient under your care will require a nasogastric (NG) tube as she is not able to maintain sufficient nutrition orally. The patient in question has a known diagnosis of Alzheimer's dementia and is often confused on the ward. She has had multiple NG tubes in the past, which she removed each time by herself. She provided consent for the previous tubes, which you find documented in the notes. You gather the equipment required for the procedure and approach the patient's bedside. As you approach, the patient says she will not have the feeding tube because it 'feels horrible' as it is inserted.

Rank in order the following actions in response to this situation (1 = Most appropriate; 5 = Least appropriate).

A Discuss the situation with her family and your consultant and insert the tube if it is deemed to be in her best interests.

B   Insert the NG tube as she lacks capacity because of her diagnosis of dementia.
C   Request a psychiatric review of the patient as she has refused feeding.
D   Return the equipment to the store, not completing the procedure, and document her refusal in the notes.
E   Undertake a capacity assessment of the patient using clear and concise information.

4.43 Depression and capacity

You are the FY1 on a cardiology ward. An elderly patient has been admitted for the treatment of a probable myocardial infarction. He was brought to hospital by his daughter, who found him breathless and pale at home. He tells you that he does not want any further investigations as he has no interest in life and wants to die. His daughter confirms that for the past few months, he has been very low in mood, difficult to engage in conversation, with a poor appetite and poor sleep.

Choose the **THREE most appropriate** actions to take in this situation.

A   Ask the patient's daughter to speak to him and encourage him to accept treatment.
B   Bleep your registrar.
C   Conduct a full mental state examination and assess his capacity to make this decision.
D   Make a referral to liaison psychiatry.
E   Start treatment with an anti-depressant.
F   Tell the patient that you cannot help them to end their life, and they therefore must accept the recommended tests and treatment.
G   Use the Mental Capacity Act to proceed with an investigation.
H   Use the Mental Health Act to proceed with an investigation.

4.44 Delirium and consent to investigation

You are the FY1 on a general medical ward. A patient with known dementia has become more unwell. She is rousable but very drowsy and not communicating at all. Normally, she is confused and agitated but can answer basic questions. Her oxygen saturations have dropped to 80% on room air. Your registrar asks you to perform an arterial blood gas (ABG) sample.

Choose the **THREE most appropriate** actions to take in this situation.

A   Ask a nurse to assist you by holding the patient's arm in position.
B   Call the patient's next of kin and ask for their consent.
C   Delay until later to see if the patient becomes communicative.
D   Document in the notes that the patient did not have capacity to consent to this procedure at the time.
E   Document in the notes that the patient does not have capacity to make decisions.
F   Start the procedure but stop if the patient becomes distressed/resists.

G Talk to the patient and explain what you are doing throughout the procedure.
H Tell your registrar you cannot perform the test as the patient cannot consent.

4.45 Child autonomy

You are the FY1 working on a paediatric ward. You have been asked to take blood from a 14-year-old boy to monitor his condition. When you go to speak to him, he says that he does not want to have the blood test because he is fed up of needles. His mother is in the room and tells you that he is being silly and you should go ahead.

Rank in order the following actions in response to this situation (1 = Most appropriate; 5 = Least appropriate).

A Attempt to carry out the blood test but stop if he physically resists.
B Call your registrar and ask them to take over dealing with the situation.
C Do not attempt the blood test and document in the notes that the patient refused.
D Explain to the boy why the blood test is important, but if he is definite that he doesn't want it, do not attempt to take it.
E Take several nurses with you to hold his arm still while you take the blood.

4.46 Withholding treatment

After finishing the ward round, one of your jobs is to cannulate a patient who needs intravenous (IV) antibiotics and fluids. However, as you tell her that you have come to insert the cannula, she tells you that she does not want the cannula or the antibiotics as she does not wish to live anymore. She had been reluctant to say this to the consultant as everyone has been so nice since she was admitted. She asks if you could not mention this to the consultant and just not prescribe the antibiotics.

Choose the **THREE most appropriate** actions to take in this situation.

A Ask the patient if you can place the cannula and only give her the fluids to keep her comfortable.
B Assess the patient using the Mental Capacity Act to see if she has the capacity to make such a decision.
C Explain to the patient that you are just the FY1 following the consultant's orders, and you will have to place the cannula.
D Refer the patient to the psychiatry team as she may be depressed.
E Tell the patient that it would be best if you ring the consultant to ask him to come back and talk to her, and ask her if she would agree to this.
F Treat the patient under section 2 of the Mental Health Act.
G Try and find out her reasons for not wanting to live to see if there is something you can do to help.
H Use the principle of best interests to treat the patient with antibiotics.

4.47 Questioning consent

While working an on-call shift on the surgical admissions unit, you attend with the registrar to consent a patient for surgery. During the consent procedure, your registrar doesn't mention some of the risks you think are associated with the procedure. The patient signs the consent form and is due to go to theatre later that evening.

Rank in order the following actions in response to this situation (1 = Most appropriate; 5 = Least appropriate).

A   Ask the registrar, while still with the patient, about the risks you were thinking of, in case they have slipped his mind.

B   Assume that you do not know the risks for the procedure and that the registrar has correctly consented the patient.

C   Revise the risks of the procedure when you finish your shift to learn them for next time.

D   Stay with the patient once the registrar has left to mention the further risks that you think you have identified.

E   Wait until you have left the patient's bedside, and then question the registrar about the risks of the procedure and suggest that they go back to the patient, if indeed there are risks that have not been mentioned.

4.48 Consultant decisions

While on the surgical ward round, your consultant is talking to a patient about surgical management for a herniated lumbar disc. The patient asks about acupuncture as an alternative to surgery for pain relief. They are concerned about surgery as a friend of theirs recently had a similar procedure and was left with little change in their pain but experienced post-operative complications. The patient would therefore rather avoid surgery if possible. Your consultant, however, disregards their views saying that holistic treatments aren't effective and will only make things worse for the patient in the long term. He does not offer any non-operative methods of treatment.

Rank in order the following actions in response to this situation (1 = Most appropriate; 5 = Least appropriate).

A   Ask your consultant, after the ward round, to explain the use of alternative treatments in cases such as this so that you can learn more about when they should be recommended.

B   Follow the consultant's plan; he is experienced and will know when treatments are and are not indicated.

C   Give the patient an information leaflet regarding alternative treatment options to read through on their own.

D   Recommend to the patient that they make a complaint about their treatment if they are dissatisfied with the options offered to them.

E   Talk to the consultant and suggest that the patient would benefit from some further explanation as to why he feels that surgical management is preferable to conservative management.

4.49 Consent for children

You are working in the paediatric surgery department when you are called to see a 15-year-old girl who was admitted for observation the previous day with suspected early appendicitis. In the last few hours, the nurses feel that she has deteriorated, and you are worried that she may need to go to theatre. The surgical registrar comes to review the patient and also decides that this may be the case; however, on trying to contact both of her parents, neither of them are answering their phones. Meanwhile, the patient is becoming tachycardic and hypotensive. The registrar feels that she needs to go to theatre immediately.

Rank in order the following actions in response to this situation (1 = Most appropriate; 5 = Least appropriate).

A Call the patient's grandmother so that she can give consent in the absence of being able to contact the parents.

B Consent the patient herself as long as she has the ability to understand and retain the information you give to her.

C Delay the operation as, without her parents' consent, the procedure cannot go ahead.

D Use the principle of best interests so that your patient can be taken to theatre without consent.

E Write in the notes that you have unsuccessfully tried to contact the parents and therefore the procedure cannot go ahead because you have been unable to gain consent for it.

4.50 Coercion

You are the FY1 working on a care of the elderly firm. One of your patients, Edith, a 77-year-old woman with sub-acute bowel obstruction, asks you to talk through her treatment options with her and her daughter-in-law. During the consultation, the daughter-in-law does not let Edith do any of the talking. She tells you that she has been researching the options online and has already talked to Edith about her options, and they have decided together that surgery is the best treatment choice for her. You, however, disagree with this in view of Edith's co-morbidities. You are worried that Edith is being coerced by her daughter-in-law since surgery would result in a quicker outcome but would involve much greater risk.

Choose the **THREE most appropriate** actions to take in this situation.

A Don't worry about this; as you are not consenting Edith for theatre, it doesn't concern you. The consultant will make the final decision.

B Explain the risks of surgical intervention and the benefits of non-operative intervention in order to highlight that non-operative intervention would be a better choice.

C Explain to the daughter-in-law that she will need to talk to the consultant before any treatment can be decided as they will be performing the treatment and therefore must help make the decision.

D   Once her daughter-in-law has left, ask Edith again what her thoughts on the situation are.

E   Remind the daughter-in-law that, since she is not Edith's next of kin, she does not have any say in the matter, and you will not discuss it further with her.

F   State that, as the FY1, you don't fully understand the treatment options and therefore are unable to offer advice; you can simply list the options.

G   Tell the daughter-in-law that, as Edith has to sign the consent form, you need to hear her opinions.

H   Tell the daughter-in-law that she is not thinking in Edith's best interests and should not help her make the decision.

4.51 Ectopic pregnancy

You are the FY1 working in the emergency department and see a 15-year-old girl who has presented with severe right-sided abdominal pain. While taking the history, she reveals that she has had unprotected sexual intercourse with her boyfriend, and this morning, she noticed some vaginal bleeding and discharge. You explain to the patient that an ectopic pregnancy needs to be excluded and ask her whether she would like you to ring her parents. She flatly refuses saying that 'they would kick me out' if they found out she was pregnant.

Rank in order the following actions in response to this situation (1 = Most appropriate; 5 = Least appropriate).

A   Ask the sister on the ward to come with you to have a longer talk with her about why she doesn't want her parents to know.

B   Discuss the situation with your clinical supervisor.

C   Keep the information confidential as you feel that the girl is competent to make this decision.

D   Phone her parents anyway and ask them to come in and have a chat with you.

E   Refuse to give her any more treatment until she agrees that you can telephone her parents.

4.52 Coercion

A 75-year-old male patient on your ward has metastatic lung cancer. He has been informed of the diagnosis and agrees that the risks of an operation are not outweighed by the potential benefits. It is now the following day, and his son is visiting the ward. He asks why you are doing nothing for his father, exclaiming that 'he's very forgetful, he doesn't know what is best for him. He needs the surgery and you are killing him without it.' When you go to see the patient before the end of your shift, he says that he wants you to arrange surgery for him as he isn't ready to die.

Rank in order the following actions in response to this situation (1 = Most appropriate; 5 = Least appropriate).

A Ask one of the nurses to come with you and talk to the son in a place of privacy.
B Discuss with the patient why he has now changed his mind.
C Explain again to the patient why surgery wouldn't be in his best interests but say that you will ask your consultant to come and discuss it with him at the earliest opportunity.
D Speak to your specialist registrar (SpR) about what the patient is now saying and ask them to come with you to discuss the reasons behind his change of decision.
E Tell the son that it would probably be best if he didn't visit his father, if he is going to cause trouble.

4.53 Terminal diagnosis

An elderly woman has been admitted with jaundice, and investigations have revealed that she has terminal cancer. She is profoundly deaf and finds it difficult to keep up with conversations. She has therefore given permission for her family to be told everything about her condition and treatment so that they can help in explaining it to her. Her family have now been told of her terminal diagnosis; however, they have asked that the patient not be told. They want to break the news to her once she is back at home because they think that she is going to be very upset and would prefer to be in a familiar environment. You feel uncomfortable that the patient has no idea of her terminal diagnosis.

Rank in order the following actions in response to this situation (1 = Most appropriate; 5 = Least appropriate).

A Ask your consultant for advice.
B Encourage the family to explain the terminal diagnosis to the patient as soon as possible.
C Explain the terminal diagnosis to the patient.
D Let the family inform the patient of her diagnosis in their own time.
E Tell the family that you will inform the patient of her diagnosis if they do not.

4.54 Cancer diagnosis disclosure

While working as an FY1 in general surgery, you are approached by a patient who is due to go for flexible sigmoidoscopy to investigate his rectal bleeding. The patient does not want his family to know if the results show that he has cancer as he does not want to distress them. You subsequently learn that the patient has a rectal tumour, and the patient opts for a conservative, non-curative approach. You are then approached by his wife, who asks you what the results are.

Rank in order the following actions in response to this situation (1 = Most appropriate; 5 = Least appropriate).

A   Advise the patient's wife to discuss this with the consultant looking after her husband.
B   Advise the patient's wife to talk to her husband about it.
C   Inform the patient's wife that you cannot disclose the information.
D   Talk to the patient and advise him to tell his wife.
E   Tell the patient's wife the diagnosis.

4.55 Relative phones ward

You are the FY1 working on a surgical ward. You answer the ward telephone because you're waiting for your registrar to respond to their bleep. The caller says that they are a patient's mother and asks you whether he is on this ward and how he is doing. The patient is a young man admitted after an accident at work. There are no concerns about his capacity or independence.

Rank in order the following actions in response to this situation (1 = Most appropriate; 5 = Least appropriate).

A   Ask the caller to hold, mute the phone and pass it over to the nurse in charge.
B   Ask the caller to hold while you go and speak to the patient and ask him whether he is happy for you to speak to his mother.
C   Confirm that the patient is on the ward, reassure her that he is doing well and give details of visiting hours.
D   Explain politely that you cannot discuss the details of how the patient is doing over the phone.
E   Tell the caller that you're waiting for a call on this line, apologise and hang up.

4.56 Giving information to relatives

You are the FY1 on a respiratory team. One of your patients has recently been diagnosed with lung cancer. The patient knows his diagnosis. The prognosis is poor, and he is likely to need a lot of care at home. During visiting hours, his daughters approach you. They are very upset that he is still so unwell and want to know what is happening and why he doesn't seem to be getting better.

Choose the **THREE most appropriate** actions to take in this situation.

A   Call your registrar and ask them to come explain the diagnosis to the daughters.
B   Carefully break the news to the daughters that their father has cancer.
C   Explain that they will need to provide a lot of care for their father when he leaves hospital.
D   Explain to the daughters that you cannot give them information about a patient's clinical condition unless the patient has given their permission.
E   Give them a leaflet about local support groups for carers.

F   Listen attentively to the daughters' concerns.
G   Refuse to discuss the situation with them and tell them to ask their father for information.
H   Talk to the patient later that day and discuss his feelings about involving his daughters.

4.57 Safeguarding

You are the FY1 working on a busy gastroenterology ward and have a 25-year-old patient with learning difficulties, who has been admitted with recurrent episodes of haematemesis. While clerking her in, you note that she is very underweight, and the nurse mentions to you that her clothes were very dirty and smelly. She still lives at home, and in the past, there have been numerous involvements with social services, who have been concerned that her parents are not looking after her properly.

Rank in order the following actions in response to this situation (1 = Most appropriate; 5 = Least appropriate).

A   Ask the nurse in charge to talk to the patient.
B   Call her parents and ask them to come in and have a chat with you about her weight.
C   Discuss with your clinical supervisor what action you should take, if any.
D   Speak to social services about your concerns.
E   Take a nurse with you and speak to the patient about your concerns, giving them an opportunity to say anything in confidence.

4.58 STI testing

You are working in the emergency department when a 14-year-old boy comes in with right-sided scrotal pain and swelling. Following your history and examination, you suspect epididymo-orchitis, and you therefore need to ask a sexual history and perform a screen for sexually transmitted infections (STIs). The patient has come in with his mother, who is very concerned for her son and doesn't seem to want to leave him alone.

Rank in order the following actions in response to this situation (1 = Most appropriate; 5 = Least appropriate).

A   Ask his mother to go home to get your patient some pyjamas as he is likely to stay in hospital. Once she is gone take the sexual history.
B   As your patient is only 14, examine him with his mother in the room because legally she has to consent to this.
C   Send a urine sample having told your patient that it is to look for a urine infection, and wait for the results before discussing a sexual history.
D   Tell his mother that you need to ask some sensitive questions and it would be better if she waited outside.
E   Wait until your registrar has reviewed your patient and then let them make the decision about whether or not to carry out an STI screening.

4.59 Mental health consent

You are on a rotation in psychiatry and have a psychiatry in-patient who also has a diagnosis of lymphoma. They confide in you that they would like to stop having active treatment for the lymphoma as it is making them feel too unwell. They are currently under a mental health section in order to be treated for their schizophrenia.

Rank in order the following actions in response to this situation (1 = Most appropriate; 5 = Least appropriate).

A Continue to give them medication for the lymphoma without their consent as they are under mental health section and therefore you don't need their consent.
B Stop giving them the treatment for lymphoma.
C Ask them to consider speaking to their haematologist about other options before withdrawing treatment altogether.
D Assume that the patient must want to end their life and move them to an increased security ward.
E Speak to your registrar about the situation.

4.60 Inappropriate images on laptop

You are an FY1 doctor working on a busy hepatology ward and decide to take a break in the doctors' mess. Upon entering the mess, you find your colleague looking at indecent images of children on the internet. After noticing that you have entered the room, your colleague closes the laptop and asks you not to tell anyone. He goes on to explain that he was researching for a presentation on child abuse. He asks you not to inform anyone about what you have seen because it could be misinterpreted and embarrassing.

Choose the **THREE most appropriate** actions to take in this situation.

A Agree with your colleague and wait to see the presentation.
B Directly telephone the police and report to them what you saw.
C Explain to your colleague that he needs to inform his clinical supervisor and if he does not you will have to.
D Inform the General Medical Council (GMC) of what you saw and ask for advice.
E Inform your clinical supervisor of what you saw and ask for help with the situation.
F Interrogate your colleague about the presentation and investigate whether he has ever been involved in child abuse.
G Investigate whether your colleague will be working with children in the future and take no further action if he is not.
H Offer to help your colleague with his presentation.

4.61 Wrong site surgery

You are an FY1 doctor, and you have been asked to assist in orthopaedic theatres with your consultant and registrar. The next patient on the operating list is a woman whom you have examined several times before. She is coming to theatre for a total hip replacement. The consultant surgeon is about to make the first incision when you realise that he is approaching the left hip. You remember that when you examined the patient she had only complained of problems with the right hip. Furthermore, you remember reading the preoperative notes documenting that the right hip is to be replaced.

Choose the **THREE most appropriate** actions to take in this situation.

A Ask the consultant to operate on the right hip as you are sure that was the one that had been troubling the patient.
B Ask the consultant to stop and discuss the issue before proceeding.
C Ask the nurse in charge to check the patient's notes.
D Ask to see the pre-operative assessment notes to check which side should be operated upon.
E Ask your consultant to re-examine the patient and review the X-ray images before proceeding.
F Assume the consultant has re-examined the patient and allow him to continue.
G Inform the specialist registrar (SpR) of your concerns.
H Inform the whole theatre staff by saying, firmly, that you have concerns over which hip is to be operated upon and that the operation should be stopped.

4.62 Chaperones

You are on call for colorectal surgery, and it is a particularly busy evening. There are no nurses available to chaperone for you while you do a digital rectal examination (DRE) on a patient presenting with constipation. The patient says that they are happy for you to examine them and don't require a chaperone.

Rank in order the following actions in response to this situation (1 = Most appropriate; 5 = Least appropriate).

A Await one of the nurses to be free to chaperone.
B Decline to perform the examination until someone is available to chaperone.
C Perform the examination, documenting that the patient is happy for you to proceed without a chaperone.
D See if a relative can come and chaperone for the patient instead.
E Document in the notes that you could not perform a DRE.

4.63 End-of-life HW

You are working in the acute admissions unit (AAU), and one of the registrars takes you with them so you can see how they discuss putting the end of life care tool into place with patients. After the consultation, you are unsure that the patient fully understood what the registrar was saying about the fact that they are entering the final stages of their illness. The registrar begins to pre-scribe the appropriate pre-emptive medicines and inform the staff about the decision. You have not met this patient before.

Rank in order the following actions in response to this situation (1 = Most appropriate; 5 = Least appropriate).

A Ask the nurse to go back and fully explain things to the patient.
B Ask the registrar to go back and explain clearly to the patient that their disease is likely to lead to death in the near future.
C Ask the registrar what they thought the patient understood by their discussion.
D Go back into the room alone and explain to the patient again exactly what is happening.
E Leave things as they are: the registrar is more experienced than you at this.

4.64 Chaperone declined

You are the FY1 working on a medical ward. One of your patients is consti-pated and needs a rectal examination for assessment of this. The patient has the necessary mental capacity to give consent to the examination. It is visiting hours, and the patient has a relative present when you go to see them. You offer for a chaperone to be present but the patient declines, saying that they will not allow you to proceed with the examination with any additional people in the room as they feel too embarrassed.

Choose the **THREE most appropriate** actions to take in this situation.

A Agree to examine the patient alone.
B Ask a nurse to remain in the room.
C Ask the patient's relative to stay in the room.
D Call your registrar and ask them to perform the examination.
E Document in the notes that a chaperone was offered and declined.
F Do not perform the examination.
G Explain fully to the patient what you are doing as you perform the examination.
H Explain to the patient that there must be a chaperone present.

4.65 HIV avoiding blood test

You are the medical FY1 on call at the weekend. A newly admitted patient urgently needs a blood test to evaluate their condition and determine further management. You know that the patient is positive for the human immunodeficiency virus (HIV), and you feel very anxious about performing the procedure in case of sustaining a needlestick injury.

Rank in order the following actions in response to this situation (1 = Most appropriate; 5 = Least appropriate).

A Call your senior house officer (SHO) and ask them to take the blood test.
B Record in the notes that you are declining to perform the examination due to personal risk.
C Carry out the blood test following standard precautions.
D Record in the notes that the patient declined the procedure.
E Hand over the job to the night team.

4.66 Unable to get a chaperone

You are working as an FY2 doctor in a GP surgery, and you are asked to go on a home visit to a pregnant patient. The nurse who has triaged the call hasn't provided you with much information on the patient, and you have not met her before. The nurse does, however, inform you that she is 32 weeks pregnant and has had some abdominal pains. When you arrive, the patient is sitting in the living room looking quite pale. She says she has 'had some blood loss from down below', but she can't explain how much blood there was. You perform a simple examination and find her to be pale and slightly tachycardic. You explain to the patient that you would like to perform a visual examination of her vagina before deciding further management, which she agrees to. Before you start, you realise that you don't have a chaperone. You are happy to carry out the examination, but you are unsure as to your ethical obligations.

Rank in order the following actions in response to this situation (1 = Most appropriate; 5 = Least appropriate).

A Call your educational supervisor for advice.
B Perform the examination as she could potentially be having a life-threatening vaginal bleed.
C Phone the GP surgery and ask for a colleague to come and act as a chaperone.
D Refuse to perform the examination and ask the patient to come into the clinic later that afternoon for a thorough, more professional examination.
E Refuse to perform the examination and ask the patient to immediately attend the maternity unit at the local hospital.

4.67 Drunk

You are an FY1 in an emergency department. A man is brought in, having been found collapsed on the pavement. He is a frequent attender of the emergency department with alcohol-related problems, and on this occasion, he is conscious on arrival, appears drunk and is verbally abusive. A nurse tells you that they usually put him in a side-room to 'sober up a bit' before he is assessed.

Choose the THREE most appropriate actions to take in this situation.

A   Ask the nurse to do regular clinical observations on the patient.
B   Ask the nurse to inform you when he has sobered up.
C   Ask the nurses to restrain the patient while you examine him.
D   Ask your senior colleague to examine the patient.
E   Carry out a clinical assessment of the patient on arrival.
F   Give the patient sedation.
G   Inform the nurse that you cannot delay his assessment or treatment.
H   Refuse the patient access to the emergency department as he is being abusive.

4.68 Keeping promises

You are an FY1 working in paediatrics. One of your patients is nearly ready to be discharged, and their parents ask whether you can help them with a problem they have. They had made a decision for their child not to have a vaccine that was offered at birth but have subsequently changed their minds. You offer to try to arrange for them to come back to the ward for their child to have it. After they leave, you ask your consultant who says that this is not a service the ward can provide.

Choose the **THREE most appropriate** actions to take in this situation.

A   Avoid the parents on the ward.
B   Call the patient's health visitor and ask them to provide the vaccine.
C   Contact the pharmacist to order the vaccine.
D   Do not arrange for the vaccine to be given on the ward.
E   Explain to the parents that vaccines should be provided in the community.
F   Explain to your consultant that you feel you have to give the vaccine now as you have made a promise to the parents.
G   Get a second opinion from a different consultant.
H   Make an appointment for the patient as a ward attender.

4.69 Keeping promise to refer to dentist

It is a Friday during your FY1 rotation on a busy respiratory ward. You are the only junior doctor looking after 16 patients. You see a patient on the ward round who tells you that he has broken one of his teeth, and it is causing him to cut his tongue and lips. You make a promise to the patient to contact the on-call maxillofacial surgeon to inform them of the situation. The patient is otherwise stable and is receiving antibiotics for a chest infection. You complete your ward round late in the day and are still completing jobs, despite it being after the time you should have finished. You suddenly remember that you have forgotten to refer your patient to the maxillofacial surgeon for review.

Choose the **THREE most appropriate** actions to take in this situation.

A   Apologise to the patient and keep them up to date with the situation.

B   Prescribe some painkillers for the patient during the weekend.

C   Telephone the on-call maxillofacial surgeon informing them of the situation.

D   Telephone your consultant and ask him for help as you are still completing jobs after hours.

E   Telephone your on-call FY1 colleague asking them to refer the patient to the surgeon.

F   Wait until Monday to refer the patient.

G   Write a letter of complaint to the human resources department informing them that you have had to stay out of hours.

H   Write a letter to your patient's dentist asking them to review him after discharge.

4.70 Drunk colleague

You are an FY1 working in respiratory medicine, and you have been scheduled to work on New Year's Day. When you arrive at work, you find your FY1 colleague looking unwell. They tell you that they have had a big night out for New Year and are feeling quite ill; in fact they stayed up all night at a party and have come straight to work.

Rank in order the following actions in response to this situation (1 = Most appropriate; 5 = Least appropriate).

A   Get your colleague a cup of coffee and assist them with their work today as they are unwell.

B   Tell your registrar that your colleague is unsafe due to their tiredness and that they may be drunk.

C   Ask your colleague to go home sick as they are not safe to work today.

D   Ignore your colleague and make a pointed remark on a social network website as to how irresponsible they have been.

E   Ignore your colleague most of the day: it is their own fault that they are unwell, and you shouldn't have to do extra work trying to sort them out.

ANSWERS

4.1 Ordering wrong test

C D A

This question deals with honesty and responsibility. You are the person who ordered the test for the wrong patient, and now you need to take responsibility for it. Any mistake made in medicine can leave patients exposed to risks that they needn't be. The best answers in this question involve apologising truthfully to the patient in question and trying to prevent this from happening again by speaking to senior staff. You shouldn't feel like bringing this mistake to light is turning yourself in, more like actively trying to protect patients in future. Other staff members are just as likely to make the same mistakes as you. Options C, D and A all involve either apologising to the patient or raising the matter with senior staff, whether clinical, your supervisors or through the incident form reporting system. The rest of the options do not attempt to prevent this situation happening again. Although option B makes an attempt to apologise to the patient, this should still be followed by you escalating your mistake to more experienced members of the clinical team. Similarly option E is also wrong since there is no acknowledgement of the error made despite ensuring that the x-ray is properly reviewed, as all tests should be. The rest of the options try and cover up the mistake by pretending it didn't happen (G), making up a false justification for the test (H) or blaming colleagues (F), which are all dishonest.

Recommended reading

General Medical Council (2012), Explanatory guidance, in *Raising and Acting on Concerns About Patient Safety*, paragraphs 11–15.
General Medical Council (2013), *Good Medical Practice*, paragraph 55.

4.2 Signing sick note

B A E D C

As an FY1 doctor you have a responsibility to communicate effectively with patients, to listen and respond to their concerns but also to be honest when signing forms or completing documentation and to take reasonable steps to ensure that what you are writing is correct. Option B is therefore the best response as it combines both these approaches. Option A may also be appropriate, although it risks delaying the care of patients who are being looked after by your team. Option E is perhaps too brusque a response, despite your being under stress; however, it is preferable to options C and D, which ignore the situation and contravene General Medical Council guidance. Since option D does not involve actively disregarding guidance on completing sick notes but does include poor patient communication, this is more favourable than option C.

Recommended reading

General Medical Council (2009), *The New Doctor*, paragraph 11.
General Medical Council (2013), *Good Medical Practice*, paragraphs 31–34, 71.
Medical Protection Society (2012), Honesty, in *MPS Guide to Ethics: A Map for the Moral Maze*, chapter 6.

4.3 End of life care

C B A E D
The consultant has given you enough information to give the patient an idea of what is going to happen to them, and you are in possession of enough surrounding knowledge of the patient to be able to be honest with her. Despite this, as an FY1, you will lack the experience in breaking bad news, so the most appropriate course of action is to give the patient an idea of what is likely to happen and wait until the consultant is available to have a frank discussion with her (C). Of the remaining options, the safest would be to decline to comment and await the consultant review for similar reasons (B), although this means that the patient will be without this information over the weekend. Option A is the next best response; if you have been caring for the patient before, it is better for the patient to receive this information from a familiar doctor rather than your SHO. Option E is better than D; although you should be honest with the patient, it is never wise to try and put a time limit on a prognosis since, as an FY1, you do not have the knowledge to give specifics to a patient in this way. Option D is clearly unacceptable because telling the patient that they will be fine is a lie.

Recommended reading

General Medical Council (2013), *Good Medical Practice*, paragraphs 14–16.
Medical Protection Society (2012), Honesty, in *MPS Guide to Ethics: A Map for the Moral Maze*, chapter 6.

4.4 Discussing options with patient

D B E A C
It is important to be open and honest with patients, which includes ensuring that they are aware of alternative options and are able to weigh these up for themselves. A CT scan involves a large dose of radiation, so it is not a procedure without risk. However, unlike consent for an operation or major procedure, this is a procedure that you should have the competency to discuss. Asking your registrar to do this (B), at considerable disruption to their other responsibilities, therefore ranks lower than doing it yourself (D). Both options E and A, which involve proceeding to request the scan, do not involve describing the alternatives to the patient. Option E is better than option A because it includes informing the patient of what is going on; whereas in option A, they may be unaware that the scan has been organised until the porter arrives to take them to the radiology department. Refusing the request on the grounds

that your consultant has not discussed it with the patient (C) is likely to make you unpopular and is not strictly true given that there are other methods of ensuring the patient is aware of their options, which is why it ranks last.

Recommended reading

General Medical Council (2008), Explanatory guidance, in *Consent: Patients and Doctors Making Decisions Together*.

Medical Protection Society (2012), Honesty, section: Consent, in *MPS Guide to Ethics: A Map for the Moral Maze*. chapter 6.

4.5 Imminent cardiac arrest

D C A B E

Cardiac arrest or peri-arrest situations can be exceedingly daunting for an FY1 doctor with little experience of these scenarios. The important factor to consider here is that the nurse is clearly very worried about the patient and believes that they may have a cardiac arrest soon. While there are scenarios where you would leave duties to the on-call team outside your shift hours, this patient quite clearly requires urgent medical attention. In this scenario, the least appropriate option would be to commence CPR (E) as the patient needs to be assessed further before deciding whether it is appropriate to commence basic life support. In this case, the patient still has a pulse and is breathing, so the most appropriate method of assessment would be the ABCDE approach (D). If the patient does suffer a cardiac arrest, CPR should be started, and the crash team must be called. In this scenario, it is clear that you are going to need the support of an on-call colleague, so initially asking the nurse to perform a full assessment (if she hasn't already) and phoning for help would be a sensible course of action (C). Even though this situation has occurred 'out of hours', if the patient is very unwell, as in this case, your knowledge of her background history and ability to immediately assess her clinical state are likely to be very useful. Leaving the scene and handing over the task would compromise patient safety and be unacceptable given what the nurse has told you; therefore, options A and B are poor choices. However, asking the nurse to make a full assessment and escalate to the necessary persons (A) is always preferable to waiting for the FY1 on call to assess the patient, which could lead to a 5–15 minute delay.

Recommended reading

General Medical Council (2013), Duties of a doctor, in *Good Medical Practice*.

4.6 Chest drain at nighttime

E B A D C

As a doctor, you need to balance your educational needs with patient safety. Inserting a chest drain is likely to be beyond your training and competence as an FY1 doctor. Doing this procedure at nighttime would be unnecessary and places your patient under increased risk due to clinician fatigue and associated decreased situational awareness as well as decreased staffing levels should a problem arise. Therefore the least appropriate option is C: doing the procedure. The most appropriate option is E, challenging your SHO about their suggestion that you perform the procedure. Junior doctors often find it difficult to challenge seniors, but this should be overcome especially in scenarios where patient safety is at risk. If your SHO refuses to acknowledge your opinion or you don't feel comfortable in challenging their decision directly, then you should advise the SHO to speak to their senior (B). The next most appropriate option would be to seek similar learning opportunities in the daytime (A). Asking the SHO to insert the chest drain while observing (D) would be putting the patient under unnecessary risk, but this is preferable to carrying out the procedure yourself when you have no previous experience (C).

Recommended reading

Medical Protection Society (2012), Duty of care, in *MPS Guide to Ethics: A Map for the Moral Maze*, chapter 4.

4.7 Poor equipment

B E D A C

Respecting patients' dignity means that intimate examinations should be undertaken in a private area where they cannot be overlooked by other staff or patients. Importantly, however, you should ask the patient what their preference is, as patients' opinions of what protects their dignity vary from person to person. The room available in this situation is not suitable for catheterising a patient, so you should not attempt to 'make do' with it. The best response is B: there is a time constraint and calling the department to let them know of a likely delay is good practice and will allow them to rearrange the patient list to ensure everyone receives their tests today. Ensuring safe and private catheterisation in a more controlled environment off the ward (E), although making the patient late, would be appropriate since it protects their dignity, which is the most important factor. Option D is the next best response as the urodynamics department will be a more private area than the room available in the day case department, and therefore, it might be necessary to send the patient down to be catheterised in the department. The last two available options attempt to use the inappropriate room; however, option A, with a chaperone (standard practice), is better than option C, without.

Recommended reading

General Medical Council (2013), Explanatory guidance, in *Maintaining Boundaries: Intimate Examinations and Chaperones*.
General Medical Council (2013), *Good Medical Practice*, paragraph 47.

4.8 Nurse prescribing

A D H

Nursing staff should never give patients regular medication without a valid prescription. 'As required' medication is prescribed and given at the nurses' and patients' discretion but can only be given within the defined parameters of the prescription. The options that are appropriate in this question protect the patient immediately from an unneccesary and potentially dangerous treatment and take steps to prevent this from happening again.

Option H is appropriate as stopping the infusion and letting the heads of both the medical and nursing team know of this serious and preventable error enables the appropriate staff to take the relevant action. Option D is also sensible as it protects the patient immediately and ensures that the incident is looked into, although perhaps some time after the event. Managerial and clinical staff are obliged to look into and follow up every incident form, so this is a useful route for reporting clinical issues. To ensure the patient's safety, it is important that you also assess the patient for any adverse effects from the heparin infusion, as in option A. This also involves apologising and explaining the mistake, which keeps the patient fully informed and shows respect, and contacting your registrar, who should be able to advise you further on how to prevent this happening again. Importantly, documenting any serious prescription errors enables other medical staff to be aware of potential adverse reactions and gives them the appropriate information to deal with any subsequent consequences. The other responses are not ideal because, although many of them do include stopping the infusion (C, E, F and G), they do not prevent the situation from happening again. Continuing the infusion for the sake of your colleague's feelings (B) is both unprofessional and unsafe.

Recommended reading
General Medical Council (2013), Explanatory guidance, in *Good Practice in Prescribing and Managing Medicines and Devices*, paragraphs 6–13.
General Medical Council (2013), *Good Medical Practice*, paragraph 16.

4.9 Staying late

D   A   E   C   B
While you should not be expected to stay late on a regular basis, you still have a duty of care to your patient, even if your shift has finished. You should review the patient and prescribe the analgesia rather than leaving them in pain. Option D is therefore the most appropriate response. If you decline to prescribe the analgesia, you have a duty to ensure that someone does. Bleeping the on-call team yourself ensures that the job has been handed over to someone before you leave. Option A is therefore preferable to E, which relies upon the nurse to hand over the task. A verbal handover is far more effective than a written request. Leaving a note in the doctor's office risks the note never being seen or a significant delay before it is seen and acted upon. Option C is therefore an unfavourable option. Ignoring the request (B) is clearly inappropriate since the patient should not be left without analgesia.

Recommended reading
General Medical Council (2013), Duties of a doctor, in *Good Medical Practice*.
Medical Protection Society (2012), Duty of care, in *MPS Guide to Ethics: A Map for the Moral Maze*, chapter 4.

4.10 Faulty equipment

B E F

Your first duty is to your patient, and you need to ensure that their urgent ECG is performed, so option B should be the immediate response. You also have a duty to ensure that any faulty equipment is repaired or replaced. Calling the medical equipment department yourself will result in timely reporting of the fault (E), while informing the ward manager ensures that someone will follow up the fault and make sure that it is resolved (F). Completing an incident form (A) is unnecessary since there has been no risk to patient safety, and you have taken steps to prevent any future risk. While putting a note on the machine (C) may be useful in informing people that it is broken, it does not actively resolve the issue. Similarly, failing to take any steps to alert the fault to others, as in option D, will not solve the issue, and taking the machine from another ward (G) will just create a problem elsewhere. Trying to fix the machine yourself (H) is potentially dangerous and not a good use of your time.

Recommended reading

General Medical Council (2013), *Good Medical Practice*, paragraphs 15b, 25b.

4.11 Child protection

C A D B E

Identifying and acting upon signs of non-accidental injury early is extremely important in the protection of children and young people. However, your first concern in this scenario should be to complete your assessment of the child to identify and address the underlying cause for her presenting complaint, which, in this case, is difficulty breathing (C). Furthermore, you may go on to find further injuries as you continue your examination. There may be a reasonable explanation as to how the bruise occurred, and indeed any explanation should be clearly documented. It is therefore important to ask the parents about it (A). Any concerns about child safety must be escalated, and a good first step would be to discuss this with the emergency consultant (D). It is usual to discuss any concerns you may have with the parents as well and to keep them informed about any investigations into their child's care. This is unless you feel that informing the parents may place the child at further risk. In this instance, there is no need to ask the parents to leave (B), and this may even be detrimental to their future cooperation. Taking a picture of the baby on your phone is completely inappropriate. You should never take pictures of patients on your phone as this breaches data protection (E). Photographic evidence of the bruise will be needed but should only be obtained by a medical photographer.

Recommended reading

General Medical Council (2011), Explanatory guidance, in *Making and Using Visual and Audio Recordings of Patients*.

General Medical Council (2012), Explanatory guidance, in *Protecting Children and Young People: The Responsibilities of all Doctors*, paragraphs 2–5, 18–22.

4.12 Abortion

E   A   D   C   B

Doctors have a right to conscientiously object to participation in abortion, fertility treatment and withdrawal of life-sustaining treatment. However, a doctor cannot discriminate against a group of patients, such as patients who have had an abortion, and cannot refuse to treat the consequences of a lifestyle choice. The patient in this scenario has made the choice to have an abortion, and you have a duty to provide the care that she now requires (E). While asking one of your colleagues to take over her care (A) is not the most suitable response, it still ensures that the patient receives appropriate care. Regardless of your beliefs, the care of your patient is your priority, and it remains your responsibility to find a means of providing that care. It is therefore inappropriate to ask the ward manager to find another doctor to care for the patient (D). There is no need to tell the patient about your beliefs in this situation, and indeed the patient may feel that she is the subject of discrimination if you were to inform her (C). Refusing to treat the patient properly is unprofessional and fails to fulfil your duty of care (B).

Recommended reading

British Medical Association, *Expressions of doctor's beliefs*, http://bma.org.uk/
practical-support-at-work/ethics/expressions-of-doctors-beliefs.
General Medical Council (2007), Explanatory guidance, in *0–18 Years: Guidance for All Doctors*, paragraph 72.
General Medical Council (2013), *Good Medical Practice*, paragraphs 52, 54, 59.

4.13 Sleeping tablets dementia

D   C   E   B   A

As a doctor, you will have pressure put on you by carers, relatives and other colleagues to take specific courses of action. It is important that you keep the patient as your main focus and make any decisions based on their best interests, while also acknowledging and respecting the opinions of your colleagues and the patient's relatives and carers. In this scenario, you should first gather more information during her stay in hospital (D) before prescribing any sedation and see whether any more help could be offered to the patient and her daughter. Telling the daughter to organise more care on discharge (C) would achieve the same effect but is less appropriate than option D. The care of the elderly department should have resources to be able to make a quick and thorough MDT assessment, and it should also prevent the situation reaching a crisis point if the patient was to be discharged without further help. The daughter may need personal support from her GP (E), but the mother is the first priority in this instance. Prescribing the patient sedatives and asking the GP to review this (B) is inappropriate as you do not have sufficient information to prescribe the sedative, which could have negative effects (such as sedation during the daytime and increasing the patient's risk of falls). However, option A is the most inappropriate response. As a doctor, you are not in a position to advise such action; you should instead offer her access to healthcare professionals who can further assess the patient and help the daughter to make informed decisions.

Recommended reading
General Medical Council (2013), Explanatory guidance, in *Good Practice in Prescribing and Managing Medicines and Devices*, paragraphs 14–16.

4.14 Group and save

D C E A B
This is a significant omission in a patient's treatment and could be viewed as a breach of your duty of care. After realising that you have made a mistake relating to a patient's management that could cause harm or distress, the General Medical Council (GMC) states that you should do three things: put matters right if possible, apologise and explain the situation, including the likely short-term and long-term effects. In this scenario, your priority is reducing harm to the patient. The most appropriate thing to do would be to inform the operating theatre staff (D) as they will be able to judge the risk of continuing the operation without readily available blood products. The operating team could potentially delay the surgery or send off an urgent sample from the theatre. Informing your SpR (C) would be the next most appropriate option as they could notify the theatre; however, this is not a task that requires their seniority, and this could cause further delays. Taking the blood test after theatre (E) could prevent harm after surgery but would leave the patient under major risk in the operating theatre. Completing an incident form (A) would be a good action after the event as processes could be put in place to avoid patients being put in this situation again. However, in the first instance, you should deal with the immediate risk to the current patient. The least appropriate response is doing nothing (B): this would be negligent, putting the patient at risk of serious harm.

Recommended reading
General Medical Council (2013), *Good Medical Practice*, paragraph 55.
Medical Protection Society (2012), Duty of care, in *MPS Guide to Ethics: A Map for the Moral Maze*, chapter 4.

4.15 Disruptive intravenous drug user patient

A D C E B
This scenario relates to your duty of care to a patient and where this may end. The patient is disruptive and taking attention away from the care of others, which subsequently affects your duty of care to your other patients. If the patient is taking recreational drugs, it makes surgical or medical care extremely difficult and potentially dangerous. The most appropriate action in this case is to seek senior input or advice from your registrar or consultant (A); it is likely that this patient will need discharging from hospital care, but as

an FY1 doctor, you should not be expected to make this decision. The next most appropriate action would be to speak to the patient about their inappropriate behaviour (D); however, it would be best to involve seniors in the first instance, as the nurses require a decision. Signposting the patient to drug misuse and addiction services (C) would be useful but is not the first priority in this situation. Telling the nurses to continue the care of the patient (E) may be appropriate but should be a senior decision; a clinician is within their rights to end a professional relationship when a breakdown of trust between themselves and the patient means that they cannot provide good clinical care. The most inappropriate response is B as this should be a senior-led decision, as previously discussed.

Recommended reading
General Medical Council (2013), *Good Medical Practice*, paragraph 62.

4.16 Waiter with diarrhoea

C   A   G

As a doctor, you have a duty of care to your patient but also to the general public. In this case, you should be concerned about someone working in a restaurant with infectious diarrhoea. The most appropriate course of action would be to obtain a stool sample to exclude infection (C), advise the patient not to take loperamide at this time (A) and tell him that he should not work until the diarrhoea has stopped (G) or an infectious cause has been excluded. Option B is a step that would reduce transmission of an infectious diarrhoea; however, he would still pose a risk to the general public. Notifying the HPA (D) would be a valid option if an infectious cause had been found or strongly suspected. Reporting the restaurant to the local newspaper (F) would be very unprofessional. Option E is inappropriate at this stage as an infectious cause has not been ruled out, and if the patient continued to work, he could cause an outbreak of infectious gastroenterititis. Advising him to get in touch with occupational health (H) is unnecessary at this point as he does not have a clear diagnosis; however, this should be considered further down the line.

Recommended reading
Medical Protection Society (2012), Duty of care, in *MPS Guide to Ethics: A Map for the Moral Maze*, chapter 4.

4.17 Hyperkalaemia and chasing blood tests

E   A   C   D   B

Making mistakes is an inevitable part of being a doctor. GPs can see up to 50 patients a day and deal with a wide range of complaints. This scenario requires a small amount of knowledge with regard to hyperkalaemia, which puts patients at risk of potentially fatal cardiac arrhythmias. While the blood sample may be haemolysed (B), causing the potassium level to be falsely high, unless this was specifically reported by the laboratory, it would not be safe to disregard what you have found. The best course of action would be to urgently repeat the results in a safe environment, which in this case would be a hospital (E). It would be appropriate to first discuss the patient case with the hospital on-call medical team and explain the situation. Asking for senior advice, particularly within a primary care setting, is vital as the experience and knowledge of a GP trainer will help you to decide your course of action (A). Booking urgent blood tests for the following day (C) would cause too much delay as the patient is in danger of a serious arrhythmia and should be seen immediately. Rechecking your other consultations (D) may be appropriate if you think you have missed something; however, your priority should be this patient as he is in danger.

Recommended reading
Nyirenda MJ, Tang JI, Padfield PL, Seckl JR. (2009), Hyperkalaemia, *BMJ*, 339, b4114.

4.18 Responsibility between teams

A   D   G

Now that you are aware of the need for monitoring, you have a responsibility to ensure that this takes place, especially as the patient is primarily under your care. You should ensure that it is easy for other members of your team to be aware of the monitoring plan by adding it to your handover sheet (A), but you should also make a more formal record in the patient's notes (G), where it will also be accessible to other professionals involved in the patient's care. It is sensible to fill in the request for the blood test now in order to ensure that it is not forgotten or delayed the next day (D), which is particularly important if you are not working then. It would be unhelpful and unsafe for the patient if you were to deny any responsibility and insist that this lies with the neurology department (H), even if you have discussed this with them (B). It would be negligent and unsafe to alter the treatment plan simply to avoid the hassle of monitoring (E). There is no point in performing the blood test now, when it is not due until the next day (F); even if you are just trying to ensure it is performed, the results will be difficult to interpret and act on. There is no reason why you would need advice urgently from your registrar in this situation (C) as you should be able to sort this out yourself.

Recommended reading
Foundation Programme Curriculum (2012), Section 1.3: Continuity of care.
Medical Protection Society (2012), Duty of care, section: Acts and omissions, in *MPS Guide to Ethics: A Map for the Moral Maze*, chapter 4.

4.19 Ensuring follow up

E   D   B   A   C

Although this is not an ideal situation for yourself or the patient, you should try to communicate the additional request to the GP as per the plan made by your team (options E and D). It is better to do this is writing (E) rather than by telephone (D), since this means that there is a formal record of you having informed them and also means that the message is less likely to get lost or misinterpreted. You have a responsibility to ensure that the necessary follow-up takes place, and it is not fair to place this entirely on the patient (B). While many patients are completely capable of managing their follow-up plan, not all will be, and by doing so, you are vulnerable to criticism if they forget or confuse your advice. Options A and C rank lowest because they alter the plan your team has made for the patient's follow-up. There are resource availability issues around organising the follow-up in a hospital setting rather than in primary care. Option A is better than option C because the burden falls on you to chase the results of the test rather than leaving your consultant to deal with this. They are likely to be incredibly unhappy that you have used up one of their clinic slots for a patient they did not need to see (C).

Recommended reading
Foundation Programme Curriculum (2012), Section 10.4: Discharge planning.
Medical Protection Society (2012), Duty of care, section: Scope, in *MPS Guide to Ethics: A Map for the Moral Maze*, chapter 4.

4.20 Negligence 1

C E D B A
Option C is the best choice here as the patient may come to harm from your omission. They therefore deserve a full explanation and will definitely need their drug levels monitored the next day. This was a simple error, but such things may be seen as negligence by the patient, and an apology can make a big difference in how they view the mistake. While options E and D are both good responses, they do not include an immediate action to explain to the patient what has happened. Option E ranks higher than option D, as you are talking to a member of your team and someone who is directly involved in the patient's care. Calling the SHO on call (B) may be helpful, but your team's registrar or a member of the microbiology department is better placed to answer your queries; therefore, it would be preferable to speak to them. Option A ranks last as this sounds like you are blaming the nurse for your mistake, and this will not help improve patient care. It will also not help you find out what to do next and may create friction within the team.

Recommended reading
General Medical Council (2013), *Good Medical Practice*, paragraph 25.

4.21 Negligence 2

C D E
In this scenario, the trust would have a protocol in place and following this (E) would give you all the advice you need for initiating treatment. In addition, it should tell you the standard of care to be followed. If you are really uncertain,

then a call for help from someone more senior is appropriate, and the SHO may be available even though the registrar is not (D). When seeing an acutely ill patient, the ABCDE approach should always be used (C) as this will help regardless of whether or not you are confident in treating the specifics of a condition. Your memory may be right on how to treat DKA (F), but following trust protocol is a far better way to manage this patient. Doing nothing and waiting for the SpR (G) is not appropriate in this case and is actually negligent. While the ward matron may be experienced in managing acutely unwell patients, they should not be your first port of call as it may have been a while since the last time they saw a similar case; therefore, option B is not appropriate. Your handbook may be outdated, therefore option H is not the best way to manage the patient; trust protocols are updated regularly and are a much better resource in this case. Asking a fellow FY1 for help (A) may give you some support, but they will also most probably have had little experience here, so it is not one of the best responses.

Recommended reading
General Medical Council (2013), *Good Medical Practice*, paragraphs 14, 18.

4.22 Challenging decisions

A   E   C   B   D

This is a difficult scenario as there may be clinical details you are not aware of explaining why the consultant made the decision. However, a raised potassium at this level is a medical emergency, and you should therefore act on it in some way. Calling the on-call registrar (A) would be a good start as they can give you advice about your next step or might be better placed to speak to the consultant themselves. Talking to the consultant directly (E), while sometimes a scary prospect, would be appropriate since this will clarify all the details. You should remember that the consultant has ultimate responsibility for the patient's care, so calling them for advice would be the next best course of action. Contacting the patient at home (C) would ensure immediate action; however, it involves going over the consultant's head and is therefore not appropriate. The remaining two responses (B and D) are the least appropriate, as both will delay care in this emergency situation. Option B is preferable to D though as this will result in the matter being raised with the consultant.

Recommended reading
General Medical Council (2013), *Good Medical Practice*, paragraphs 24, 25.
Medical Protection Society (2012), Duty of care, in *MPS Guide to Ethics: A Map for the Moral Maze*, chapter 4.

4.23 Breaking bad news

E   B   A   C   D

The patient is under the consultant's care, and you do not have the knowledge to give the patient an adequate understanding of what the results will mean for the treatment and prognosis of the patient; therefore, it is inappropriate for you to discuss them with the patient (E). This will be a very difficult subject for the patient, and for continuity of care, it is better that the consultant tells the patient themselves. Option B is the next best response because, although the registrar is not directly linked to the patient's care, they will know a lot more about the disease and will be able to adequately counsel the patient on the results. Option A is not ideal, but the FY2 is more experienced than you and therefore better placed to discuss the results with the patient, if you feel unable to. Option C is preferable to D, as it involves making the patient aware of the limitation of your competencies, and you would not be giving the patient any false information. Retrieving information from the internet (D) is not always reliable or fully up to date, especially in the field of oncology where there are often new treatments being trialled.

Recommended reading
General Medical Council (2009), *Tomorrow's Doctors*, paragraph 133.
General Medical Council (2013), Duties of a doctor, in *Good Medical Practice*.
General Medical Council (2013), *Good Medical Practice*, paragraph 25c.
Medical Protection Society (2012), Personal conduct, in *MPS Guide to Ethics: A Map for the Moral Maze*, chapter 12, p. 91.

4.24 Analgesia

B G F
This is a difficult set of options as some of the best responses are conflicting. Option B is appropriate, as you are letting the correct member of the team know that a job needs doing and maintaining patient care. Option G is also a good response as many doctors consider leaving a patient in pain to be inappropriate, and you are qualified to prescribe basic analgesia as an FY1. If you are to prescribe analgesia, you should always review the patient first to see if they have tried any analgesics previously and if they have any allergies or intolerances. Option F, while it does not involve giving any pain relief, is also appropriate since during the day, a member of the patient's team should be available to prescribe analgesia for their patients, and this patient is not under your care. Options A and H are not the best options here as they leave the responsibility solely with the nurses to resolve the issue. Options C, D and E, while resulting in the patient receiving analgesia, are not safe as they do not involve you actually seeing the patient. It should be recognised that simply looking through a patient's notes (C) is not a replacement for seeing them. Also, simply prescribing paracetamol (E) may not be adequate analgesia, while prescribing a variety of analgesics (D) is not appropriate as it leaves the decision to the nurse over what to give.

Recommended reading
General Medical Council (2010), Explanatory guidance, in *Treatment and Care Towards the End of Life: Good Practice in Decision Making*.

4.25 MRSA patient

D C A B E

This question deals with a situation in which your actions may influence the health and safety of both your patient and the other patients and staff on the ward. Option D is therefore the most appropriate response. You should inform the nurse in charge in a timely manner, in case they are unaware of the results, so that suitable safety measures can be implemented. This aims to decrease the risk of transmission among people on the ward and contribute to maintaining patient safety. Option C is also a courteous action to take and maintains good patient–doctor communication; however, this should be done after the sister has been informed so that, in the meantime, arrangements for a side room can be underway. Option E, on the other hand, demonstrates conscious neglect of patient care. While it may be true that the nurses arrange the infection control measures, this shows poor communication with colleagues and could put the health of patients and staff at risk. In matters such as this, your registrar should not be the first person you call, and therefore, option B is also unsuitable; you are wasting both your time and that of your senior, consequently delaying important patient care. Asking one of the other nurses to contact the ward sister to organise the move of the patient while you deal with their abnormal blood results (A) is more appropriate and may be necessary if you couldn't find the nurse in charge and were called to a sick patient. However, when relying on another member of staff, you cannot be sure when or if the message was relayed.

Recommended reading

General Medical Council (2012), Explanatory guidance, in *Raising and Acting on Concerns About Patient Safety*.
General Medical Council (2013), Duties of a doctor, in *Good Medical Practice*.
General Medical Council (2013), *Good Medical Practice*, paragraphs 25, 35.
Medical Protection Society (2012), Duty of care, in *MPS Guide to Ethics: A Map for the Moral Maze*, chapter 4.

4.26 Arranging follow up

D F G

This question is concerned with ensuring you uphold a duty of care toward your patients while maintaining good professional relationships. As an FY1, it is your responsibility to ensure that discharge letters and follow-up arrangements are in accordance with seniors' advice, and although it may not have been your job to complete the discharge letter, you have a duty to voice any concerns that may impact patient care. Option D is appropriate as it shows good communication skills and humility (unlike H), which is important, especially as you are not certain of what you remember. To change the discharge letter yourself without discussion (B) would show a lack of respect for your colleague, and in this scenario, you have not checked whether your memory of the conversation is accurate. As there is some dispute about the information on the current discharge letter, option F is advisable; however, you should also confirm your decision by speaking to the consultant themselves (G). Option C is less appropriate as your colleague may not remember the correct information either. Asking the patient (A) is not advisable as there is the chance that she may not correctly remember what advice the consultant had given and may negatively affect her future care. Similarly, option E may adversely impact her outcome and is inappropriate: ensuring that the correct follow-up is in place for your patients after discharge is part of your remit as an FY1.

Recommended reading

General Medical Council (2013), Duties of a doctor, in *Good Medical Practice*.
General Medical Council (2013), *Good Medical Practice*, paragraphs 15, 25, 35, 36, 44.
Medical Protection Society (2012), Duty of care, in *MPS Guide to Ethics: A Map for the Moral Maze*, chapter 4.

4.27 Antibiotic guidelines

A B D C E
This question is assessing your ability to adhere to local clinical guidelines and remain up to date with practices in your specialty. It is important that this patient receives effective timely treatment, while also minimising the risk of eliciting antibiotic resistance. Option A is the preferred response as you are complying with the guidance that is recommended by your hospital. Although asking for advice (B) may also be appropriate, this is information that, as an FY1, you should at least endeavour to find yourself before troubling other colleagues. Using the old guidelines (D) is unlikely to cause harm to your patient and may well be effective. You are also ensuring regular monitoring of your patient. However, this action fails to demonstrate compliance with local policies. Option E is the least advisable, as it not only demonstrates a shirking of responsibility but also delays the antibiotics, a key action in the management of sepsis. For this reason, option C is slightly more appropriate. Although your handbook may be out of date, beginning empirical antibiotic treatment after taking cultures is more proactive than failing to do anything.

Recommended reading

General Medical Council (2013), Duties of a doctor, in *Good Medical Practice*.
General Medical Council (2013), *Good Medical Practice*, paragraphs 8, 11, 16, 18.
Medical Protection Society (2012), Duty of care, in *MPS Guide to Ethics: A Map for the Moral Maze*, chapter 4.
www.survivingsepsis.org

4.28 ABG competence

A B E

The correct answers in this question immediately correct the error and prevent the patient from bleeding or bruising badly. Nursing staff can often perform this task if you need to process the sample immediately, so option A is one of the appropriate responses. If you are confident that the patient themselves can apply pressure, it can be appropriate for the patient to do so, although you should give them full instructions and check on them in a few minutes (B). Option E is also an appropriate response, as putting pressure on the area yourself ensures that it is done promptly and well. The inappropriate responses are those that involve leaving the patient bleeding, such as option C, when you go off to call back the FY2, and option D, when you ignore the situation to learn how to use the analyser. Options F and G involve an attempt to prevent this situation happening again, either through personal reflection or discussing the FY2's incompetence with their supervisor; however, neither detail an immediate response to the potentially bleeding patient. The final inappropriate answer is H, which attempts to remove blame from you by detailing the FY2's fault in the notes, thereby doing little in the immediate situation. This would also likely damage your professional relationship with your colleague, so it is unsuitable.

Recommended reading
General Medical Council (2013), *Good Medical Practice*, paragraphs 22–30.

4.29 Keeping up to date

D B A C E

The most appropriate response in this scenario is to discuss the matter with someone more senior than yourself. This is perhaps best done as a reflection with your educational supervisor (D), providing that the management plan as set out by your consultant will not lead to patients coming to harm. Option B is the next best response as this again involves discussing the matter with someone more senior than yourself, with more experience; however, it is not ideal as you will not be making your thoughts about patient management known to your consultant. While option A seems like a sensible response, the consultant may not take kindly to an FY1 questioning their judgements, and the teaching session may not provide an opportunity to ask. Options C and E are both not appropriate; in the case of option C this leaves your concerns unreported and is therefore not helping the situation. It is better than option E, however, since, as an FY1, you should not be going over the consultant to change management plans.

Recommended reading
General Medical Council (2012), Explanatory guidance, in *Raising and Acting on Concerns About Patient Safety*, part 1, paragraphs 7, 13.
General Medical Council (2013), *Good Medical Practice*, paragraphs 11, 12, 13.

4.30 Clinical skills

C B D A E

It is important to remember that, as an FY1 doctor, you should always ask for help if you are unsure of your competencies. Option C is therefore best as you have performed the procedure before and probably just need reassurance that you can still do so. Option B is the next most appropriate action as this still results in both the patient being catheterised and a learning experience for you. Option D is the third best as, if you do not feel competent and the nurse is not trained, it is not appropriate to try and fumble your way through the procedure together (A). It should be remembered, however, that the continence nurse should only be called in cases of difficult catheterisation; therefore, this is not an appropriate referral. Option E is inferior as simply booking a clinical skills session will not help your patient in the immediate situation.

Recommended reading

General Medical Council (2009), Practical procedures for graduates, in *Tomorrow's Doctors*, appendix 1.

General Medical Council (2013), *Good Medical Practice*, paragraphs 14, 15, 16.

Medical Protection Society (2012), Competence, sections: Acquiring and developing new skills, in *MPS Guide to Ethics: A Map for the Moral Maze*, Referrals, chapter 10.

4.31 Incident reporting

C D G

In this scenario, the patient has become increasingly unwell because he has not received the antibiotics he needs. Your first priority should therefore be to ensure that the antibiotics are made available as soon as possible. The best way to do this is via the pharmacy (C) rather than taking them from another ward (A). The antibiotics may either be unavailable or needed by other patients on other wards. Although prescribing the readily available second line antibiotic may be easier (E), you should only use second line drugs once first line agents have failed. A further priority is to ensure that this error is investigated and addressed to ensure that it does not happen again. The best method for incident reporting is by using an incident form (D), although you should also inform the ward manager since they are responsible for the running of the ward (G). Although it may be appropriate to make the consultant aware of the incident (F), this is not an immediate priority, and they are not best placed to deal with the problem. While the nurse should be made aware of why drugs need to be given as prescribed (H), it is not your place to do this. The need for further education or training will be identified and acted upon through proper incident reporting.

Recommended reading

General Medical Council (2013), Explanatory guidance, in *Good Practice in Prescribing and Managing Medicines and Devices*, paragraphs 17–19.

4.32 Patient handover

B E A D C

This question tests your ability to prioritise patient care despite the potential for conflict between work and personal commitments. As an FY1, you should make sure that patient safety is put first while also delegating where appropriate, so long as you can ensure a safe handover. Option C is clearly the least sensible in this scenario as you have not responded to a colleague's request for help and, without assessing the patient, are potentially jeopardising patient care. It is also worth remembering that posting jobs on an electronic handover system may alter the perceived urgency of addressing tasks. The most appropriate response to this situation is to fully assess the patient (as you would at any time of day) and ensure that any necessary investigations are ordered (options B and E). It would be sensible to hand over the chasing of outstanding results to the evening team (a verbal as well as written handover is often safest) so that you can leave work and get enough rest before your next shift (B) and also potentially attend part of your social engagement. Waiting for the results to come back is unnecessary (E) as long as you facilitate a safe handover. Option A, while initially demonstrating professional behaviour by undertaking a clinical review of the patient, lays subsequent responsibility on your colleagues, but it would be safer and more courteous to initiate tests and management yourself. Option D is unprofessional because, although your investigation may be appropriate, you should always assess a sick patient in the same way: through history and examination first. This demonstrates a shirking of responsibilities and is only slightly more preferable to option C because you are initiating management (albeit blindly).

Recommended reading

General Medical Council (2009), *The New Doctor*, paragraph 6.
General Medical Council (2013), *Good Medical Practice*, paragraphs 15, 26, 35, 44, 45.

4.33 Non-accidental injury

C E F

Child protection is a vital part of working with children and young people, and every professional has a responsibility to raise concerns if they are worried that a child may be at risk. In this case, it is possible that the child received these injuries as a result of physical abuse. The welfare of the child is paramount and continuing to take a history, examining the child and treating their burns would be the first priority (F). Raising concerns with parents can often be difficult particularly for junior staff, but it is your responsibility (regardless of seniority) to flag children who are potentially at risk to the appropriate person. In this case, the most important person to discuss your concerns with is the consultant in charge of the emergency department (E). The consultant will have the experience and knowledge to guide you through the relevant procedures and will likely take a central role in the case. In the majority of cases, it is appropriate to inform parents or guardians if you have concerns over their child's safety (C). This transparency can avoid conflict in the future and maintains an honest relationship. There are certain situations where not informing the parents may be appropriate, for example if there were concerns that this would put the child at further risk; but this is not the case here. While asking for the help of a senior doctor is not wrong, you would be expected to perform the initial history and examination in your role as a junior doctor; therefore, option A is inappropriate. The fear of offending parents is not a reason to forgo informing them of your concerns (B), while inflammatory comments such as those in option D are unlikely to help the situation. While the police are likely to be involved at some stage of the investigation (options G and H), your immediate priority involves treating the child and information gathering and sharing, which should be done with the support of the consultant in charge of the department.

Recommended reading

General Medical Council (2012), Explanatory guidance, in *Protecting Children and Young People: The Responsibilities of all Doctors.*

4.34 GP treatment final

D E A B C

This situation refers to giving patients the knowledge they need to make informed and autonomous decisions about their own care. Empowering patients in this way helps to increase compliance with treatment. This is a difficult situation because you are not one of the members of the team in this setting, and it is harder to interject as an outsider. However, it is important for improved patient care that this issue is flagged, even though you do not have a direct duty of care for the patients. Therefore, the best response here would be to raise your concerns with the GP (D) so that you can gain further information and understand his reasoning for the way in which the consultation was conducted. The next best response would be to raise the issue with the practice manager (E) so that they can investigate the matter further. Discussing the topic informally with the practice staff (A) ranks higher than the remaining two options, but it may be misconstrued as gossiping about the GP in question. The worst option would be to do nothing (C) as this means that nothing will change. Asking to learn from another GP (B) would be equally ineffective, although, by doing this, you would at least be improving your own learning so as to benefit patients in the future, which is why this is the fourth ranking option.

Recommended reading

General Medical Council (2013), *What to Expect from Your Doctor: A Guide for Patients.*

Medical Protection Society (2012), Patient autonomy and consent, in *MPS Guide to Ethics: A Map for the Moral Maze*, chapter 8.

4.35 Consent for blood test

E   B   A   C   D

This scenario poses a number of issues surrounding consent, capacity and your duty of care to your patients as well as ensuring that you are acting in your patients' best interests. In order to have capacity, a person must be able to understand and retain information given to them about a course of action, use this to weigh up their decision and then be able to communicate their decision to the relevant practitioner. It is important to remember that patients who have an established diagnosis of a cognitive deficit (such as Alzheimer's disease) should not be assumed to lack capacity. In this scenario, a repeat blood sample is clinically imperative, particularly if the patient is at risk of sustaining a significant bleed from a fall. For this reason, omitting the repeat sample is unacceptable and outright negligent, so option D comes last. Patients with dementia are often disorientated, particularly in new environments, so it would be appropriate in this situation to wait a while before attempting to assess capacity to take the sample (E). Escalating this to your registrar would be sensible if you were struggling with this lady's care (C); however, you should be able to determine yourself whether your patient has the capacity, at this point in time, to decline the blood test. Therefore, option B ranks second. Nursing staff can be very successful in calming down agitated patients, so it would be reasonable to ask them for help as your next course of action (A), before your registrar who is most likely tied up with other patients.

Recommended reading

General Medical Council (2008), Explanatory guidance, in *Consent: Patients and Doctors Making Decisions Together*, paragraph 75–76.
Mental Capacity Act (2005), chapter 9, pp. 5–6.

4.36 Jehovah's Witness

C   E   G

Adults can refuse any aspect of treatments if they have the capacity to do so. One of the more common causes for refusal of treatments is religion, and a typical example is the refusal of blood products by Jehovah's Witnesses. Different people interpret their religion in different ways, and it is important to assess exactly what the patient would accept and not accept well in advance of any surgery. The correct responses here include option E: to let the theatre staff know in advance of the patient's wishes so that they can accommodate them and prepare alternative equipment if needed. Similarly, letting the consultant who is performing the surgery know in advance (G) allows them time to prepare alternative operative methods. The patient's expressed refusal of treatment should additionally be written down, and hospitals often have special forms for this (C); these prompt the correct questions and allow you to go through all of the available options with the patient. It is not necessary for the patient to get a legal document to refuse blood products (B), although it is safer from a medico-legal point of view to get a signed and witnessed declaration from them. Simply documenting the patient's decision in their medical notes (H) is not sufficient as such important details might easily be overlooked in the notes, and they may inadvertently receive blood unwillingly. Ignoring the patient's requests and giving blood (F) can amount to grievous bodily harm, prosecutable in the criminal courts of England, so this is entirely unacceptable. Asking a patient to give monetary compensation for their different beliefs (D) is unprofessional and goes against much of what the National Health Service stands for. Finally, option A is also inappropriate; as an FY1, advising patients on surgical options for serious conditions is beyond your competence and is best left to more senior doctors.

Recommended reading

General Medical Council (2008), Explanatory guidance, in *Consent: Patients and Doctors Making Decisions Together*, paragraphs 44–50.

Joint UK Blood Transfusion and Tissue Transplantation Services: www. transfusionguidelines.org.uk.

Mental Capacity Act 2005, Advanced decision to refuse specified medical treatment.

4.37 Advanced directive

B D A C E

Advanced directives allow people to make decisions about their medical care should they lack the capacity to do so in the future. Like wills, they do not need to be signed by a lawyer, but it adds to their credibility if they are. They should as a minimum be signed by the patient and by a witness. Relatives are not allowed to overrule the advanced directive unless they have lasting power of attorney (whereby the patient signs over their power for decision-making to someone else in case of lack of capacity). The patient can overrule the advanced directive themselves if they retain capacity. It would be appropriate in cases where there is conflict over the statements in the advanced directive to contact the lawyer who has countersigned it to check its legal validity (B). The second best option is D, which also includes getting more help and information, this time from a medico-legal point of view. Your malpractice insurer is there to offer advice and guidance on the legality of complex ethical and legal scenarios. The next best responses are to talk sympathetically with the patient's wife (options A and C). Your registrar probably has more experience with advanced directives and should ideally speak to the patient's wife with you (A), rather than you alone (C). The only truly inappropriate response here is to treat the patient with antibiotics without further investigation into the validity of the advanced directive (E). This can amount to assault. There are some circumstances when you can challenge the validity of an advanced directive; if treatment options have significantly improved since the directive, which they do not specify in the document, if the person's religion has changed to be one that forbids declining treatment or if you believe that the patient may have been coerced or entered into the advanced directive without sound mind.

Your medico-legal insurer would be able to give you advice on how to challenge an advanced directive, should you feel the need to do so.

Recommended reading
Mental Capacity Act 2005.

4.38 Refusal of treatment

C   A   E
Adults who have capacity have the right to refuse treatment. Any decisions that they make must be respected, even if this may result in their death. It is therefore important in this scenario to establish whether this patient has the capacity to decide whether she wishes to receive oxygen (C). This is a difficult situation, and assessing capacity can be difficult. It would therefore be prudent to ask for support from someone more senior, such as your registrar and/or your consultant (options A and E). It would be inappropriate at this stage to complete a DNACPR form (B), given that capacity has not yet been established. Similarly, it would be inappropriate to leave the oxygen off indefinitely (G) or to sedate the patient against her wishes without any assessment of capacity (H). A seemingly irrational decision is not necessarily an indication of mental illness, so seeking advice from a psychiatrist is not necessary (F). Calling the crash team is also unnecessary at this stage (D). The solution to the deterioration in the patient's condition is oxygen, which you are equipped to provide, if appropriate, without the help of the crash team.

Recommended reading
General Medical Council (2008), Explanatory guidance, in *Consent: Patients and Doctors Making Decisions Together*, paragraph 5, 43; Legal annex.

4.39 Capacity

E   B   A   C   D
In order for a patient's consent to be valid, the patient must have the capacity to make a decision about the proposed investigation or treatment. Capacity may fluctuate and can be affected by factors such as pain, confusion or problems with memory. In this scenario, it is important to discuss your observations with your consultant (E). The issues surrounding capacity and consent can be difficult and should ideally be handled by a senior. In addition, the consultant may have felt that, at the time of gaining consent, the patient had the capacity to make the decision, although she may have subsequently forgotten some of what was discussed. Assessing the patient's capacity yourself is also a suitable response (B). The patient may simply need some extra assistance, such as a written explanation of the procedure to keep as a reminder. The nursing staff should have a good insight into the patient's normal state and may be able to give you information about whether they feel that the patient has deteriorated (A). However, even if the patient has deteriorated, she may still have capacity, which is why option B is preferable. Cancelling the colonoscopy at this

point (C) is inappropriate since you have not assessed the patient's capacity. To continue with the colonoscopy without addressing your concerns (D) goes against your duty as a doctor and therefore ranks last.

Recommended reading
General Medical Council (2008), Explanatory guidance, in *Consent: Patients and Doctors Making Decisions Together*, paragraphs 62–74.

4.40 Patient unsafe at home

C D B A E

In this scenario, your first priority should be to establish whether the patient has capacity to make this decision (C). Regardless of whether the patient has capacity or not, you should try and reduce the patient's risk of falls and contemplate whether the patient may be safe if they have increased care and help at home (D). Getting the patient's family involved (B) would be very useful; however, the decision ultimately rests with the patient and the healthcare professionals involved in their care. Asking a psychiatrist to assess capacity (A) should only be an option when you and your seniors have attempted this yourself and are not confident about reaching a decision. Telling a patient that they are unable to return home (E) would be a deprivation of their liberty and should only be carried out if they are deemed not to have capacity, and subsequent measures to increase safety at home have failed.

Recommended reading
Medical Protection Society (2012), Patient autonomy and consent, in *MPS Guide to Ethics: A Map for the Moral Maze*, chapter 8.

4.41 Family disagreement

E D B A C

Sometimes it can be difficult to take on board the concerns and beliefs of relatives as well as the patient. You should bear in mind that, on the whole, they are also putting the patient's safety and well-being first. In this situation, the most appropriate action to take would be option E. This would enable the family to speak to all professionals concerned with their mother's care and would give them the chance to voice their opinions and concerns. Informing the therapy team and asking them to carry out further assessments (D) may prove useful as they could bear in mind the family's concerns and may come to a different conclusion. Advising the family to discuss this with your consultant (B) would not be as useful as an MDT meeting as your consultant would be unlikely to be able to provide information about physiotherapy and occupational therapy findings. Option A would be unhelpful and inappropriate as you should be considerate to those close to your patient. Telling the patient to go into nursing care (C) would be highly inappropriate, and you should not coerce a patient into making a decision.

Recommended reading
General Medical Council (2013), *Good Medical Practice*, paragraph 33.

4.42 Dementia and capacity

E   A   C   D   B

Dementia is a common illness and will be seen frequently during the foundation years. Patients with dementia can often be confused or disorientated. Capacity to give consent and mental illness are therefore common problems that are faced. The cardinal rule, which must be remembered, is outlined in Section 1 of the Mental Capacity Act (MCA) 2005: 'a person must be assumed to have capacity unless it is established that they lack capacity'. A diagnosis of dementia does not mean that a patient lacks capacity to make decisions. Furthermore, it is important to remember that capacity is decision-specific and time-specific, making the previous consent documents in this case irrelevant. The best course of action would be to attempt to assess the patient's capacity (E). This should be a skill an FY1 doctor can complete, and the results of the assessment would then be discussed with your senior colleagues before taking further action. Discussing the situation with her family and your consultant (A) would be the next most appropriate course of action. The patient may be at risk of malnutrition, and an NG feeding tube may be in her best interests. Requesting a psychiatric review (C) may prove to be helpful; however, a competent FY1 doctor should be able to carry out a capacity assessment alone. While abandoning the procedure (D) would avoid violating the patient's rights, it would also not help to solve her nutritional needs. The least appropriate response would be to assume she lacks capacity (B), which is clearly contradicted by the MCA.

Recommended reading
General Medical Council (2008), Explanatory guidance, in *Consent: Patients and Doctors Making Decisions Together*, paragraph 71.
Mental Capacity Act (2005), chapter 9, pp. 5–6.

4.43 Depression and capacity

B   C   D

This is a complex situation that involves issues of mental illness, free will and possibly capacity. You would not be expected to try to make any decision yourself about the use of the law here (options G and H). Indeed, you cannot treat medical conditions under the Mental Health Act (H) in any case, and full assessment would be needed before using the Mental Capacity Act (G). Option F is inappropriate as patients must be assumed to have capacity to make a decision until proved otherwise and making an unwise or life-threatening decision does not indicate lack of capacity. It would be unfair to put the responsibility on the daughter to convince her father (A). Indeed, if she were to coerce him in any way, his consent would be invalid. Firstly, you should carry out a full mental and physical assessment of the patient (C).

Once you are prepared with this information, you should then refer him to liaison psychiatry (D). Given the need to involve psychiatry, you should leave any decision to start anti-depressant treatment to them (E). You will also need senior support from within your team, so your registrar should be involved (B).

Recommended reading
General Medical Council (2008), Explanatory guidance, in *Consent: Patients and Doctors Making Decisions Together*, Part 3, paragraphs 62–76.

4.44 Delirium and consent to investigation

A D G

In this situation, it is clear that the ABG is in the patient's best interests. Delirium is a medical emergency and assessing the gas partial pressures and acid–base status of the patient is vital. Options which involve either delaying (C) or declining to perform the procedure (H) are not appropriate. Likewise, abandoning the test if the patient is distressed (F) is not one of the best answers because the results will not be obtained, and an ABG is well recognised to be a painful test; therefore, it is inevitable that some distress will be caused. Next of kin do not have a right to consent for patients who lack capacity to make a decision (B); the responsibility for choosing the action in the patient's best interests lies with the medical team. While it is not desirable to have to restrain the patient, this is important for both your safety and theirs during the test and can be achieved gently and safely (A). You should document in the notes that you performed the test without consent, why the patient was unable to consent and why it was necessary to proceed (D). Lack of capacity is decision-specific and time-specific, so you should never declare a patient to be globally lacking in capacity (E). Even if you don't think the patient can understand, you should always treat them with respect and kindness and explain what you are doing throughout the procedure (G).

Recommended reading
General Medical Council (2008), Explanatory guidance, in *Consent: Patients and Doctors Making Decisions Together*, Part 3, paragraphs 62–76.
Medical Protection Society (2012), Patient autonomy and consent, section: Capacity, The 'best interest' principle, in *MPS Guide to Ethics: A Map for the Moral Maze*, chapter 8.

4.45 Child autonomy

D B C A E

If a patient initially declines a procedure, you should try to verbally persuade them to provide informed consent by ensuring they understand what is involved and the risks and benefits involved (D). It would be inappropriate to forcefully perform the blood test in a normally developing child of this age (E) as they should be allowed to take decisions about their care as much as is safe. Although option A is better because it does not use physical force, it is still an attempt to perform the test without the child's consent, and it could be dangerous if they were to physically resist. Option C is better than A because it is safe; however, you should try to tackle the problem proactively rather than just accepting and recording the refusal. Deferring to your registrar (B) actively ensures that the issue is dealt with but is not as good as trying to resolve it yourself. However, if this fails, it may be reasonable to escalate, given the complex capacity issues in question.

Recommended reading
General Medical Council (2007), Explanatory guidance, in *0–18 Years: Guidance for all Doctors*, paragraphs 22–41.

4.46 Withholding treatment

B E G

The Mental Capacity Act states that, even if this decision does not seem to be in their best interests, patients are within their rights to refuse treatment as long as they have the capacity to make the decision. In this case, the first thing that you should do is assess the patient's capacity to refuse treatment (B). Option G should also be high on your list of priorities as, by trying to find out the reasons for refusing treatment, you may find something you can help with. Despite the patient asking you not to tell your consultant, this is not something that, as an FY1, you should be dealing with alone, and therefore, asking your consultant for help is important (E). Simply carrying on with the cannula against the patient's wishes (C) could be seen as assault and should not be attempted. Option D maybe necessary once you have assessed the patient, but if she has an acute infection requiring IV antibiotics, a referral to psychiatry will not be useful in the short term, and she may well be suffering from delirium that will most likely resolve on treatment. Placing the cannula purely for hydration (A) is something that can be considered if she does decline treatment but should not be your first course of action. Neither options F nor H should be used in this instance as, if the patient is assessed to have capacity, it is her right to refuse treatment, and section 2 of the Mental Health Act can only be used for assessment and treatment of psychiatric disorders, not for physical disease.

Recommended reading
General Medical Council (2013), *Good Medical Practice*, paragraphs 31–33.
Medical Protection Society (2012), Patient autonomy and consent, in *MPS Guide to Ethics: A Map for the Moral Maze*, chapter 8.
Mental Capacity Act (2005), http://www.legislation.gov.uk/ukpga/2005/9/section/1

4.47 Questioning consent

E A D C B

It is crucial that the patient is fully informed about any treatment they are consenting to. Therefore, the best response here is option E as hopefully in doing this, you will either learn that you were in fact mistaken, or the registrar will be prompted to go back to the patient and add to the list of risks of the procedure already discussed. This also avoids undermining the registrar in front of the patient, which will not only damage your professional relationship but could also risk the patient losing trust in their clinical ability. While openly challenging the registrar (A) seems confrontational, it is better than option D since, as an FY1, you are not trained to consent people for theatre. It is better that the registrar is reminded of their omissions in front of the patient so that they can amend the consent form, than you doing this without their knowledge. If you stay behind to further consent the patient, this won't be recorded on the consent form, leaving the surgeon with the possibility of legal action if any of these risks occur. Using this as an opportunity to do further research (C) ranks higher than ignoring your concerns (B) as, although not helping this patient, at least you will be able to apply this knowledge to similar situations in the future.

Recommended reading

General Medical Council (2008), Explanatory guidance, in *Consent: Patients and Doctors Making Decisions Together*, paragraphs 47–49.

Medical Protection Society (2012), Patient autonomy and consent, in *MPS Guide to Ethics: A Map for the Moral Maze*, chapter 8.

4.48 Consultant decisions

E A B C D

Option E ranks highest since consultants still need guidance as to how they work to aid their continuing professional development. In addition, under the General Medical Council's (GMC) consent guidance, doctors *must* listen to and respect their patient's views and share all information with patients to facilitate their decision-making. This is key to gaining informed consent. Asking your consultant to further explain the management of the condition to you and why he recommends surgery over other therapies to aid your understanding (A) is good practice, but it will not help the patient in the first instance. Option B, while potentially looking like you are not helping the situation, is better than C and D since, in these responses, you are overstepping your knowledge and responsibility as an FY1. This could be seen as undermining your consultant, which has the potential to make your working environment very difficult. In particular, suggesting that the patient makes a complaint about your consultant (D) is wholly inappropriate.

Recommended reading

General Medical Council (2008), Explanatory guidance, in *Consent: Patients and Doctors Making Decisions Together*, paragraphs 1, 2.

Medical Protection Society (2012), Patient autonomy and consent, in *MPS Guide to Ethics: A Map for the Moral Maze*, chapter 8.

4.49 Consent for children

B D A E C

Consent in children is a difficult area for doctors, and it is always important to consult more senior colleagues. In this patient, at the age of 15, she could be deemed able to consent as long as you can prove that she is Gillick competent, making option B the best response here. Gillick competency is a medico-legal term that applies to treatment decisions in patients under 16 years of age. If a minor is deemed competent to retain the necessary information and use it to weigh up the pros and cons of a decision, they are said to be Gillick competent, and a procedure can continue without the parents' consent. If she is deemed to be unable to give consent, in an emergency, you can still operate on her without her parents' consent under the principle of best interests (D). Trying to get consent from another relative (A) is not desirable as, if they do not have direct caring rights for the child, they are not usually allowed to consent the patient. However, this may be the only option available to you and should be considered if all other avenues have been exhausted. Waiting for the parents to make contact (options C and E) is not plausible as this patient urgently needs an operation, and it would risk further deterioration. Recording in the notes the reasons why you could not consent the patient is important (E), but it still leaves you doing nothing to address the underlying reason for why the patient requires to go to theatre.

Recommended reading

General Medical Council (2008), Explanatory guidance, in *Consent: Patients and Doctors Making Decisions Together*, paragraph 79.

Medical Protection Society (July 2012), Factsheet, in *Consent – Children and Young People*.

4.50 Coercion

C D G

In this scenario, as the FY1, you can only advise Edith and her daughter-in-law about the treatment options and alert the consultant to your concerns; you are not in a position to make any decisions for her regarding the optimal treatment. Giving basic treatment information and deferring the decisive component of the conversation to your consultant (C) therefore encompasses all of these things. Option G is true: Edith is the person who will sign the consent form, therefore, ultimately the method of treatment has to be her choice. Option D is also appropriate as this will allow you to find out Edith's ideas and concerns without the worry of upsetting her daughter-in-law. Ignoring your analysis of the situation (A) is unprofessional as this does not make the patient's care your first concern and therefore goes against one of your duties as a doctor. Option B involves only communicating the risks of one procedure and the benefits of another. This would give a biased view of the possible treatment options, which, conversely is as bad as, if not worse than, the daughter-in-law deciding the best course of action for your patient. Options E and H are also not appropriate as you risk antagonising the daughter-in-law. Option F is true in that, as an FY1, you can only suggest treatment options; however, saying you don't fully understand them would be lying and is therefore deceitful.

Recommended reading
General Medical Council (2008), Explanatory guidance, in *Consent Guidance: Patients and Doctors Making Decisions Together*, paragraphs 41, 42.
General Medical Council (2013), Duties of a doctor, in *Good Medical Practice*.
Medical Protection Society (2012), Patient autonomy and consent, in *MPS Guide to Ethics: A Map for the Moral Maze*, chapter 8.

4.51 Ectopic pregnancy

A C B D E
This is a question of assessing whether a patient has sufficient capacity to make a decision. It is generally accepted that if a person under 16 is deemed 'Gillick competent' (i.e. able to fully rationalise the advantages and disadvantages of a decision), then they are able to make their own decisions, and you have to respect their right to confidentiality, provided that you do not believe them to be at risk. In this situation, you may deem the patient to be Gillick competent, but you should try gently to persuade her that she should tell her parents first (A). A nurse is often a good source of non-threatening support in these situations. If the patient still flatly refuses, maintaining confidentiality at this stage would be acceptable too (C). It would not be wrong to discuss this situation with your clinical supervisor (B); however, this is an acute situation, and doing this may delay urgent treatment and investigations. Option D would be inappropriate if you deem her competent as this would be going against the patient's wishes; however, at 15 years old, she is still regarded as a child in the eyes of the law, so it would be more appropriate than refusing medical treatment (E).

Recommended reading
General Medical Council (2008), Explanatory guidance, in *Consent: Patients and Doctors Making Decisions Together*; Legal annex.
General Medical Council (2013), Duties of a doctor, in *Good Medical Practice*.
General Medical Council (2013), *Good Medical Practice*, paragraphs 17, 31, 47, 49, 50.
Medical Protection Society (2012), Patient autonomy and consent, in *MPS Guide to Ethics: A Map for the Moral Maze*, chapter 8.
Wheeler R. (2006), Gillick or Fraser? A plea for consistency over competence in children, *BMJ*, 332, 807.

4.52 Coercion

D C B A E
While doctors are required to respect patients' autonomy, it is also important that you ensure decisions are made of their own free will. In the case

of a competent adult who changes their mind, it is necessary to explore the reasons why. Option D is the best response in this scenario as, in cases like this, it is firstly important to maintain good communication within your team, and as an FY1, it is a good idea to ask someone more senior, with more experience of treating the patient's condition, to come with you to talk to them. This is why option D is preferable to C; however, being party to these discussions can be a valuable learning opportunity for junior doctors. Option C also ensures that the patient receives the information they need and would demonstrate good communication skills on your part, which should be maintained at all times. As previously mentioned, it is important to explore why he has changed his mind (B) and to ensure that it is definitely his decision, with no overt pressure or coercion from his son. Talking to the son may be appropriate and taking a nurse with you is often a good idea (A); however, your first priority should be to talk to the patient. Option E would be inappropriate and demonstrates both unprofessional behaviour and a lack of respect for the son.

Recommended reading

General Medical Council (2008), Explanatory guidance, in *Consent: Patients and Doctors Making Decisions Together*.

General Medical Council (2009), *The New Doctor*, paragraphs 6, 9, 10.

General Medical Council (2013), Duties of a doctor, in *Good Medical Practice*.

General Medical Council (2013), *Good Medical Practice*, paragraphs 14–17, 27, 31, 33–36, 44, 46–49, 68.

Medical Protection Society (2012), Patient autonomy and consent, in *MPS Guide to Ethics: A Map for the Moral Maze*, chapter 8.

4.53 Terminal diagnosis

A   B   E   C   D

No one else can make decisions for a competent adult, unless they specifically indicate that they do not want to be involved in their treatment. Furthermore, you should not withhold information from patients, unless you think that the information may cause real harm to the patient. 'Harm' should be more than the patient becoming upset, and you should not be influenced by what a patient's relatives ask you to do. In this scenario, the patient has a right to know about her terminal diagnosis as soon as possible. This is a complicated and delicate situation, however, and is probably best handled by someone more senior, such as your consultant (A). It is also appropriate to encourage the family to tell the patient about her condition themselves (B). While option E also gives the family the opportunity to tell the patient, giving them an ultimatum risks damaging your relationship with them and would be unprofessional. To tell the patient yourself, without consulting the patient's family (C), is inappropriate and would certainly damage your relationship with them. Failing to ensure that the patient is informed about her terminal diagnosis (D) does not fulfil your responsibility to the patient and is therefore unacceptable.

Recommended reading

General Medical Council (2008), Explanatory guidance, in *Consent: Patients and Doctors Making Decisions Together*, paragraphs 13–17.

4.54 Cancer diagnosis disclosure

C   B   D   A   E

This question relates to the underlying principles of confidentiality. If the patient has specifically asked for this information not to be disclosed to his family, his wishes should be kept (C). It would also be appropriate to advise the wife to talk to her husband about this issue (B). Option D is less appropriate as the patient has already expressed his wishes; he may, however, change his mind if he realises that the current situation of his family not knowing his diagnosis may be causing them more distress. Option A is not appropriate as the consultant would only say the same things that you can, so passing on a difficult situation that you can handle yourself is not ideal. It may be unavoidable, however, if the situation escalates, and the patient's wife cannot be placated by a conversation with you. Option E is the least appropriate response as this involves breaching patient confidentiality against the patient's specific wishes.

Recommended reading

General Medical Council (2009), Explanatory guidance, in *Confidentiality*, paragraph 6.

4.55 Relative phones ward

B   A   E   D   C

It is tempting to provide information in this context because the caller claims to be a close relative and the questions asked are very basic. However, you do not know what the patient's relationship with his mother is like and whether he would even want her to know where he is. Ideally this dilemma would be solved by speaking to the patient yourself and asking him how he would like the situation to be handled (B). The next best responses involve not disclosing any information at all. The nurse in charge would be a good person to involve if you had concerns (A), although it would be better to handle it yourself. Option E is quite rude and unhelpful but at least does not involve disclosing any confidential information. By stating that you cannot discuss how the patient is doing (D), you have acknowledged that he is your patient and is on the ward, which is a fact he may not wish to be disclosed. The worst action in this situation is to answer the caller's questions (C) since, without the patient's permission, this breaches their confidentiality.

Recommended reading

General Medical Council (2009), Explanatory guidance, in *Confidentiality*, paragraphs 9, 64.

4.56 Giving information to relatives

D F H

The daughters must not be given any information about their father's condition without explicitly seeking his consent for this. It would be inappropriate to inform them that their father has cancer (B), even if this conversation were to take place with a more senior doctor (A). It is also inappropriate to indicate the level of care he will require or to assume that he would want to be cared for by them (options C and E). However, it is rude to refuse to speak to the daughters and would cause conflict with their father if you suggest that he has information he has not shared with them (G). You should therefore listen politely and attentively to their concerns (F) before explaining that you are not able to give the information they are asking for (D). It would be helpful to discuss the situation with the patient to find out his wishes and offer support in disclosing the information to them if he wanted to (H).

Recommended reading

General Medical Council (2009), Explanatory guidance, in *Confidentiality*, paragraphs 6–11.
General Medical Council (2013), *Good Medical Practice*, paragraphs 46–48.

4.57 Safeguarding

C E D A B

This question requires you to maintain patient confidentiality in a situation that may have safeguarding implications. You should meet your professional duties in the context of an FY1 doctor; therefore, it would be appropriate to seek advice from a senior colleague. Your clinical supervisor would be the best-placed person for this (C). Maintaining a trusting relationship and open communication with the patient is very important and a skill that is expected of all doctors; therefore, it may be wise to talk to the patient (a competent adult) to make sure that there is nothing else she wishes to disclose in confidence (E). If you are concerned about the welfare of one of your patients, the General Medical Council (GMC) states that disclosing patient information is appropriate if failing to do so may put the patient or others at serious risk or if it is likely to help in the prevention or detection of a serious crime. Social services may be useful if the patient is known to them already or simply as a source of advice on further action (D). While nurses are very good at talking to patients and it may be helpful to have them present during difficult conversations, you should not shirk your professional responsibility to protect your patient by passing on all responsibility to uncover the information you need to another colleague (A). Speaking to the parents may, in fact, put the patient at risk of more harm and you should seek advice from senior colleagues or those with more experience in dealing with such manners first (B).

Recommended reading

General Medical Council (2012), Explanatory guidance, in *Protecting Children and Young People: The Responsibility of all Doctors*.
General Medical Council (2013), Duties of a doctor, in *Good Medical Practice*.
General Medical Council (2013), *Good Medical Practice*, paragraphs 12, 14, 15, 16, 23, 25, 27, 31, 50, 73.
Medical Protection Society (2012), Confidentiality, in *MPS Guide to Ethics: A Map for the Moral Maze*, chapter 9.

4.58 STI testing

D E A B C
This is an ethically interesting question because, although your patient is below the age of consent, he could still be sexually active; however, you cannot make any assumptions, so you will have to ask some difficult questions.

Option D, to ask his mother to wait outside while you take the appropriate history, is the most suitable response as it is important to collect all the relevant medical information, and you are unlikely to get this with his mother in the room. Stalling until your registrar is available to review the patient (E) is a good option if you are unhappy about asking such sensitive questions; however, the registrar may not be happy that you left this task to them. Ignoring the patient's autonomy and proceeding to the examination, asking the mother for consent (B), is not appropriate when considering the Gillick principles. Even though this is not an encounter about contraception, if you think that your patient has the capacity to consent to sex, you should apply the same principles here, which therefore means that your patient deserves confidentiality. Lying to the patient and his mother about the reason for a urine test (C) is wholly inappropriate.

Recommended reading

General Medical Council (2007), Explanatory guidance, in *0–18 Years: Guidance for all Doctors*, paragraph 42–45, 64–73.

4.59 Mental health consent

C E B D A
If patients are kept in hospital under section for treatment of a mental health illness (section 3), this applies to treatment of the mental health illness only. As part of their mental health illness, they are deemed not to have the capacity to refuse treatment for their mental health illness. They may, however, have capacity to make decisions about other illnesses they have. The best option is to try and consider some other avenues of treatment as you would with any patient who was suffering side effects from treatment. So arranging a follow-up appointment with their haematologist (C) is the best response. Seeking advice from a senior doctor would also be appropriate (E). This is a potentially life-threatening decision that the patient is making, so it shouldn't be made lightly. Your registrar would probably want to speak to the patient themselves about their change of heart. Option B is ranked third; if a patient withdraws consent for treatment you

cannot continue that treatment unless they are proven to lack the capacity to make that decision, in which case it can then be given in their best interests. Until a formal capacity assessment is made, you cannot continue to treat this patient against their will. Thinking about the end of life and making plans regarding end of life should not be considered suicidal ideation, so moving your patient to a more secure ward (D) is unfair to your patient, and this option is ranked low. The least appropriate answer is option A, which involves continuing to treat your patient without their consent because they are under section 3. As mentioned earlier, you cannot treat patients under section 3 against their will for anything but their mental health disorder, unless you also have proof that they lack capacity. Treating without consent a competent adult amounts to assault.

Recommended reading
General Medical Council (2013), Legal annex, Common law: Refusal of treatment, in *Consent*.

4.60 Inappropriate images on laptop

B D E

This is a serious situation to be faced with, and one which raises a number of difficult issues, the most important being concerns about your colleague's fitness to practise. Informing your own clinical supervisor (E) will ensure that you have the necessary support for taking steps to deal with the issue you have come across. This is an illegal activity, so although it seems drastic, the police should be involved (B). It would also be necessary to contact the GMC (D) as they will be able to determine the best course of action regarding your colleague's professional licence. The other options, while mostly sensible, will therefore rank lower than these three, which are the most appropriate responses. Ideally, your colleague needs to face the situation and inform his clinical supervisor himself, but if needs be, you will have to report the issue yourself (C). While investigation into whether your colleague will have contact with children in the workplace might help you decide how urgent the issue is (G), you will still have to report it regardless of whether this is likely to happen. Agreeing with (A) or even offering to help (H) your colleague would involve not reporting the issue, so these options are inappropriate. You may even be implicated yourself by carrying out either of these courses of action. It is not your place to interrogate your colleague (F), and this should be left to your senior colleagues, the GMC and the police.

Recommended reading
General Medical Council (2013), *Good Medical Practice*, paragraph 25.

4.61 Wrong site surgery

B E H

Wrong site surgery is a National Patient Safety Agency 'never event'. In this situation, your duty of care lies with the patient, and you should not be afraid

302 Chapter 4: Patient Focus

to raise your concerns despite your consultant's seniority. Your priority in this situation would be to postpone or delay the operation until the correct site has been confirmed. Options B and E, asking the consultant to stop and discuss or to review the x-rays, would allow you to delay the operation until the documentation has been checked. Option H would also be a safe option as it would announce your concerns to the whole surgical team. Informing the SpR (G) of your concerns would not necessarily prevent a potential wrong site surgery as they may not relay these concerns to the consultant operating on the patient. Although the consultant will have examined the woman before operating on her, allowing him to continue (F) would not be appropriate if you have concerns. Asking to see the pre-operative notes (D) or asking the nurse to view the patient's notes (C) will identify the correct site for the operation, but these responses might not delay the initial incision. Asking the consultant to operate on the other limb without checking any documentation or images (A) is potentially dangerous and is not good practice.

Recommended reading
National Patient Safety Agency, *Never Events Framework 2009/10*.

4.62 Chaperones

B A C E D
This situation is difficult because a DRE should be part of the examination of any patient presenting with lower abdominal pain, constipation or a history of lower or upper gastrointestinal bleeding. Therefore, if you feel that there is a clinical need, the examination should always be performed. However, this examination can sometimes wait if the patient is not acutely unwell. In this scenario, the patient is not acutely unwell, and therefore, the examination could wait, making option B the most appropriate response to ensure that you are practising safely. Awaiting one of the nurses to be free to chaperone for you is sensible (A), although this may be difficult if the shift is busy. If the patient does not wish to be chaperoned (and they are deemed to have capacity), then you can perform the examination, but it is vital that you make sure that this is documented clearly in the notes for legal reasons (C). If there is no one to chaperone at all, and you do not feel comfortable performing the examination, then document this clearly in the notes, and the day team can perform the examination tomorrow (E). Relatives should not be used as chaperones under any circumstances, so this is the least appropriate response (D).

Recommended reading
General Medical Council (2013), Explanatory guidance, *Intimate Examinations and Chaperones*.
Medical Protection Society (2012), Morality and decency, section: Chaperones, in *MPS Guide to Ethics: A Map for the Moral Maze*, chapter 5.

4.63 End-of-life HW

B C D A E

In this scenario, you need to ensure that the patient understands the full implications of their situation and that they are not just 'being made as comfortable as possible'. The best thing to do therefore is to ask the registrar to go and re-explain the situation to the patient, to make absolutely sure that they understand (B). The next best response is to discuss the consultation with the registrar (C) as this may prompt them to return to the patient. Following this, it is best if a doctor who was present at the initial conversation re-explains the situation, so this could be you (D), although ideally your registrar should be the one to do this as they have more clinical experience. In addition, you must be careful that your actions are not construed as being undermining. Asking a nurse to have this conversation (A) is not appropriate as the nurse should not be left to explain things about the end of life to a patient. However, this would be better than failing to act on your concerns (E), which would be both unprofessional and unethical.

Recommended reading

Balaban RB. (March 2000), A physician's guide to talking about end-of-life care, *Journal of General Internal Medicine*, 15, 3.

4.64 Chaperone declined

A E G

It would be potentially detrimental to the patient's health to omit the examination, so you should agree to examine them alone (A) as long as you don't have a personal objection to this. It would be against their wishes to insist on a chaperone being present (H). Having a nurse in the room (B) would therefore make the experience distressing and undermine the patient's trust in you. As you don't know the nature of the patient's relationship with the relative present, it could cause extreme embarrassment if you asked them to observe the examination (C). The examination is important for the patient's care, so it should not be avoided if at all possible (F). It is unnecessary to ask a senior to perform the examination instead of you (D), and it will only cause delay and is therefore inappropriate. It is of vital importance that you document formally that a chaperone was offered and declined (E) in order to protect yourself against any allegation that you intentionally examined the patient unsupervised. It is important in all examinations or procedures to explain step-by-step what you are doing, but this is especially the case for intimate examinations (G).

Recommended reading

General Medical Council (2013), Explanatory guidance, in *Intimate Examinations and Chaperones*.

Medical Protection Society (2012), Morality and decency, section: Chaperones, *MPS Guide to Ethics: A Map for the Moral Maze*, chapter 5.

The UK Foundation Programme Curriculum (2012), Section 7.2: History and examination.

4.65 HIV avoiding blood test

C A E B D

You should not refuse treatment to a patient on the grounds of personal risk. The most appropriate response is therefore to carry out the procedure (C). The next best course of action would be to ask a colleague to do this for you (A) as that would still ensure that the patient received the test they need. However, it is arguably selfish to expect a colleague to expose themselves to a risk that you are unwilling to take on yourself. Handing the task over to the night team (E) is less appropriate than option A because it will delay the test unnecessarily, and it is also dishonest as it implies that you did not have time to carry out the test before the end of your shift. Options B and D rank lowest because neither make any attempt to ensure the test is performed. Documenting that you are declining to perform the test (B) is more appropriate, however, than claiming that the patient has refused the test (D), because the latter is dishonest and therefore deeply unprofessional.

Recommended reading

General Medical Council (2013), *Good Medical Practice*, paragraph 10.

4.66 Unable to get a chaperone

B A C E D

This is potentially a very serious situation and one that a foundation doctor may be faced with while working in the community. There is clear guidance produced by the General Medical Council (GMC) about intimate examinations and chaperones. The guidance suggests that a chaperone should always be offered to the patient prior to an intimate examination. If a chaperone is not available or if the patient doesn't want a chaperone, it is possible to delay the examination or refer them to a more appropriate colleague. However, with both of these courses of action, it is important to consider whether a delay in examination could adversely affect the patient's health. In this scenario, the patient could potentially be suffering from a severe haemorrhage and an examination is urgently required to assess whether she needs acute hospital admission. Therefore, as long as the patient is happy for the examination to continue, you should do so without waiting for a chaperone (B). This situation puts you in a difficult situation, so asking for support from an educational supervisor (who has more experience in similar scenarios) would be the next best response (A). Asking for a colleague to come to the patient's house (C) would ensure the examination is carried out, but it could delay her receiving the treatment she requires. Refusing to perform the examination and delaying her treatment is potentially life-threatening. However, given the choice of asking the patient to attend the clinic that afternoon (D) or immediately attend the hospital (E), attending the hospital would ensure any necessary treatment was available earlier.

Recommended reading
General Medical Council (2013), Explanatory guidance, in *Intimate Examinations and Chaperones.*

4.67 Drunk

A E G

In all areas of medicine, you are likely to encounter patients under the influence of alcohol or recreational substances. It is important not to discriminate against these patients by refusing or delaying treatment. Therefore, in this scenario, you should carry out a clinical assessment of the patient without delay (E) and to the best of your ability. This may be difficult if the patient continues being abusive, and you should make absolutely sure that your safety is always considered a priority. Making sure that the patient has regular clinical observations (A) until he is examined would also ensure that the patient is not being discriminated against and would make sure that any deterioration, which could indicate a serious injury or illness, is noticed. You should also challenge the nurse's comment (G), making them aware that in doing this they would be discriminating against the patient and informing them of the reasons why you need to examine the patient promptly. Examining the patient when they have sobered up (B) is unacceptable as this would delay their treatment, which could potentially be detrimental to their clinical care. Asking the nurses to restrain the patient (C) is unnecessary and likely to be counter-productive by antagonising the patient. Healthcare professionals can restrain a patient without capacity under common law only in an emergency situation if it is deemed to be absolutely necessary. Asking a senior colleague to examine the patient (D) would only be appropriate once you have tried to examine the patient yourself and encountered difficulty. Giving the patient sedation (F) would be dangerous before you have examined them and also unnecessary unless the patient poses an immediate threat to others or himself. Refusing to allow the patient access to emergency services (H) would be immoral and illegal; however, the department would be within their rights to discharge an abusive patient once serious pathology has been excluded.

Recommended reading
General Medical Council (2013), *Good Medical Practice*, paragraphs 57 and 59.
Malone D, Friedman T. (2005), Drunken patients in the general hospital: their care and management, *Postgraduate Medical Journal*, 81, 953.

4.68 Keeping promises

B D E

Your consultant has told you that the ward should not provide this service, and you must respect this decision (D). The consultant has to consider service planning and funding issues, which are important. Standing up to your consultant (F) is likely to cause unnecessary conflict between you because there are other solutions to this situation. It would also be disrespectful to your consultant if you try to get approval from a different consultant (G) when they have already told you not to provide the vaccine. You should not go against their advice and arrange to give the vaccine on the ward (options C and H). This would be unprofessional, and it is not necessary to keep your promise literally. As long as you try to make alternative arrangements for the parents (B), you are not letting them down. You should be honest and tell the parents the situation (E) rather than being avoidant and leaving them feeling that you have either forgotten or broken your promise (A).

Recommended reading

General Medical Council (2013), Duties of a doctor, in *Good Medical Practice.*
Medical Protection Society (2012), Professionalism and integrity, section:
    Keeping promises, in *MPS Guide to Ethics: A Map for the Moral Maze,*
    chapter 3.

4.69 Keeping promise to refer to dentist

A   C   E

This scenario raises a number of issues: working out of hours, referring patients and making promises. In this scenario, although it may seem that the patient has a fairly trivial issue, it could have great implications for his care. Not only are necrotic teeth a potential source of infection, they are also likely to be preventing him from eating a normal diet. The best course of action would be to make sure that the referral is made. It would be appropriate for either yourself (C) or your on-call FY1 colleague (E) to make the referral. This would ensure that your patient is reviewed and your promise has not been broken. Apologising to the patient ensures good communication, which could avoid any misunderstandings (A). Waiting until Monday (F) is not appropriate for the clinical reasons already stated. Despite the fact that painkillers will probably be appropriate (B), the referral to the maxillofacial surgeon is more important as it will offer senior definitive management. Informing the patient's dentist will also be necessary prior to discharge (H), but the priority here is to tackle the current issue of his broken tooth. Asking the consultant for help (D) would be appropriate for an unwell patient or for a patient who needed a senior review, but for day-to-day tasks this is not advised. Informing the human resources department could be appropriate if staying beyond your paid hours is an ongoing issue (G), but this is not the priority in this scenario.

Recommended reading

Medical Protection Society (2012), Professionalism and Integrity, section:
    Keeping promises, in *MPS Guide to Ethics: A Map for the Moral Maze,*
    chapter 3.

4.70 Drunk colleague

C   B   A   E   D

Part of the General Medical Council's (GMC) fitness to practise literally deals with physical fitness to practise medicine. If you are drunk or overtired, you are not safe to be treating patients. The best response here is to try and deal with things at source and advise your colleague to go home (C). Reporting this incident to a senior, such as your registrar, is the next most appropriate course of action (B). An overtired and possibly drunk FY1 puts patient safety at risk, and the team leader should be informed if one of their doctors is unfit to work. Option A is the third best response since, if you know that something about another doctor's practice is unsafe, it is your duty to do something about it, even if this means going above and beyond what you are usually expected to achieve in a day. Options that involve doing nothing are the least appropriate in this question (options D and E); however, doing nothing and then making the situation public on the internet (D) is worse than simply doing nothing at all (E).

Recommended reading

General Medical Council (2009), Explanatory guidance, in *Confidentiality*, Principles.

General Medical Council (2015), Declaration of fitness to practice: Guidance on declaring health issues.

Chapter 5

WORKING EFFECTIVELY AS PART OF A TEAM

QUESTIONS

5.1 Extra on-calls

You are an FY1 in orthopaedics. You notice that your colleague is doing many more on-call shifts than you and the rest of your colleagues on the rota.

Rank in order the following actions in response to this situation (1 = Most appropriate; 5 = Least appropriate).

A Alert your colleague and tell them to go and see the rota organiser.
B Do nothing.
C Tell your colleague that you can do half of their extra on-call shifts.
D Tell your colleague to contact the British Medical Association (BMA) to alert them that they are exceeding the European Working Time Directive (EWTD).
E Wait until a point in your rota where you will not be able to do many of their extra on-calls and then inform your colleague of the unequal work-load and offer to share their shifts.

5.2 Colleague faking illness

You are an FY1 in general medicine working a weekend on-call shift. Your colleague calls in sick, so you have to cover both on-call bleeps. Consequently, your shift is very busy. Later, you see pictures on a social media site of your colleague at a music festival, which you know took place on the weekend of your on-call shifts.

Rank in order the following actions in response to this situation (1 = Most appropriate; 5 = Least appropriate).

A Call in sick the next time that you do an on-call shift with your colleague.
B Confront them about where they were over the weekend.
C Discuss the situation with your colleague's consultant.
D Do nothing: it is easier to leave it alone.
E Tell them that you won't tell anyone if they do two of your next on-call shifts.

5.3 Colleague deleting records

You are an FY1 doctor working an on-call shift. You are reviewing several patients on the same ward. In each of the patients' medical notes, you notice that some of the previous entries have been erased from the notes with a permanent pen. It is not possible to read what the entries say, but they are all signed by an FY1 colleague of yours. The patients are stable and improving and you identify no issues with their care.

Rank in order the following actions in response to this situation (1 = Most appropriate; 5 = Least appropriate).

A   Confront your colleague and his team during the ward round.
B   Ignore the entries as they have clearly been deleted.
C   Inform your educational supervisor about what you have seen and ask for advice.
D   Investigate further to see whether you can decipher what has been erased and only take action if there is anything serious deleted.
E   Speak to your colleague in private about your concerns.

5.4 Failing to escalate care

You are an FY2 working in a hospital on a medical night shift. A nurse runs up to you and says that your FY1 colleague requires your help. She tells you that he has been dealing with an unwell patient for over an hour. She says she offered to telephone some senior for help over half an hour ago, but he refused help saying 'I've got everything under control'. You arrive to find your colleague attempting to insert a cannula. You briefly read through the management plan he has written and notice several omissions. You believe that the patient is likely to be suffering from sepsis, yet your colleague hasn't prescribed any empirical antibiotics. When you offer to help, your colleague refuses and asks you to leave.

Rank in order the following actions in response to this situation (1 = Most appropriate; 5 = Least appropriate).

A   Inform the medical registrar on nights that you have concerns about the patient.
B   Justify the rationale for your suggestions to the FY1 and offer to discuss the case further if required.
C   Raise your concerns with your colleague's educational supervisor at a future date.
D   Submit a formal complaint to your employer after your shift about your colleague's rudeness.
E   Tell your colleague to leave and take over the care of the patient immediately.

5.5 Registrar prescribing against protocol

You are an FY1 working on a medical team. One of your patients develops an infection. Your registrar tells you to prescribe two antibiotics. However, you know from previous cases that the hospital anti-microbial protocol describes a different treatment regimen.

Rank in order the following actions in response to this situation (1 = Most appropriate; 5 = Least appropriate).

A Discuss the protocol with your registrar, and go ahead and prescribe whichever option they decide on.
B Discuss the protocol with your registrar, and only make the prescription yourself if the registrar agrees to the protocol antibiotics.
C Don't discuss your concerns with your registrar, and prescribe the antibiotics that they had requested.
D Don't discuss your concerns with your registrar, and prescribe the protocol antibiotics.
E Tell your registrar that their choice is against hospital protocol and you are therefore not prepared to write the prescription they have suggested.

5.6 Getting help when beyond limits of skills

You are an FY1 working on a medical ward at night. One of the patients has become acutely psychotic overnight, making delusional statements and being physically threatening towards staff, including hitting one of the nurses. Your registrar asks you to get psychiatric assistance immediately, prior to being urgently called away to a cardiac arrest. However, when you bleep the on-call psychiatrist, they decline to come see the patient until the following morning, telling you to use an emergency holding order to keep the patient in hospital until then, if necessary.

Choose the **THREE most appropriate** actions to take in this situation.

A Barricade the patient in their room.
B Call hospital security.
C Call the police.
D Call your consultant at home for advice.
E Fast-bleep your registrar and ask them to come back to the ward.
F Get senior nursing support from the site manager.
G Give an injection of anti-psychotic medication to calm the patient down.
H Make sure the nurse is alright and administer first aid if required.

5.7 Sick patients

You are working on a general medical ward. One of your patients, a 45-year-old woman, has been complaining of haematemesis for the last 12 hours, vomiting small amounts of blood on a regular basis. She has no previous history of this. You review her, and although she feels well clinically, you notice her systolic blood pressure is only 85 mmHg, and her full blood count shows a drop in haemoglobin by 2 g/dL in the last 48 hours. You feel that she needs an endoscopy, so you contact your specialist registrar for advice, but they disagree.

Rank in order the following actions in response to this situation (1 = Most appropriate; 5 = Least appropriate).

A   Ask your senior house officer (SHO) who is also currently on the ward.
B   Contact your consultant for advice and voice your concerns.
C   Follow the advice of the registrar.
D   Leave the matter for now but go back and review the patient in an hour to see if they are still feeling well.
E   Refer the patient for an upper GI endoscopy, despite the advice of the registrar.

5.8 Inadequate equipment

You are working a night shift covering medicine and are contacted to assess a patient whose oxygen saturations have fallen to 75%. You adopt an ABCDE approach and decide to give the patient oxygen, take an arterial blood gas (ABG) and some blood tests and arrange an electrocardiogram (ECG). However, you cannot find the equipment necessary for obtaining an arterial blood sample, and the nurses on the ward are also unable to help you locate this.

Rank in order the following actions in response to this situation (1 = Most appropriate; 5 = Least appropriate).

A   Ask a nurse to ring around other nearby wards to try and locate the equipment while you stay with the patient.
B   Ask one of your senior house officers (SHO) to stay with the patient while you locate the ABG equipment you need.
C   Contact the on-call medical registrar and explain the situation to them to get advice.
D   Decide not to do the ABG as you can't find the necessary equipment but tell the nurses to get back in contact with you if the patient deteriorates further.
E   Go to the other wards and try to locate the ABG equipment yourself.

5.9 Leaving sick patients

It is 10 minutes until your FY1 on-call shift finishes, and you are asked to see an unwell patient who has acute chest pain and has become tachycardic and tachypnoeic. You assess the patient and decide that they need an echocardiogram (ECG), a full set of bloods, an arterial blood gas (ABG) and a chest x-ray. After your full assessment, you realise that your shift should have finished 20 minutes ago, but your plan needs to be commenced.

Choose the **THREE most appropriate** actions to take in this situation.

A   Ask the clinical support workers to take the bloods and ECG while you do the other jobs.
B   Ask the nurses to pass on the message to the on-call doctors to complete the task; then go home.

C Inform the evening senior house officer (SHO) of this patient and ask them to complete the required jobs.

D Inform the on-call registrar of this patient and ask them to complete the required jobs.

E Inform the SHO of the patient and offer to complete the jobs if they are currently looking after other acutely ill patients.

F Put out a crash call to summon senior doctors quickly to look after this patient; then leave.

G Stay late to complete the jobs yourself and escalate the situation if necessary.

H Write a message on the handover board and leave without verbally handing over the remaining jobs.

5.10 Competence

You are working at an ENT (ear, nose and throat) firm and are caring for a patient who has had a severe nosebleed. The patient also has a mitral valve replacement, and your registrar requests on the ward round that you put the patient on prophylactic antibiotics to protect them from bacterial endocarditis. You have recently read some guidance from the National Institute for Health and Care Excellence (NICE) that recommended that antibiotics should not be routinely used for prophylaxis in patients with prosthetic valves and should only be used to treat suspected infection in this cohort.

Choose the **THREE most appropriate** actions to take in this situation.

A Ask your FY1 colleague to prescribe the antibiotics as you don't want to take the blame for incorrect prescribing.

B Discuss the need for antibiotics with microbiology and act according to their advice.

C Don't prescribe the antibiotics and neglect to tell your registrar why, to save his embarrassment at this mistake.

D Inform the registrar of the NICE guidance during the ward round in front of the patient.

E Mention the NICE guidance after the ward round and discuss with your registrar whether the patient really needs the antibiotics.

F Prescribe the antibiotics and suggest that you have a teaching session on anti-microbials at your next departmental meeting.

G Prescribe the antibiotics and then telephone your consultant to check if this is the right course of action.

H Prescribe the antibiotics without mentioning the new guidelines to your registrar.

5.11 Consultant advice

You are working as an FY1 in the emergency department. You clerk a patient complaining of chest pain, who has an abnormal electrocardiogram (ECG). You are unsure of the exact management plan and ask a consultant for advice. He tells you not to worry about the ECG changes and advises you to discharge the patient. You are worried that the consultant has given you the wrong advice and feel that the patient needs to be admitted instead.

Rank in order the following actions in response to this situation (1 = Most appropriate; 5 = Least appropriate).

A   Arrange for the patient to be admitted.
B   Ask another consultant for a second opinion.
C   Ask a registrar for their advice.
D   Discuss your concerns with the consultant.
E   Ignore your worries as the consultant probably knows what he is doing.

5.12 Referral to another specialty

You are an FY1 on a care of the elderly ward. One of your patients has been confused and, therefore, has had a computed tomography (CT) scan of their brain. The scan shows that your patient has bilateral subdural haematomas, and the report recommends seeking a neurosurgical opinion. Your patient is stable. You find the neurosurgical team intimidating, and they have rudely rejected one of your referrals before. You do not wish to make the referral yourself, but your senior specialist registrar (SpR) is in clinic and your senior house officer (SHO) is not at work today.

Rank in order the following actions in response to this situation (1 = Most appropriate; 5 = Least appropriate).

A   Ask the evening on-call team to make the referral.
B   Leave it until tomorrow to make the referral when your seniors are on the ward.
C   Make a referral to the neurosurgical team yourself.
D   Ring your SpR in clinic and ask them to make the referral.
E   Tell the patient that there is no treatment available, without speaking to the neurosurgical team.

5.13 Nurse questions your competence

You are an FY1 working on a busy gastroenterology ward and are asked to prescribe anti-emetics for a patient who is persistently vomiting. You take an appropriate history from the patient and perform a full examination. You decide that the appropriate course of action is to prescribe some anti-emetic medication and give some intravenous fluids. After you have completed your management plan, the nurse who is caring for the patient reads it and says that she disagrees. She refuses to give the prescribed medications.

Choose the **THREE most appropriate** actions to take in this situation.

A   Ask another nurse to give the medications you have prescribed.
B   Ask the nurse what her concerns are about the prescription.
C   Ask your senior house officer (SHO) to review your management plan.
D   Change the prescription to a different anti-emetic and ask her to administer that instead.

E Complain to the ward sister about the nurse in question.
F Explain your rationale for prescribing the medications to the nurse.
G Omit the anti-emetic and just give the intravenous fluid.
H Return to the patient and repeat your history and examination in case you missed something.

5.14 Colleague wants to be a surgeon

You are working as an FY1 on a general surgery ward with a fellow FY1 colleague. Your day includes completing the ward round, taking the blood tests and completing the jobs list. Your colleague has repeatedly stressed her desire to become a surgeon. You have discussed your career preferences several times with her, and you have said that you don't know what career path you would like to take. After four weeks in the job, you notice your FY1 colleague is leaving the ward most days at 1.30 pm to go to theatre to practise skin suturing. When you ask your colleague about this she says, 'I should go to theatre. Anyway, you don't want to do surgery.'

Rank in order the following actions in response to this situation (1 = Most appropriate; 5 = Least appropriate).

A Allow your FY1 colleague to attend theatre, completing the jobs list on the ward yourself.
B Ask your senior house officer (SHO) one day if they could complete the jobs list so you can attend theatre.
C Attend theatre with your colleague.
D Inform your clinical supervisor that you are not getting to spend any time in theatre.
E Inform your colleague that, although you are unsure of your career choice, you would also like the opportunity to attend theatre while she stays on the ward.

5.15 Colleague not competent with ABGs

You are working as an FY1 in a busy respiratory firm. As part of your job, many patients require arterial blood gases (ABGs) to be done. Usually you have five or six ABGs to complete each day. You have noticed that your FY1 colleague always asks you to do the ABGs while she completes other tasks. You now feel very competent at doing ABGs. After several weeks, you overhear your colleague saying to your senior that she doesn't like doing ABGs because she finds them 'too hard'.

Rank in order the following actions in response to this situation (1 = Most appropriate; 5 = Least appropriate).

A Discuss the situation with your colleague and explore her reasons for avoiding doing ABGs.
B Discuss the situation with your colleague's educational supervisor.
C Offer to complete all of the ABGs on the ward so that your colleague doesn't feel embarrassed.

D   Offer to teach your colleague your technique and give advice about how to carry out the procedure.

E   Refuse to carry out any further ABGs in the hope that this will force your colleague to develop her skills.

5.16 Training

You are the FY1 on a busy respiratory team. You have a long job list, including inserting several cannulas and completing three discharge summaries. Your registrar bleeps you and asks if you can insert a pleural drain in a patient as this needs to be done in the next few hours, and he is occupied in clinic for the foreseeable future. You have never inserted a pleural drain before, but you have observed the procedure when you were a medical student. You are aware that the FY2 on your team has carried out the procedure several times since starting this job.

Rank in order the following actions in response to this situation (1 = Most appropriate; 5 = Least appropriate).

A   Agree that you will insert the drain if the FY2 is available to supervise you.

B   Agree to insert the pleural drain and ask an experienced nurse to assist you.

C   Politely request that the registrar leaves clinic to supervise you inserting the drain.

D   Refuse to insert the pleural drain and continue with your ward jobs.

E   Refuse to insert the pleural drain but offer to contact the FY2 and arrange for them to carry out the procedure.

5.17 Registrar illness

You are the FY1 on a cardiology team. You notice that your specialist registrar (SpR) seems to be extremely tired and is having difficulty concentrating during consultations with patients on the ward round. You are concerned that this may affect their decision-making as well as their relationship with patients.

Choose the **THREE most appropriate** actions to take in this situation.

A   Approach the registrar, ask if everything is ok, explain your concerns and suggest they discuss the matter with their clinical supervisor.

B   Ask the consultant to review all the recent decisions the registrar has made.

C   Contact your consultant immediately and explain your concerns.

D   Do nothing now as no direct patient harm has occurred and observe the situation from now on.

E   Keep an eye on the decisions the registrar makes and discuss any concerns with them.

F   Offer to take over the ward round to give the registrar a break.

G   Suggest that the registrar visits their GP.

H   Tell the registrar that they need to go home if they aren't well enough to work.

5.18 Referring appropriately

You are the FY1 on a general surgical ward. You are called by the nursing staff to see a post-operative patient who is experiencing palpitations. The nurse has already performed an electrocardiogram (ECG), which you review when you arrive. This shows fast atrial fibrillation. You know the treatment options for this condition from medical school but have not managed it before in practice. The patient is otherwise stable.

Rank in order the following actions in response to this situation (1 = Most appropriate; 5 = Least appropriate).

A Bleep the intensive care outreach team and ask them to come help you with a sick patient.

B Examine the patient fully, review the notes, then call the on-call medical registrar, give them a summary of the case and ask them to come see the patient.

C Examine the patient fully, review the notes and then go to theatre to speak to your surgical registrar for advice.

D Get your FY1 colleague from the neighbouring ward to come help you assess the patient and initiate a management plan.

E Go to the cardiology clinic to speak to the cardiology consultant for advice.

5.19 Attending teaching

You are the FY1 working on a general surgical ward. The job is busy, and the day when you are due to attend your FY1 teaching sessions is your consultant's theatre day. This results in both your specialist registrar (SpR) and senior house officer (SHO) wanting to be in theatre as well, leaving you alone on the ward. You know that your teaching is mandatory and that it may affect your ability to progress from FY1 if you do not attend the required amount of teaching sessions.

Rank in order the following actions in response to this situation (1 = Most appropriate; 5 = Least appropriate).

A Ask a fellow FY1 friend to give you their notes from the teaching so that you stay up to date.

B Ask the FY2 covering the neighbouring ward if they can cover for you while you attend your teaching.

C Ask your SHO if there is any way they can help you get through the jobs on the ward on your teaching days before they attend the theatre session.

D Bring this matter up with the consultant and ask if there is anyway the SHO can be let out of theatre during the hours you are meant to be in teaching to cover the ward.

E Continue to miss the teaching sessions, and let the teaching coordinator know that it is because you are too busy on the ward.

5.20 Thorough clinical examination

You are an FY1 working on an orthopaedic ward and have just returned from your annual leave. You have arrived early at work to review the patient notes ahead of the consultant ward round. The last entry in the notes for one patient is from a physiotherapist who had noticed that the patient had a foot drop and weakness in both her legs. The consultant had written that a full neurological examination should be carried out followed by a referral to the neurologist on call. You approach your FY1 colleague and ask him whether he has done this yet. He replies that he saw the patient quickly last night but did not fully examine her and that he doesn't agree with the physiotherapist's findings.

Rank in order the following actions in response to this situation (1 = Most appropriate; 5 = Least appropriate).

A   Book a magnetic resonance imaging (MRI) scan of the patient's spine without examining them.
B   Suggest that you examine the patient while your colleague joins the consultant ward round and then report your findings to the consultant.
C   Suggest to your colleague that you both go and examine the patient again while the consultant does the ward round alone.
D   Tell the consultant that the physiotherapist was wrong and that there is no need for further investigation.
E   Tut under your breath and leave your FY1 colleague to do the consultant ward round while you proceed to examine the patient.

5.21 Depressed colleague

You are one of the doctors working on the medical admissions unit (MAU), and over the past few weeks, you have noticed that one of your FY1 colleagues has stopped socialising with your team, has been turning up late for work and doesn't seem to be able to concentrate. No one else seems to have noticed any change in his behaviour, but you suspect that something might be troubling him.

Choose the **THREE most appropriate** actions to take in this situation.

A   Approach your colleague when you are alone and voice your concerns.
B   Make an appointment with your educational supervisor to get some advice on how you should handle the situation.
C   Send your colleague an anonymous text message with some advice on where to seek help for depression.
D   Speak to your colleague's housemates about your concerns and tell them to look after him.
E   Speak to another FY1 colleague at a different firm about your concerns.
F   Suggest that your colleague speaks to his educational supervisor about any problems he may be having that are affecting his work.
G   Talk to your colleague about your observations while on the ward round so that your consultant knows about your worries as well.
H   Tell your colleague that he isn't doing his job properly and that patient care is being put at risk as a result of his careless attitude.

5.22 OGD consent

You are an FY1 working on a gastrointestinal ward, and you are increasingly being asked to consent patients who are due to undergo an oesophago-gastro-duodenoscopy (OGD). You have always declined since you know little about the procedure and have never seen it performed. Your refusal has, however, caused delays in some instances.

Rank in order the following actions in response to this situation (1 = Most appropriate; 5 = Least appropriate).

A Continue to decline when asked to consent.
B Do some reading about the procedure so that you can consent in the future.
C Make your team aware that you are not willing to consent for this procedure.
D Observe a colleague consenting a patient for the procedure so that you can consent in the future.
E Observe a morning endoscopy list and discuss the risks of the procedure with the endoscopist so that you can obtain informed consent from patients in the future.

5.23 Treatment options

You are the FY1 on a medical admissions unit and have just clerked a patient presenting with a severe flare-up of his inflammatory bowel disease. During a team discussion, your consultant asks you to refer him to the surgeons for a bowel resection as he feels that this would be more appropriate than medical management at this stage. Looking back in the patient's notes, you see that, since his diagnosis, he has only been on steroid therapy.

Rank in order the following actions in response to this situation (1 = Most appropriate; 5 = Least appropriate).

A Do not refer the patient or make any further management plans until you talk to your consultant after the ward round tomorrow.
B Have a discussion with your consultant about other medical therapies and the patient's past drug history, and ask him to clarify why he thinks further medical management should not be explored first.
C Speak to your educational supervisor about your concerns.
D Talk to your registrar about the consultant's decision and explain that you feel he may benefit from a gastroenterology opinion with regards to further medical management.
E Tell the patient that he needs to have an operation in order to control his disease and say that you will refer him to the general surgeons for further care.

5.24 FY1 ward round

You are one of three FY1s working in respiratory medicine. As a team, you take it in turns to cover the post-take ward round each day. However, during the second month of your job, you notice that one of the other FY1s regularly seems to come up with reasons why they cannot do the ward round as often as you and your other colleague.

Rank in order the following actions in response to this situation (1 = Most appropriate; 5 = Least appropriate).

A Ask your consultant to speak to the FY1 as you think this behaviour is unfair.
B Ask the other FY1 if they too have noticed the absence.
C Discuss this with the FY1's educational supervisor.
D Do not mention it further as the current situation means that you do not have to cover the post-take ward round every day.
E Speak to the FY1 yourself and ensure that they are coping with their workload and not struggling.

5.25 Colleague not coping with bleeps

You are working as an FY1 doctor in a district general hospital on call for medicine at the weekend. You are covering half the hospital, and an FY1 colleague is covering the other half. Throughout the day you receive several calls from nurses on the wards your colleague should be covering. They inform you that they have bleeped your colleague several times, and he hasn't replied. They say that they have several jobs that need completing on their wards.

Rank in order the following actions in response to this situation (1 = Most appropriate; 5 = Least appropriate).

A Attempt to contact your on-call FY1 colleague and enquire whether he needs further support.
B Complete an incident form and raise the issue at the next junior doctors' forum.
C Discuss the situation with the on-call medical registrar.
D Go to your colleague's wards and complete the jobs that need doing.
E Tell the nurses to continue to bleep your FY1 colleague as you are not responsible for his patients.

5.26 Working as a team

You are the FY1 on a busy medical admissions unit, and you are finishing off your morning jobs before you join your colleagues for lunch. As you are leaving the ward, a nurse shouts for a doctor as one of her epileptic patients is having a seizure. There is only you and two medical students on the ward.

Choose the **THREE most appropriate** actions to take in this situation.

A Ask one of the nearby support workers to record a set of observations on the patient.
B Ask the medical students to get some oxygen and an airway adjunct in case you need it.

C   Ask the medical students to go and see what the nurse needs and ask them to bleep you if they need to.
D   Ask the nurse to help you protect the patient from any danger but do not hold them down.
E   Immediately go to the drug cupboard to draw up some intravenous (IV) lorazepam.
F   Obtain a history and background from the nurse before attending to the patient.
G   Pretend not to hear the call for help and continue walking to lunch.
H   Start chest compressions on the patient.

5.27 Negligence

You have just started your morning shift and a colleague comes to see you. She is clearly agitated and tells you that she thinks that she has accidentally pre-scribed an antibiotic containing penicillin for a patient with a penicillin allergy during yesterday evening's on-call shift.

Choose the **THREE most appropriate** actions to take in this situation.

A   Advise your colleague to review the patient immediately.
B   Ensure that the antibiotic has been stopped.
C   Fill out an incident form.
D   Offer your help in dealing with the situation.
E   Review the patient yourself.
F   Speak to microbiology to find a suitable alternative antibiotic.
G   Tell the patient what has happened.
H   Tell your colleague's consultant about the incident.

5.28 Registrar leaving patient list

You are a surgical FY1. You notice that your registrar has been leaving his patient list lying around on the ward. On several occasions, he has left it in a patient's bed area, and this morning, the nursing staff informed you that a patient had read their entry on a list left on their bedside table. They had become upset about the fact that this information about them was so readily available.

Rank in order the following actions in response to this situation (1 = Most appropriate; 5 = Least appropriate).

A   Apologise to the patient and let your registrar know about it the next time you get an opportunity to speak to him privately.
B   Apologise to the patient, discuss with your fellow FY1s and agree to keep a careful eye on the registrar to try to notice when he leaves his list around.
C   Call your registrar and explain what has happened, asking him to come back to the ward and talk to the patient.
D   Discuss your concerns with your clinical supervisor.
E   Put the list in question in the confidential waste bin and let the nursing staff handle the patient's complaint.

5.29 Nurse vs SpR

You are working in the orthopaedic firm, and you notice that one of the registrars on the ward, while friendly to you, does not interact with the nursing staff. The nurses feel that the registrar does not listen appropriately to their concerns and questions, and he is therefore compromising patient care. They would like you to discuss this with the registrar.

Choose the **THREE most appropriate** actions to take in this situation.

A Ask the nurses to communicate the details of their concerns to you so that you can raise them appropriately with the registrar.
B Ask the ward sister to raise the issue as an advocate for the nurses.
C Discuss with the nurses the registrar who is causing a problem and how you have noticed this also.
D Do nothing as it does not impact you directly.
E Let the registrar know that the nurses are unhappy with his patient care.
F Recommend to the nurses that, while you appreciate their concerns, it would be better placed coming from them rather than through you.
G Tell the nurses that you have not noticed such a problem.
H Tell the registrar after tomorrow's morning trauma meeting that the nursing staff are worried that he is not listening to their concerns about the patients.

5.30 Colleague's inappropriate comments

You are the FY1 working on a surgical ward. A patient has decided that they do not wish to have surgery, even though this means they are likely to die. One of your FY1 colleagues has been making comments such as 'Why are we even bothering to see them, they turned down our help' and calling the patient 'an idiot' and 'attention-seeking'. They never make these comments when patients or staff members outside the FY1 team might hear them.

Rank in order the following actions in response to this situation (1 = Most appropriate; 5 = Least appropriate).

A Discuss your concerns with other FY1s on the ward.
B Inform the foundation programme director about your concerns.
C Explain to the FY1 that they need to respect the patient and their decision.
D Inform the FY1's educational supervisor about your concerns.
E Don't agree with the FY1 but don't say anything further.

5.31 Nurse conflict

You are the FY1 working on an acute admissions unit. There is a shortage of beds in the hospital, and the entire team is under a lot of pressure to discharge when possible. The medical team have decided that a young man with pneumonia is not well enough to go home. However, the senior nurse approaches you and says that she feels he would be fine to be discharged and marks him as a planned discharge on the bed manager's board.

Rank in order the following actions in response to this situation (1 = Most appropriate; 5 = Least appropriate).

A Complete the discharge paperwork for the patient.
B Change the information on the board yourself so that the patient is not marked for discharge.
C Ask your registrar to speak to the nurse to clarify the situation.
D Explain to the nurse why the patient is not fit for discharge and ask if she can change the information on the board.
E Do nothing.

5.32 Poor discharge summaries

You are working as an FY2 doctor on a respiratory ward and receive a phone call from a GP. The GP reports that he has received a number of discharge summaries from the ward with very little information about the patients' stay in hospital and incorrectly prescribed medications. The discharge summaries in question have been completed by your FY1 colleague. This is not the first time that the issue has come to your attention as you have previously found his summaries to be of poor quality.

Rank in order the following actions in response to this situation (1 = Most appropriate; 5 = Least appropriate).

A Apologise to the GP and take no further action so as not to embarrass your colleague.
B Edit your colleague's summaries after he has completed them to amend any mistakes.
C Inform your colleague's educational supervisor about your concerns.
D Offer to complete all of your colleague's summaries for him.
E Offer to help your colleague by supervising him writing a number of summaries to improve his performance.

5.33 Colleague alcohol

You are an FY1 on a medical ward. You notice that your FY1 colleague often arrives late to work and smells of stale alcohol. You feel that his performance is being affected by this.

Rank in order the following actions in response to this situation (1 = Most appropriate; 5 = Least appropriate).

A Inform your medical consultant.
B Advise your colleague to go to his GP.
C Inform the General Medical Council (GMC).
D Write an anonymous letter to the local newspaper about your colleague.
E Ask your colleague to give a blood sample to test his blood alcohol levels.

5.34 Colleague dispute

You are an FY1 working on a busy medical ward. The senior house officer (SHO) on your team often leaves work early, meaning that you end up leaving late. You also feel like they aren't 'pulling their own weight'. One day you become angry and challenge your colleague directly. Now your colleague will not speak to you.

Rank in order the following actions in response to this situation (1 = Most appropriate; 5 = Least appropriate).

A Ask to switch medical teams.
B Agree to divide the patients between you and your SHO so as to avoid working together.
C Inform your registrar about the dispute and ask them to mediate.
D Apologise to your colleague and discuss your concerns.
E Relay messages in the future to your colleague through the nursing staff.

5.35 DNACPR

You are working as an FY1 on call over the weekend. You and a senior house officer (SHO) review an elderly patient who has pneumonia and multiple co-morbidities and is deteriorating despite antibiotics and IV fluids. The patient's son is at his bedside and says that he thinks his father is dying. He also says that his father has previously expressed a wish not to have cardiopulmonary resuscitation (CPR). The patient is too unwell and drowsy to discuss CPR. Your SHO refuses to sign a Do Not Attempt CPR (DNACPR) form as he isn't comfortable doing so without speaking to the patient. You disagree with your SHO and think that a DNACPR should be written.

Rank in order the following actions in response to this situation (1 = Most appropriate; 5 = Least appropriate).

A Inform the SHO's clinical supervisor about the event.
B Explain to your SHO why you disagree and suggest that he talks to a senior about it.
C Ask the nursing staff not to call the arrest team if the patient arrests.
D Speak to the on-call specialist registrar (SpR) and ask them to write a DNACPR for the patient.
E Document your concerns in the notes and leave the patient without a DNACPR card.

5.36 Radiologist

You are an FY1 on a general surgical job. On a post-take ward you see a patient with symptoms and x-ray imaging that suggest bowel obstruction. Your specialist registrar (SpR) asks you to request an abdominal computed tomography (CT) scan by speaking to the duty radiologist. You explain the situation to the radiologist, who rudely refuses and asks you to 'get one of your seniors to speak to me so that we can have a proper conversation'.

Rank in order the following actions in response to this situation (1 = Most appropriate; 5 = Least appropriate).

A Inform your registrar and ask them to call the radiologist.
B Tell the radiologist that you are the surgical registrar.
C Reiterate the reasons why you want the scan and that your registrar has requested it.
D Inform your clinical supervisor about the rudeness of this radiologist and say that you would like to make a complaint.
E Refuse to escalate to your seniors as they will say exactly the same thing as yourself.

5.37 Rude colleague

You are working as an FY1 on a general surgical ward. You are reviewing a patient on an outlying ward when you receive a bleep from a staff nurse, on your usual ward, asking you to review a patient that she is concerned about. You return to review the patient and then notice that one of your FY1 colleagues is on the ward. You ask the staff nurse why they did not approach your colleague instead of you, to which they reply that he is rude and patronising to the nursing staff.

Choose the **THREE most appropriate** actions to take in this situation.

A Agree to review all the patients that the nursing staff are concerned about.
B Ask other nursing staff if they have found your colleague's behaviour to be a problem.
C Inform the matron about your colleague's behaviour.
D Inform your colleague's educational supervisor.
E Refuse to get involved.
F Speak to your FY1 colleague about his relationship with the nurses.
G Tell the nurse that she should discuss her issues with the FY1 in question directly.
H Turn off your bleep.

5.38 Tearful colleague

You are an FY1 working on a busy general surgery ward. Your FY1 colleague is often tearful and is struggling to cope. She has been asking you to do a lot of her work for the past two weeks.

Choose the **THREE most appropriate** actions to take in this situation.

A Advise her to see her GP.
B Ask another FY1 to help you out with the workload.
C Ask your registrar to speak to her.

D   Carry on sharing her workload and wait for her difficulties to resolve.
E   Speak to her about her issues.
F   Suggest that she finds a different profession.
G   Tell her that you cannot go on sharing her workload.
H   Tell her to speak to her supervisor.

5.39 Argument

You have been working on a busy surgical ward for three months. You and your fellow FY1 have had a particularly busy morning looking after two patients who have become unwell. That afternoon you overhear your registrar shouting at your FY1 colleague because she has not ordered a scan which they had asked for during the morning's ward round. Your colleague is visibly upset.

Rank in order the following actions in response to this situation (1 = Most appropriate; 5 = Least appropriate).

A   Advise your colleague to discuss the altercation with her educational supervisor.
B   Pretend you have not overheard.
C   Advise your colleague to tell the registrar that she was upset by what was said.
D   Ask the registrar to apologise to your colleague.
E   Tell your colleague that she shouldn't take things so personally in future.

5.40 Colleague's incompetence

You have just started work as an FY1. You notice that your FY1 colleague working on the same ward avoids performing practical procedures such as cannulation. You are concerned that in some instances patient treatment may have been delayed as a result of you having to perform these procedures for them instead.

Rank in order the following actions in response to this situation (1 = Most appropriate; 5 = Least appropriate).

A   Do nothing and keep an eye on the situation to see if patient care is compromised.
B   Ask other members of staff on the ward whether they have similar concerns.
C   Speak directly to your FY1 colleague about your concerns.
D   Discuss the situation with the registrar on the ward.
E   Suggest to your colleague's educational supervisor that your colleague attends remedial teaching on practical procedures such as cannulation.

5.41 Consultant kiss

You are coming to the end of your job on the medical admissions unit when your consultant offers to give you some extra teaching. You are alone in his office one evening when he leans across and tries to kiss you. You move away and ask him to stop, which he does immediately.

Choose the **THREE most appropriate** actions to take in this situation.

A Avoid the consultant from now on.
B Call the police and report your consultant for sexual harassment.
C Complete the remaining time in the job.
D Discuss the event in confidence with your educational supervisor.
E Discuss with your educational supervisor the option of moving jobs for the remaining time of the placement.
F Take annual leave so that you do not have to work the remaining time in the job.
G Tell your consultant that, while you are flattered, you feel that it would be inappropriate to pursue a relationship.
H Warn your female colleagues not to go to the consultant's office alone.

5.42 Supporting a colleague

You and an FY1 colleague work together on a medical ward. One day a week you are both required to review the patients together on a ward round without your consultant since she runs a clinic all day. Your consultant has suggested that you and your colleague alternate reviewing the patients so that you gain equal experience. Over the weeks, you notice that your colleague lacks confidence in reviewing the patients and encourages you to see them instead.

Rank in order the following actions in response to this situation (1 = Most appropriate; 5 = Least appropriate).

A Discuss your observations with your colleague and encourage him to try and improve his confidence.
B Do nothing since there is no compromise in patient safety.
C Encourage your colleague to review more of the patients.
D Offer to give your colleague some teaching after work.
E Raise your concerns with your consultant.

5.43 Struggling colleague

One of your FY1 colleagues has been making frequent mistakes on the ward, such as forgetting to fill in clerking booklets fully, not keeping notes up to date and failing to request important blood tests for patients in a timely manner. You and your colleagues are feeling increasingly put upon by the nursing staff, who prefer to ask you to complete tasks because you are more reliable.

Choose the **THREE most appropriate** actions to take in this situation.

A Ask medical personnel to get a locum doctor to cover the extra work you have to do.
B Ask the nurses to come to you first and avoid giving work to your colleague.

C Ask your registrar to speak with your colleague regarding remedial training.
D Get the rest of your FY1 colleagues together so that you can raise your grievances to your seniors as soon as possible.
E Have a private word with your colleague to ask if they are struggling.
F Inform your colleague's educational supervisor of their incompetence.
G Keep working hard as you will change jobs on rotation soon, so you won't have to work with them again.
H Offer to teach your colleague some of the basics again.

5.44 Physiotherapist date

You are an FY1 working in a district general hospital. During your second attachment, you work with a physiotherapist whom you get on well with. You feel that there is a romantic spark between you. One day, you see them in the corridor, and they ask you if you would go on a date with them.

Rank in order the following actions in response to this situation (1 = Most appropriate; 5 = Least appropriate).

A Refuse to give an answer, and avoid the physiotherapist as much as possible in future.
B Decline and explain to them that you can't date somebody you work with.
C Report the physiotherapist to their manager for inappropriate behaviour.
D Accept but say that you'd want to delay the date until you've moved on to a new rotation.
E Accept and arrange for next week.

5.45 Respecting authority

You are working with another FY1 on a busy respiratory ward. This week your consultant is away on holiday, so the specialist registrar (SpR) is conducting the daily ward rounds. You notice that your FY1 colleague is not coming in as early to prepare the patient list with you, nor is he completing his fair share of the jobs during the day. When you raise your concerns with him that lunchtime, he says, 'I don't agree with the decisions the SpR is making, and he isn't the consultant, so I can't be bothered to make an effort.'

Choose the **THREE most appropriate** actions to take in this situation.

A Explain to your colleague that his attitude could potentially impact patient safety and that he should think about the wider implications of his behaviour.
B Get advice from one of your FY1 friends on another ward.
C Listen to your colleague but don't make any remarks about his comments.
D Raise your concerns about your colleague with the SpR in question.
E Speak in confidence to his educational supervisor about his attitudes.
F Suggest that he raises any issues he has with the SpR so that he can learn the reasons why those decisions have been made.

G   Tactfully explain that, as an FY1, he should respect all staff members, particularly those in positions of authority.

H   Tell your colleague to help you out more as you feel he is not pulling his weight.

5.46 Anticoagulating patients

You are the FY1 working on a general surgical ward caring for a post-operative patient having had a bowel resection for colorectal carcinoma. As per the protocol, you have prescribed prophylactic low molecular weight heparin for the patient, although his dose is higher than normal as he is obese. That evening, the surgical registrar walks towards the ward holding the patient's drug card and says loudly at the nurses' station: 'Which idiot prescribed this anticoagulation; do they want him to bleed out from his bowel resection?!' The nursing staff point out that it was you.

Choose the **THREE most appropriate** actions to take in this situation.

A   Ask the registrar to perform a case-based discussion with you about the role of post-operative anticoagulation.

B   Ask the registrar to publicly apologise for being rude about you in front of the team.

C   Ask the on-call haematology registrar to come and explain to the surgical registrar why you were correct.

D   Cross out your prescription and leave the patient without anticoagulation.

E   Explain to the registrar, in a voice as loud as the one he used, that you were following the hospital protocol, so if the patient bleeds, it is not your fault.

F   Inform the registrar that you were following the protocol but that you will change the prescription if that is what they think is appropriate.

G   Let the registrar know the next day that you were upset by their publicly calling you an idiot.

H   Ring the consultant and ask their opinion on prophylactic anticoagulation.

5.47 Punctuality

You work in a team of five FY1s. Over a period of time, you have realised that one of your colleagues is late to work most days, which puts a lot of pressure on you for the ward round as you have fewer people to help carry the notes, write down the management plan and subsequently action any jobs generated. You think your other colleagues have also noticed this.

Rank in order the following actions in response to this situation (1 = Most appropriate; 5 = Least appropriate).

A   As a group, make the decision to come in earlier to get organised for the ward round.

B   As a group, organise a meeting with the FY1 and explain how you think it is unfair that they are late so often.

C   Contact the FY1's educational supervisor.
D   Continue as you are; it is only for four months.
E   Inform the consultant of the problem.

5.48 Colleague not arrived for handover

You are an FY1 in a small district general hospital. You are working a weekend on call covering the surgical wards. On Saturday evening, your FY1 colleague who is working the night shift does not arrive for handover. The senior members of your team are all in theatre attending an emergency case.

Choose the **THREE most appropriate** actions to take in this situation.

A   Ask an FY1 on another ward to hold the surgical bleep until the FY1 arrives, in case of an emergency arising.
B   Call the FY1's clinical supervisor at home.
C   Call your colleague to find out whether they are coming and when.
D   Go home.
E   Inform your seniors in theatre of the problem.
F   Stay and be available for any emergency issues.
G   Stay and continue with routine jobs.
H   Wait in the doctors' mess for your colleague in order to give them a handover when they arrive.

5.49 Consultant acting unprofessionally

You are an FY1 working on a trauma and orthopaedics team. You are shadowing one of the consultants in his clinic as he has offered to provide you with some teaching. Your consultant is seeing a patient who has osteoarthritis of his knee and would benefit from a total knee replacement. While discussing the options for his operation, your consultant suggests that the patient should go to a local private hospital for private healthcare. To your own knowledge, the patient had not previously mentioned wanting to have private surgery, and you know that your consultant does a private clinic at the hospital that he recommended.

Rank in order the following actions in response to this situation (1 = Most appropriate; 5 = Least appropriate).

A   After the patient has left the room, ask your consultant why he suggested private healthcare.
B   After the patient has left the room, challenge your consultant, asking him if there is a conflict of interest.
C   Inform the patient during the consultation that your consultant is acting unprofessionally and that he may be trying to profit from the situation.
D   Say nothing because your consultant didn't suggest that the patient should necessarily attend his own clinic.
E   Seek the advice of a senior colleague.

5.50 Receiving and acting on feedback

You are working as an FY1 doctor doing an on-call night shift. You are asked to see a patient who is tachycardic and is feeling unwell. You assess the patient and believe that they are dehydrated. You document your findings in the notes, take some blood tests and initiate some intravenous fluids. Two hours later, your senior house officer (SHO) calls you to say that they have just seen the same patient. The SHO informs you that your fluid prescription was wrong, but the patient is now improving because they have 'sorted them out'. They inform you that they have formulated a management plan and will review the patient again later in the shift.

Rank in order the following actions in response to this situation (1 = Most appropriate; 5 = Least appropriate).

A Do nothing as the patient is now stable.
B Go and see the patient and reassess the situation.
C Make a note of the circumstances of the case and complete an e-learning package on intravenous fluid prescription at a further date.
D Immediately ask your SHO to provide more feedback.
E Wait until the end of the shift and ask the SHO to provide you with some feedback about your management of the case.

5.51 Derogatory comments on a social media site

You are an FY1, and an FY1 colleague of yours has written several public derogatory comments about nursing staff on a social media site. You think that this is unprofessional and inappropriate as it may be construed as the general opinion of the medical profession.

Rank in order the following actions in response to this situation (1 = Most appropriate; 5 = Least appropriate).

A Confront your colleague and tell them that this is inappropriate.
B Do nothing; everyone is entitled to their own opinion.
C Inform their consultant.
D Ask a mutual friend to speak to them about it.
E Write a comment on the social media site in response to one of the comments, saying that you disagree with it and highlight that this is not the general opinion of doctors.

5.52 Annual leave

Before you started work as an FY1, you booked flights for a holiday that is scheduled for during your second FY1 rotation. It is six weeks until your planned holiday, and you submit an annual leave request. The rota coordinator contacts you and tells you that unfortunately there is not enough ward cover for you to take your annual leave.

Rank in order the following actions in response to this situation (1 = Most appropriate; 5 = Least appropriate).

A Ask another FY1 whether they will swap shifts to cover your ward while you go on holiday.
B Ask the rota coordinator to arrange a locum to cover the ward while you go on holiday.
C Cancel your holiday.
D Inform the rota coordinator that, since you booked the holiday before you started your job, you intend to go on the holiday even if the ward will be left understaffed.
E Plan to call in sick so that you can continue with your holiday.

5.53 UTI

You are an FY1 halfway through a week of long shifts. You start to develop the symptoms of a urinary tract infection (UTI). You have had similar symptoms before which were successfully treated with antibiotics. You do not have any time off for a few days, so you will not be able to go to your GP for a prescription.

Choose the **THREE most appropriate** actions to take in this situation.

A Ask a fellow FY1 to write a hospital prescription for you and take it to the hospital pharmacy.
B Ask a nurse to give you the keys to the medicine cupboard so that you can take some antibiotics.
C Ask your registrar to write an outpatient prescription for you and take it to your local pharmacy.
D Explain your situation to your consultant and ask for a few hours off so that you can attend a GP appointment.
E Swap a shift with a fellow FY1 so that you can attend a GP appointment.
F Take an afternoon off as sick leave and attend a GP appointment.
G Wait until you next get a day off before attending a GP appointment.
H Write an outpatient prescription for yourself and take it to your local pharmacy.

5.54 Unprofessional behaviour

You are eating lunch in the doctors' mess when you overhear some FY1 colleagues laughing about one of the patients on your ward because they are overweight. They are making rude comments, and one of them is performing an over-the-top impression of the patient, while the others are in fits of laughter.

Rank in order the following actions in response to this situation (1 = Most appropriate; 5 = Least appropriate).

A Join in with your colleagues; this is a private joke and means no harm.
B Ask your senior house officer (SHO) for advice on how to deal with this situation.

C Go over to your colleagues and reprimand them for their unprofessional behaviour.
D Speak to the individuals involved in the joke privately, after the incident, about the way they discuss patients in future.
E Eat your lunch and say and do nothing.

5.55 Leaving on time

You are an FY1 on general surgery, and you are supposed to be meeting your partner for dinner after work. Your shift finishes at 6 pm, but the evening cover FY1 is late and has called to say that they will only arrive at 7 pm. There are some jobs left over from the day that you want to hand over.

Choose the **THREE most appropriate** actions to take in this situation.

A Ask one of the senior nurses on the ward to complete some of your jobs for you so that you can leave on time.
B Call the registrar on evening cover to complain about the late FY1.
C Call your partner to tell them that you will be an hour late.
D Continue working through the jobs until the evening cover arrives and you can hand over the rest.
E Hand over your jobs to the evening registrar.
F Leave at your designated time and complete the jobs tomorrow a day late.
G Phone up the FY1 to do a quick handover and leave on time.
H Write a list of all the jobs and leave it at the nurses' station on the ward.

5.56 Discriminating against colleagues

You are the FY1 working on a busy colorectal ward. The ward sister approaches you and says that one of the male nurses has come to her in confidence complaining that your FY1 colleague was overheard making derogatory remarks about a nurse's sexuality. The sister wants you to do something about it.

Choose the **THREE most appropriate** actions to take in this situation.

A Ask the sister whether there is any evidence that this has happened before.
B Politely explain that it is not your place to get involved in the situation.
C Say to the sister that you have never heard your colleague make any such remarks.
D Speak to your educational supervisor about the sister's concerns.
E Speak to your senior house officer (SHO) and registrar and ask whether they have ever heard your colleague make comments such as this before.
F Suggest that the sister speaks to the FY1 in question herself.
G Tell the sister that the nurse in question should speak to your colleague's educational supervisor and make a formal complaint.
H Tell the sister that you will speak to the FY1 in question for her.

ANSWERS

5.1 Extra on-calls

A D C E B

This question relates to honesty, integrity and your personal conduct. The most appropriate answer is option A, alerting your colleague to the unfairness of the rota and suggesting that they take matters further. Telling your colleague to contact the BMA about their working hours (D) would be appropriate but only after they have raised it locally with the rota organiser. Option C would be a generous offer, but work should be shared out evenly between everyone on the rota and should be coordinated by the rota organiser. Option E would be dishonourable and unfair. Doing nothing (B) would be the least appropriate response as your colleague is unfairly doing more hours (which may subsequently adversely affect patient care) and may be unaware of this.

Recommended reading

Medical Protection Society (2012), Honesty, in *MPS Guide to Ethics: A Map for the Moral Maze*, chapter 6.

5.2 Colleague faking illness

B C D A E

This scenario relates to personal conduct and your relationship with colleagues. You must make sure that you remain level-headed and not respond in an equally unprofessional way. The most appropriate option would be to confront them calmly (B) and make them aware that this is deeply unprofessional behaviour and cannot happen again. Telling their consultant (C) is less appropriate; in the first instance, you should speak to your colleague yourself before involving seniors. However, you may find that this is a recurring problem or one of many issues surrounding your colleague, in which case you should seek senior help. Doing nothing (D) would be less appropriate as you should try to prevent the situation from happening to either you or a colleague again. Option A would be responding to the incident in an equally unacceptable manner and would compromise patient safety by decreasing doctor staffing numbers. Option E is bribery and is therefore the least appropriate option.

Recommended reading

Medical Protection Society (2012), Chapters 6: Honesty, Chapter 11: Relating to colleagues, in *MPS Guide to Ethics: A Map for the Moral Maze*.

5.3 Colleague deleting records

E C A D B

Medical records are legal documents and should not be edited in a way that is dishonest or deceitful. To delete mistakes, a single line should be placed

across the record with an explanation as to why you have made the deletion and a signature. Your FY1 colleague has acted incorrectly in this scenario by blacking out entries in the medical notes, and you need to raise the
issue regardless of the content of the deleted notes, which is why options D
and B are inappropriate. The only reason why option D is preferable to B is
that attempting to read the deletion may help to identify issues relevant to
patient care and allow you to minimise potential dangers to the patients you
are reviewing. The best way to raise your concerns would be in a discreet
fashion in a private setting, in order to remain professional and to avoid
embarrassment for your colleague (E). Involving senior support would be sensible as they will be able to advise you appropriately (C); however, you should
attempt to speak to your colleague first to see whether the matter could be
more easily resolved. Approaching your colleague during a ward round (A) is
overly confrontational and could lead to humiliation and a poor professional
relationship.

Recommended reading
Medical Protection Society (2012), Honesty, section: Records, in *MPS Guide to
Ethics: A Map for the Moral Maze*, chapter 6.

5.4 Failing to escalate care

B   A   E   C   D
Above all else, when working as a doctor, you have a duty of care to all
patients you come across. This is a difficult situation and one you may often
find yourself in when making the transition to a more senior member of the
medical team. The best option in this scenario would be to discuss the case
with your colleague and try to explain what you think is most important for
the patient and why (B). In doing so, you will be able to raise your concerns
while ensuring patient safety. If you believe that patient safety is at risk, you
have a duty to raise your concerns there and then. Omitting antibiotics in
a patient who is potentially suffering from sepsis could be life-threatening.
For this reason, raising your concerns after the shift is least appropriate
(C and D). However, if patient safety had been ensured first, raising your
concerns with your colleague's educational supervisor (C) may be more constructive than complaining to your employer about your colleague's rudeness
(D). In this scenario, if you have serious concerns about patient safety and
your colleague refuses to listen, the medical registrar should be contacted
immediately to discuss the situation (A). Asking your colleague to leave
(E) may result in you being able to provide the care you believe the patient
requires; however, you will be losing a valuable source of information and
a pair of 'extra hands' as well as potentially damaging your professional
relationship.

Recommended reading
General Medical Council (2013), *Good Medical Practice*, paragraph 6.

5.5 Registrar prescribing against protocol

B   E   A   D   C

It is important that you bring the issue to the attention of your registrar in case they are not aware of the protocol and so that you can understand their reasoning (options A, B and E). You are putting yourself in a potentially risky position by prescribing out of line with local protocol as this is difficult to defend in cases that end up in medico-legal proceedings. It is therefore better to ask the registrar to prescribe the antibiotics if they still wish to go against the guidelines issued by the microbiology department (options B and E). Option E ranks lower than B because it is likely to sound accusatory and does not facilitate further discussion. The next most appropriate course of action would be to adhere to your registrar's decision after discussion (A) as you may discover that there were important clinical reasons why they recommended against the protocol antibiotics for this patient. You should always discuss with a senior if you have concerns or questions about a decision they are making, and this means D and C rank last. Option D involves not being open with your registrar: going against their instructions in secret is more likely to cause significant problems than doing it openly. Option C is the worst course of action here because you are both prescribing against protocol and neglecting to share your knowledge of the protocol with the registrar.

Recommended reading

Foundation Programme Curriculum (2012), Section 6.2: Evidence, guidelines, care protocols and research; Section 7.5: Safe prescribing.

Medical Protection Society (2012), Duty of care, section: Scope, in *MPS Guide to Ethics: A Map for the Moral Maze*, chapter 4.

5.6 Getting help when beyond limits of skills

B   D   H

The most important initial action is to check on the nurse who has been injured (H); you now have a duty to provide care to them as well as the patient. This relates to your obligation to provide assistance in any emergency that you witness. With regard to the patient, you are out of your depth trying to manage them, and it is therefore important to get senior help. Your registrar is unavailable; you know that they are dealing with a more time-critical emergency, and you should not try to pull them away from this (E). In a situation such as this, it is appropriate to call a consultant directly for advice, even though it is out of normal working hours (D). They are in a much more powerful position to deal with the psychiatrist's refusal and to insist that they attend the ward to help with the situation. Alternatively, they may decide to call in another registrar or to attend themselves. In the meantime, you need to get hospital security to the ward to ensure that the staff and other patients are kept safe (B). Involving the site manager would be a good decision (F); however, your consultant is more likely to facilitate definitive senior medical help in this situation, and security are well placed to protect everyone who is involved. It is unethical and illegal to imprison a patient against their will (A) or to force treatment without their consent (G). Trying to give an injection in this circumstance would be dangerous for everyone involved, including you.

Recommended reading
Foundation Programme Curriculum (2012), Section 8.6: Manages acute mental
    disorder and self-harm.
General Medical Council (2013), *Good Medical Practice*, paragraph 14.

5.7 Sick patients

A B E D C

This sounds like a patient who is clinically unwell, and while your registrar has more experience than you, if you are uncomfortable in managing the patient, you should always ask for help. This makes asking your SHO (A) the most appropriate action to help you manage the patient. Going over your registrar to contact your consultant (B) is not ideal as it may affect your relationship with the registrar in future; however, this is the chain of command and therefore would be an appropriate step. Option E would be potentially difficult as referrals from FY1s are not usually accepted without prior assessment from a more senior doctor; however, this is the last option remaining where you are taking immediate action, so it is therefore appropriate here. Option D, while still maintaining care of the patient, is not ideal because leaving a potentially unstable patient, whom you are worried about, is not advisable. Option C is the least appropriate because, although the registrar is more qualified than you, they have not seen the patient, and you must treat the patient in such a way that you feel confident that you have fulfilled your duty of care.

Recommended reading
General Medical Council (2013), *Good Medical Practice*, paragraphs 16b, 16d, 18.

5.8 Inadequate equipment

A B C E D

This question focuses on a situation when a patient's care may be affected as a result of poor equipment or facilities. When presented with a hypoxic patient, an ABG is an invaluable bedside test to further assess their clinical status. Not doing an ABG because you cannot immediately find the equipment necessary (D) would be negligent since you are denying your patient an important investigation that will inform future management. In this situation, it would be sensible to ask a nurse to try and locate what you need while you stay with the patient and reassess them (A). Option B is also sensible; however, your SHO may be busy with other cases, so it is a less favourable response than option A. Option C is certainly important as it is wise to make your seniors aware of sick patients; however, there are initial steps that can be taken first to get more information for the registrar about the patient's clinical status, so this isn't the first step. Going to another ward to try and find the ABG equipment (E) is sensible; however, ideally you should not leave an acutely unwell patient without a doctor. You should instead aim to use your colleagues effectively.

Recommended reading
General Medical Council (2009), *The New Doctor*, paragraph 6.
General Medical Council (2013), *Good Medical Practice*, paragraphs 15, 16, 18.
Medical Protection Society (2012), Duty of care, *MPS Guide to Ethics: A Map for the Moral Maze*, chapter 4.

5.9 Leaving sick patients

A   D   E

If one of your patients becomes unwell within your scheduled working hours, you need to assess them fully, even if this is just before your shift finishes. At an appropriate and safe break, you can then consider handing over jobs to the on-call team. Option A is one of the most appropriate responses: delegation is an important part of an FY1's job, and you will be very busy if you do not use the support staff to help you complete your jobs. Delegating some of the work in this scenario means that you can focus on the tasks that only a doctor can do, which would make the rest of the management of the patient much swifter. Option A, followed by an effective verbal handover, would be one of the best responses. Another one of the most appropriate responses is option D, to inform the on-call registrar if there is no one else available to call. They may not complete the outstanding jobs, but they would need to be informed of this acutely unwell patient and should come to review them as well. The third most appropriate response is option E: informing the on-call SHO to hand over jobs is appropriate, but on-call teams can be very busy, and you should make yourself available to stay late to ensure they are performed timely. The inappropriate options include poor methods of handover, such as leaving a message with the nursing staff (B) or writing a message on the on-call message board (H) – both could lead to misunderstandings. A handover board is appropriate for routine jobs but is not appropriate for handing over acutely unwell patients. Option C, handing over the jobs to the SHO, is technically an appropriate response, but offering your help to complete the jobs is more conscientious and responsible, so option E is preferable. Knowingly putting out a crash call for a patient who is not peri-arrest or having a cardiac arrest (F) is dangerous and could mean that the team misses a true arrest. Staying late to complete the work yourself without considering handover (G) is an inappropriate answer as this could lead to overwork and tiredness the next day. It is the on-call team's job to review sick patients out of hours, and you should use them to protect your own work/life balance.

Recommended reading
British Medical Association (2015), *Safe Handover, Safe patients*.
Medical Protection Society, *New Doctor*, vol. 3, no. 1 (2010), What drives a good handover.

5.10 Competence

B E F

Treatments and methods in medicine are constantly evolving, and if you are aware of a new protocol for treatment, it can be useful for your own learning as well as the whole team to discuss whether it is applicable to your field. However, you need to consider an appropriate time to discuss new methods with seniors so as not to undermine their knowledge in front of others. After the ward round and away from the patient's bedside may be a good time to discuss the new guidelines and how they may apply to your practice (E). Option B is also appropriate: the microbiology department will be able to weigh up the different aspects of this patient's case and will know whether the guidelines should be followed. Although delaying learning about the new guidelines to a later teaching session, in option F the whole team will be able to study the new guidelines in detail and determine whether they are appropriate for clinical practice. Option C is inappropriate as you may have misunderstood the clinical situation, and deciding not to prescribe the antibiotics without further discussion may mean that the patient is treated incorrectly. Bringing up the new guidelines in front of the patient (D) undermines the registrar's treatment plan and may concern the patient and is therefore inappropriate. Saying nothing (H) is clearly unsuitable as it would mean that the team cannot learn from this new guidance. Option G is also inappropriate as you should discuss the pros and cons of antibiotics with the registrar before going straight to the consultant; they will have expected you to do this first. Option A is the final inappropriate response in this scenario: if you believe something that you have been asked to do is incorrect, you shouldn't pass the blame on to somebody else and ask them to do it for you.

Recommended reading
General Medical Council (2013), *Good Medical Practice*, paragraphs 11, 12, 35, 36.

5.11 Consultant advice

D B C A E

You should never feel afraid to challenge a senior's opinion, particularly if you think that patient safety may be compromised. It is most appropriate, however, to discuss you concerns with the person in question initially (D). They may reconsider their decision or provide a good justification for it. It would also be appropriate to seek a second opinion from another consultant (B). In this scenario, asking a second opinion from another consultant is more favourable than asking advice from a registrar (C) since this may be seen as undermining the consultant in question, and a consultant would have more experience interpreting such tests than a registrar. You should avoid going against a consultant's advice without first seeking a second opinion (A), but to ignore your concern about patient safety is completely inappropriate (E).

Recommended reading

General Medical Council (2013), *Good Medical Practice*, paragraphs 24, 25.

5.12 Referral to another specialty

C D A B E

As an FY1, you are expected to make telephone referrals for patients to other colleagues and specialties. This can be a difficult technique to learn, and you may have to speak to some challenging or intimidating colleagues. As with all skills, the more experience you gain, the more proficient you will be. Option C is therefore the most appropriate course of action. If you find that you are not being listened to, you could ask your senior colleague to try themself. Ringing your senior SpR and asking them to make the referral from their clinic (D) is a sensible option; however, it may prove difficult as your SpR is likely to be busy and is unlikely to have all the relevant patient information at their disposal in clinic. Option A is less appropriate since this is a situation that should be dealt with in normal working hours and by the patient's own team of doctors. Your on-call colleagues may be extremely busy, and the referral may not be completed due to more pressing clinical issues and a lack of relevant staff to take the referral. Leaving the referral until tomorrow (B) would not be optimal management for the patient and would result in a delay. However, the least professional response would be option E as this would be negligent and is therefore completely unacceptable.

Recommended reading

General Medical Council (2013), *Good Medical Practice*, paragraphs 15–16.
Medical Protection Society (2012), Competence, *MPS Guide to Ethics: A Map for the Moral Maze*, chapter 10.

5.13 Nurse questions your competence

B C F

Disagreements are an inevitable part of medicine and how to deal with them is an important skill to learn. In this scenario, the nurse may be questioning your competence and decision-making. The key here is to gather information from the nurse and use that to support your decisions. Asking the nurse about her concerns (B) and offering an explanation for your plan (F) may raise issues that you must address or may reassure the nurse that your actions are appropriate. If this fails to allay her fears, you should not be afraid to ask for a second opinion (C). Often, as a junior FY1 doctor, you will lack experience in dealing with scenarios and asking for help is not a sign of incompetence. Bypassing the nurse by asking another nurse to give the medications (A) would not display good interpersonal skills, and you may miss an important point that the nurse might have been trying to make. Switching the prescription without first discussing this with the nurse (D) would be inappropriate. Without a good reason to change your original prescription, you should not do so. Omitting the prescription (G) when you have assessed the patient as requiring an anti-emetic may lead to unnecessary suffering for the patient and is therefore inappropriate. Complaining to the ward sister (E) is not a constructive course of action at this stage and will impact negatively upon your professional relationship with the nurse in question. Repeating your history and examination (H) may be appropriate if the nurse raises an issue that you have not thought about; however, this should only be done after discussing the situation with the nurse.

Recommended reading
General Medical Council (2012), Explanatory guidance, in *Leadership and Management for all Doctors*, paragraphs 2, 6.

5.14 Colleague wants to be a surgeon

E   D   B   A   C
Attending theatre as an FY1 is not an obligatory task and many FY1s struggle to find the opportunity to do this. Operating theatres can be very valuable learning environments regardless of your future career choice (particularly for skin suturing). In this scenario, your colleague is clearly not taking an equal share of the workload or learning opportunities. The best course of action here would be to politely ask your colleague if you could attend theatre (E). You have to remember that your primary role is to look after the patients on the ward, and you must both ensure that someone is completing that task. This is why attending theatre with your colleague and thus both of you leaving the ward would be inappropriate (C). If your colleague does not respond to your polite approach, the next best response would be to discuss this with your clinical supervisor (D). They would be able to suggest an appropriate course of action. Asking your SHO to complete the list (B) could be an appropriate response; however, not as appropriate as options E or D. This is because, as an FY1, you have a training need to spend time in theatre assisting in operations. Finally, simply allowing the situation to continue while you stay on the ward (A) is not a productive response and would not tackle the issue of your lack of theatre experience.

Recommended reading
Foundation Programme Curriculum (2012), section 12: Procedures.

5.15 Colleague not competent with ABGs

A   D   B   C   E
Doctors of all levels of training will have different skill sets and different strengths and weaknesses. As a doctor, you are working as part of a team that is responsible for providing good clinical care to your patients. The key to this scenario is that you lack the appropriate information to take action. Therefore, information gathering must be your priority. Option A would allow you to approach the topic with tact and get more of an idea as to why your colleague has been avoiding ABGs. It may be that you can offer your colleague teaching and advice about ABGs (D) since you have had more experience, and this is a good way for teams to help each other develop. Option A is preferable to D as

information gathering will prevent you from causing any unnecessary offence or embarrassment to your colleague. Refusing to carry out ABGs (E) may result in your patients receiving suboptimal care and could be potentially dangerous, making this the least appropriate response. Offering to complete all the ABGs (C) will ensure that the patients have the correct investigations; however, there will be times when your colleague must perform these skills on her own, so it is vital that you help to assess her learning needs. Discussing the situation with her educational supervisor (B) may be appropriate, but firstly you should approach your colleague about the issue.

Recommended reading
Foundation Programme Curriculum (2012), Core procedures.

5.16 Training

C E D A B

Option C is the best initial choice. It is important to take opportunities to acquire new skills. Learning skills specific to your rotation, such as pleural drainage, is included in the foundation curriculum. Routine ward jobs should not prevent you from doing this. The registrar is the most appropriate person to supervise a skill of this nature, and they are obligated to make themselves available to their trainees whenever possible. Options E and D are the next best choices as they protect patient safety. You are not competent in this skill, so you should not carry out the procedure without adequate supervision. Option E is better than D because it offers to assist the registrar in getting the procedure arranged, which is important in building a positive working relationship. Options A and B are the worst responses because they involve you carrying out the pleural drain under a less than adequate level of supervision. Option B is the inferior of the two because, although the nurse is experienced, she is not competent in completing the procedure herself and therefore cannot instruct you. Supervision by the FY2 (A), though better than supervision by the nurse, is still inadequate as the FY2 has only carried out the skill a few times. It is therefore less appropriate than refusing to carry out the skill on the basis of protecting patient safety.

Recommended reading
Foundation Programme Curriculum (2012), section 12: procedures.
General Medical Council (2011), *The Trainee Doctor*, paragraphs 1.2, 1.3, 40.
General Medical Council (2013), *Good Medical Practice*, paragraph 9.
Medical Protection Society (2012), Competence, section: Acquiring and developing new skills, in *MPS Guide to Ethics: A Map for the Moral Maze*, chapter 10.

5.17 Registrar illness

A E G

You are concerned that the SpR's competence may be affected by their tiredness, perhaps related to physical illness or personal stress. You need to take some action; option D is therefore not one of the best answers. It is always best to approach the person concerned and discuss the situation sensitively (A). It would be unkind to go straight to the consultant without having spoken to the SpR first (C), and this could undermine your future working relationship. It would also be unproductive to 'tell off' the SpR (H), which will cause both conflict and resentment. You must consider whether there has been any risk to patient safety, and it is therefore a good idea to consider their past and future decisions in case you notice any which you think are out of place (E). It would be an overreaction, however, to ask the consultant to do this (B). While you should be able to spot any important mistakes the registrar has made, you are not competent to be running a senior ward round entirely yourself, so option F is not appropriate. If the SpR is having problems with their health, it is extremely important that they go to see their own GP for investigation and support (G).

Recommended reading
General Medical Council (2013), *Good Medical Practice*, paragraph 28.
Medical Protection Society (2012), Competence, section: Maintaining competence, *MPS Guide to Ethics: A Map for the Moral Maze*, chapter 10.

5.18 Referring appropriately

B C D A E
The best person to help you with the management of an acute medical condition is the on-call medical registrar regardless of whether the patient is admitted under medicine or surgery (B). It is likely that, if you speak to your surgical registrar (C), they will simply advise you to bleep the medical registrar. Therefore, although it is usually best to escalate within your team first, in this situation, it is reasonable to refer directly yourself as this will ensure the patient receives appropriate treatment as quickly as possible. It is possible that your FY1 colleague will have more experience of the condition or may be able to guide you on which senior to contact (D). However, this response is likely to be slower in terms of getting definitive treatment or may lead to continuation of the patient being managed solely by FY1s without senior help. Intensive care outreach usually consists of experienced nurses who can assist with stabilising sick patients and help with decisions about escalating to higher levels of care. However, the patient in this scenario is said to be stable apart from their arrhythmia, which is not the area of expertise for the outreach team; therefore, option A is inappropriate. The worst response would be going to the cardiology clinic because this bypasses all of the conventional processes of referral, will delay the clinic and consequently anger the consultant (E).

Recommended reading
Foundation Programme Curriculum (2012), Section 8.1: Promptly assesses the acutely ill, collapsed or unconscious patient.
Medical Protection Society (2012), Competence, section: Referrals, in *MPS Guide to Ethics: A Map for the Moral Maze*, chapter 10.

5.19 Attending teaching

C D B E A

Teaching as an FY1 is mandatory, and while you are allowed to miss a few sessions due to holidays and night shifts, you do need to attend a set amount in order to be able to complete the requirements of FY1. It is a difficult situation to manage if you are the only FY1 on a team and the SHO is in theatre, as they also have to attend a required amount of theatre sessions as part of their surgical training. It is best to address the situation initially with the SHO if you feel you need help (C). Theatre lists tend to start after 9 am, once the patient has been seen by the consultant and then been through the anaesthetic process, and therefore they may have time to help you before the list starts. The consultant should also be willing to aid you in attending your teaching; therefore, if you raise the matter with them directly (D), they may be able to provide support for you on the ward while you attend your teaching. Asking the FY2 on another ward to help (B) may be a good idea, but this is not ideal as they will not know the patients, and it places an extra burden on them. While getting the notes from a fellow FY1 (A) will enable you to keep up with what happens in the teaching, it will not account for your absence; therefore, you still will not have been recorded as having attended the teaching. It is, therefore, better to contact the coordinator and explain your reasons for missing the teaching (E) because they can then either assist you to be present in the future, or at the very least, they will now have a record of why you have been absent.

Recommended reading

General Medical Council (2009), *The New Doctor*, paragraphs 59–67.
Medical Protection Society (2012), Competence, *MPS Guide to Ethics: A Map for the Moral Maze*, chapter 10.

5.20 Thorough clinical examination

B C E A D

This question requires you to show the clinical competence that is required at FY1 level: putting patient care first while maintaining good professional relationships. If you suspect that patient safety is being compromised, you should act without delay. Option B is therefore the most appropriate as this ensures that the patient is reviewed immediately but does not hold up the consultant's ward round, which would potentially affect the care of other patients. In doing this, you are also being courteous by communicating your idea to your FY1 colleague. Options C and E are less appropriate as C involves unnecessarily delaying the ward round, and it probably does not require two doctors to carry out a neurological examination. Making it plain to your colleague that you disapprove of their actions before undertaking the neurological examination (E) may be acting in the patient's best interests, but your behaviour is not conducive to maintaining good working relationships. Option D is the least suitable in this instance as you have not examined the patient and therefore cannot assume that no further investigation is required; you would be negligent if you were not proactive when you suspected that patient care was being compromised. Organising an MRI scan (A) may be suitable following a full neurological examination, but it is important that you have a clear indication when requesting tests. You should complete the plan as documented by your consultant first and then discuss with your seniors if needs be.

Recommended reading

General Medical Council (2009), *The New Doctor*, paragraphs 6, 10.
General Medical Council (2013), Duties of a doctor, in *Good Medical Practice*.
General Medical Council (2013), *Good Medical Practice*, paragraphs 7, 15, 16, 25, 35, 36, 56, 57.
Medical Protection Society (2012), Competence, in *MPS Guide to Ethics: A Map for the Moral Maze*, chapter 10.

5.21 Depressed colleague

A B F

This question focuses on your responsibility to act if you suspect that you or someone else's health may be adversely affecting patient care. It is important to maintain healthy, supportive working relationships, while also making the care of your patients your first concern. In this scenario, it would be wise to talk to your colleague in a non-confrontational, private setting to see whether they want to talk about anything that may be bothering them (A). Broaching the subject in front of others before you are sure of what is going on (G) is not conducive to maintaining good professional relationships and may cause both parties embarrassment. If you are worried about your colleague and the effect that their health may be having on patients, it would be more appropriate to talk in confidence to your own educational supervisor (B), before you talk to your peers (E), since your supervisor will be more experienced to handle the issue. If an FY1 is experiencing personal problems that are impacting their work, they should contact their educational supervisor to discuss it, and this would therefore be good advice to give to your colleague (F). While option C is also non-confrontational, it does not proactively address the issue that may be jeopardising patient safety. Option H would be an inappropriate way to speak to your colleague and would not provide support for him or protection for patients.

Recommended reading

General Medical Council (2009), *The New Doctor*, paragraphs 6, 10, 12.
General Medical Council (2013), Duties of a doctor, in *Good Medical Practice*.
General Medical Council (2013), *Good Medical Practice*, paragraphs 1, 24, 25, 36, 43.
Medical Protection Society (2012), Competence, in *MPS Guide to Ethics: A Map for the Moral Maze*, chapter 10.

5.22 OGD consent

E   C   A   B   D

It is the responsibility of the person doing the procedure to discuss it with the patient and gain consent. However, that person can delegate this responsibility to someone else as long as that person is suitably qualified. The consenting doctor should have observed the procedure, understand what it entails and have a good knowledge of the risks but does not necessarily need to be qualified to undertake the procedure. In this scenario, you could avoid delays in patient care by taking responsibility for consenting. Ideally, you should gain the necessary experience through observing the procedure and learning about its risks (E). That said, you are not obliged to take this responsibility, so it is also appropriate to inform your team that you do not wish to take consent for OGDs (C). Clarifying your position with your team is preferable to simply declining when next asked (A). While reading about the procedure may give you some of the necessary knowledge for the consent process (B), you should have observed the procedure in order to fully understand what is entailed. Similarly, observing a colleague consenting assumes that they have the appropriate knowledge and again you have not observed the procedure (D).

Recommended reading

General Medical Council (2013), Explanatory guidance, in *Consent: Patients and Doctors Making Decisions Together*, paragraph 26.

5.23 Treatment options

B   D   A   C   E

This question highlights the importance of providing all possible treatment options to a patient before gaining consent. This is one criterion of fully informed consent. It also highlights the need to maintain respect for colleagues and to communicate professionally if you have reason to question someone else's decision. Despite being junior, it is important to voice any concerns you may have about patient care to your seniors. Option B is therefore the most appropriate action to take since, by doing this, you are proactively voicing a concern and using the experience as a learning opportunity. Similarly, it would be appropriate to speak to your registrar (D), although your consultant should be the first person you endeavor to talk to, if possible, as ultimately they are in charge of the patient's care. For this reason, delaying the referral until you can discuss this with your consultant the following day is also appropriate (A), although this is less preferable as it would delay patient care without resolving the situation in the meantime. Telling the patient what has been decided about his management (E) is the least appropriate response as the patient has not been given information about alternative treatments, nor has he been invited to discuss his options for future management with a specialist. Your educational supervisor can be a source of help and advice in tricky situations (C);

however, it is unlikely that you would be able to discuss the matter as promptly as necessary, and as highlighted earlier, the consultant should ideally be the person with whom you address your concerns.

Recommended reading

General Medical Council (2008), Explanatory guidance, in *Consent: Patients and Doctors Making Decisions Together.*

General Medical Council (2013), Duties of a doctor, in *Good Medical Practice.*

General Medical Council (2013), *Good Medical Practice*, paragraphs 15, 16, 24, 25, 32, 35, 36, 47, 49, 57, 68.

Medical Protection Society (2012), Patient autonomy and consent, *MPS Guide to Ethics: A Map for the Moral Maze*, chapter 8.

5.24 FY1 ward round

E B A C D

This may be a simple mistake or there may be an honest reason why the other FY1 is not covering the ward round; however, you should make sure they are not struggling and should also bear in mind that it is not fair if they are not doing their equal share of the teams' workload. The best response therefore is to speak to the FY1 yourself and see if they are managing at work (E). The next best response is to discuss it with your other FY1 colleague (B) because, if they have not noticed anything, it may not be a significant problem. Option A is the next most appropriate as it would be best to talk to your team's consultant initially rather than their educational supervisor (C), whom you may not know. The least appropriate response would be to ignore the situation (D) because if it is causing you worry, then it may interfere with how you interact as a team, and you may end up overlooking a problem if the FY1 is having difficulties.

Recommended reading

General Medical Council (2013), *Good Medical Practice*, paragraphs 35–37.

5.25 Colleague not coping with bleeps

A C D B E

One of the busiest times for a junior doctor is working out of hours on the wards. At weekends, nights and bank holidays, the hospital has fewer doctors to cover the same number of patients. During these periods, teamwork becomes incredibly important with a small number of doctors supporting the care of many patients. In this scenario, discussing the situation with your FY1 colleague is the most appropriate course of action (A). This will allow you not only to identify any issues he is having but also to relay the information you have received from the nurses. Seeking support from a senior colleague (C) may mean they can put in measures to alleviate the pressure on your FY1 colleague, so this is the most appropriate next option. Your aim here is to solve the problem that has arisen; asking the nurses to continue to bleep your colleague (E) doesn't assist the situation and may cause further stress for your colleague and the nurses. While completing the jobs for your colleague may be helpful (D), you may be neglecting the care of the patients you are responsible for yourself. However, assisting with jobs is more appropriate than completing an incident form (B) as it offers a more immediate solution to the problem. Completing an incident form may be important in the long term, but this is not your primary priority.

Recommended reading

General Medical Council (2012), Working with colleagues, in *Leadership and Management for Doctors*.

5.26 Working as a team

A   B   D

This question is testing your ability to work well under pressure and to be an effective team player. Although you are the only doctor on the ward, there are other members of staff and medical students around who would be able to help. It is paramount to the success of an emergency situation that all people involved work as a team. Options A and B are therefore sensible as the students and support worker can be arranging help while you are clinically assessing the patient. To prevent the patient from further harm is also important (D) as this not only shows leadership but also demonstrates good clinical care. Commencing chest compressions (H) is not appropriate unless you have assessed that a patient does not have a pulse. Pretending not to hear the shout for help or shirking your responsibility to attend (options C and G) are unprofessional responses and could jeopardise the patient's health and safety. Option E should not be one of your initial responses. It may well be sensible to ask one of the nurses to draw up some lorazepam just in case you need to use it, but you should utilise other team members for this so that you can assess the patient. Obtaining a background history (F) is important after the emergency has been managed and before documentation, but it should be secondary care in this scenario. Additionally, you may well be able to obtain the most important parts of the history during the process of assessing the patient.

Recommended reading

General Medical Council (2013), Duties of a doctor, in *Good Medical Practice*.
General Medical Council (2013), *Good Medical Practice*, paragraphs 15, 16, 26, 35 and 39.

5.27 Negligence

A   B   D

This question involves patient safety, relationships with colleagues and issues around confidentiality. Patient safety is your first and foremost concern, so you should make sure that the antibiotic has been stopped (B); the patient also needs to be reviewed immediately. It would be best if your colleague did this (A) as she has already met the patient, and this would be useful for the professional development of your colleague. As your colleague has come to you with this information, it is likely that she would like your advice and/or help (D). Reviewing the patient yourself (E) may be necessary, but as discussed earlier, it would be more beneficial to your colleague to do this herself. Telling the patient yourself (G) may also be necessary; however, it would be better for your colleague to do this. It would give your colleague the chance to explain their actions and apologise, thus hopefully reducing the damage to their doctor–patient relationship. Option C is not dealing with the immediate issue. Option H is not appropriate in this isolated incident and will compromise the trust of your colleague. Speaking to microbiology (F), while important to consider further down the line, is not one of your first priorities.

Recommended reading
General Medical Council (2013), *Good Medical Practice*, paragraphs 25–26.

5.28 Registrar leaving patient list

C A B D E

When you, your colleagues or patients have concerns, it is best in the first instance to raise them with the person involved. Calling the registrar straight away (C) gives him the opportunity to apologise for his own mistake as well as learning from it. Delaying the discussion with the registrar (A) may mean that the conversation never happens, and the chance for him to repair the damage for himself is lost. Option B is also appropriate because it includes an apology to the patient and shows a proactive effort to improve the situation. However, it is less suitable than options C or A because it does not involve the registrar at all. Your clinical supervisor can help with this sort of problem (D), but it may be an overreaction to go straight to them without any prior discussion with the registrar and is likely to damage your working relationship. The worst response is to ignore the problem. Option E makes no attempt to address the issue and unfairly leaves the nursing staff to handle the consequences, when this was a mistake made by the medical team.

Recommended reading
General Medical Council (2009), Explanatory guidance, in *Confidentiality*, paragraphs 12–16.

5.29 Nurse vs SpR

B F H

This is a common situation to find yourself in: where the nurses feel that the more senior members of the team are not appropriately responding to their concerns. Often this is because the registrars don't see a problem themselves and are too time pressured to explain this to the nurses. However, you should try and improve the situation so that all team members feel valued and listened to. Options B, F and H are therefore the best responses here as they result in the concerns being communicated to the team in an appropriate and non-confrontational way. It would be best if the nurses communicated this themselves, but in your position you are well placed to help the nursing staff. While relaying the nursing staff's concerns to the registrar (A) could result in communication of the problem, you have no active involvement in the issue, and it would therefore be more appropriate for the message to come directly from the aggrieved persons. This would also avoid your registrar feeling as if you were taking the nurses' side. To collaborate with the nurses and discuss your opinions about individual team members (C) would not solve the problem and is unprofessional on your behalf. Ignoring the issue (D) is obviously not appropriate here as the team needs to work together to provide optimum patient care. Although in option E you would be making it clear that the nursing staff are unhappy with the care delivered, this should ideally come from the nursing staff themselves, and it does nothing to further clarify the details of the complaint to the registrar. Option H is not appropriate as again simply ignoring the problem will not make it disappear, but it is also untrue as you have noticed the rift between your colleagues.

Recommended reading

General Medical Council (2013), *Good Medical Practice*, paragraphs 35–37.
Medical Protection Society (2012), Relating to colleagues, in *MPS Guide to Ethics: A Map for the Moral Maze*, chapter 11.

5.30 Colleague's inappropriate comments

C A D B E
This is a difficult situation since in this scenario your colleague is clearly acting in an unprofessional manner. You should let them know that their attitude is not appropriate, which can best be achieved with an explanation (C). If you do not feel confident about doing this, it could be useful to get some peer support and analysis of the situation from the other FY1s on the ward (A). It would be an overreaction to immediately escalate this to involve seniors (options D and B). But, if you were to involve seniors, the FY1's educational supervisor (D) would be a more appropriate starting point than the programme director (B). The worst response in this situation would be not to take any action (E) as the FY1 is behaving inappropriately, and you have a responsibility to intervene.

Recommended reading

Medical Protection Society (2012), Respect, section: Putting patients first, in *MPS Guide to Ethics: A Map for the Moral Maze*, chapter 7.
The UK Foundation Programme Curriculum (2012), section 2: Relationship and communication with patients.

5.31 Nurse conflict

D C B E A
It is important here that you remember to act in the patient's best interests, not according to what the nurse would like you to do. The best option is to

engage in a discussion with the nurse (D). Option D also includes ensuring the information on the board is changed, which is important for clarity within the wider team. It is better to deal with the issue yourself than to involve your seniors (C) as it is something you should be able to address successfully. Option C is better than option B, however, because it allows discussion and opportunity for the nurse to contribute her opinion rather than just overriding her (B). Doing nothing (E) would not be constructive in this situation as there will be confusion over the plan for the patient. However, it would be worse to complete the discharge paperwork (A) as the patient is not medically fit to leave; it is not the nurse's role to make this decision.

Recommended reading

General Medical Council (2011), Working with colleagues, in *The Trainee Doctor*, paragraph 40.
General Medical Council (2013), *Good Medical Practice*, paragraph 41.

5.32 Poor discharge summaries

C E D B A

Writing discharge summaries is a common task for foundation year doctors. Accurate and informative summaries help to ensure good continuity of care and ensure good communication between healthcare professionals. In this situation, your primary focus should be to ensure patient safety. The best person who can support your colleague is their educational supervisor (C), who can work with the doctor to address the issues raised. Offering to help your colleague (E) may be a short-term 'fix', but it may not ensure the quality of their discharge summaries in the future. While option D would ensure that good-quality discharge summaries are produced, writing the summaries yourself would not aid your colleague's education. Similarly, editing the summaries yourself (B) fails to address the issue with your colleague and is also a waste of your valuable time. Apologising and taking no further action (A) will not result in any change in your colleague's performance and will mean poor-quality discharge summaries will continue to be produced, so option A ranks last.

Recommended reading

General Medical Council (2013), *Good Medical Practice*, paragraph 44.

5.33 Colleague alcohol

A C B E D

It is your duty as a doctor to raise a concern when patient safety or care is, or could be, compromised. Therefore the most appropriate response in this case is option A: you should escalate this concern quickly to the person leading your team. If you feel that your concern is not being dealt with satisfactorily or you do not feel you can raise it within your team, you should contact a regulatory body such as the GMC (C). Advising your colleague to attend his GP (B) may be useful for your colleague, but raising your concern to someone more senior should be a priority. Option E may be helpful in gathering evidence for your colleague's misconduct, but it is not necessary to gain proof before raising a concern, and it may risk damaging your relationship with them. Reasonable belief justifies raising a concern even if you are mistaken. Option D is the most inappropriate response in this case. The GMC states that you can make a concern public if you have done all you can to raise a concern through local and/or appropriate external bodies and have good reason to believe that patients are still at risk, provided you maintain patient confidentiality. In this situation, the concern has not yet been raised through the primary levels. You should also seek help and advice through external bodies (e.g., the GMC or the British Medical Association (BMA)) before contemplating making a concern public.

Recommended reading
General Medical Council (2012), Explanatory guidance, in *Raising and Acting on Concerns About Patient Safety*, paragraphs 7, 10–18.

5.34 Colleague dispute

D C A B E

The most appropriate course of action is option D: apologising and discussing your concerns in a more controlled manner should 'clear the air' and hopefully allow resolution. Involving a senior (C) may be necessary to resolve the dispute but may make you look unprofessional and a little childish. Asking to switch medical teams (A) would not resolve your issues and is likely to make you appear unprofessional. This is also true of option B, dividing the patients between you, but most importantly, it may compromise patient safety and the management of their care due to poor team communication, so this option is ranked less favourably. Relaying messages to your colleague through the nursing staff (E) is the least appropriate response as it would be very unprofessional and could also compromise patient safety.

Recommended reading
General Medical Council (2013), *Good Medical Practice*, paragraphs 35–37.
Medical Protection Society (2012), Relating to colleagues, *MPS Guide to Ethics: A Map for the Moral Maze*, chapter 11.

5.35 DNACPR

B D E A C

In this case, it is important to balance treating a colleague with respect and keeping your duty of care to the patient. Talking to your colleague about the situation and suggesting that he discuss it with seniors if he is not confident is the best response (B). This is a difficult situation and may need senior input to reach a decision. Option D is therefore the next appropriate response if your SHO does not wish to speak to the SpR themselves. Documenting your concerns (E) may help other clinicians in reaching a decision but doesn't help the patient and his son in the immediate situation while he is deteriorating.

General Medical Council (GMC) guidance states that decisions about CPR should be made as early as possible. Informing the SHO's clinical supervisor (A) is inappropriate as it is likely to damage your relationship with your colleague and will not help in the immediate situation with your patient. Option C is the least appropriate response as nursing staff have a legal obligation to make an arrest call and a verbal request is not legally binding.

Recommended reading
General Medical Council (2010), *Treatment and Care Towards the End of Life: Good Practice in Decision Making*, paragraphs 128–134.

5.36 Radiologist

C A D B E

This question relates to your relationship with colleagues. It can be extremely hard to stay calm when a colleague is being rude and you feel that comments about you are personal. In this case, your first priorities are patient safety and duty of care to the patient, in other words ensuring that the patient undergoes the necessary imaging. Option C is therefore the most appropriate course of action as you may be able to give a better explanation for the rationale for the imaging request while remaining professional. If this fails, you should then escalate the issue to your senior (A), who will have more knowledge about the pathology and CT scanning rationale and should also be able to use their seniority to add more gravitas to their wishes. Ensuring that the attitude of the radiologist is made known to your clinical supervisor (D) is appropriate but doesn't deal with the current clinical situation. Options B and E are both inappropriate. Option B, telling the radiologist that you are the registrar, is outright lying and is therefore deeply unprofessional; however, option E, refusing to escalate the issue, is worse as the patient's management, and therefore safety, is being compromised.

Recommended reading
Medical Protection Society (2012), Chapter 4: Duty of care; Chapter 11: Relating to colleagues, in *MPS Guide to Ethics: A Map for the Moral Maze*.

5.37 Rude colleague

B F G

When working in a large team, you will find that disagreements are very common. As part of a team, you should do your best to help maintain efficiency and ensure patient safety. This situation does not appear to compromise patient safety but does affect your workload and therefore affects team efficiency. Ignoring the situation (E) is inappropriate as helping to smooth over differences between colleagues is likely to increase team productivity and better your own working environment. Turning off your bleep (H) would be unprofessional and would leave nursing staff and colleagues unsupported. To review all patients yourself from this point forwards (A) is unfeasible and would result in an unbalanced and likely unsustainable workload. Informing the ward matron (C) or your colleague's educational supervisor (D) would both be inappropriate at this stage, before approaching your colleague yourself.

You should discuss the issue with your colleague (F); it may be that your colleague is not aware of how he appears to the nursing staff. On the other hand, your colleague may be struggling in general with his work and may need your help or even more senior support. Option B would help to gather further information before speaking to your FY1 colleague. As well as discussing issues with your colleague, you should encourage the nurse to speak to your colleague herself (G).

Recommended reading

General Medical Council (2013), *Good Medical Practice*, paragraphs 35–37.
Medical Protection Society (2012), *MPS Guide to Ethics: A Map for the Moral Maze*, chapter 11.

5.38 Tearful colleague

E   G   H

This situation is not sustainable as you cannot continue doing the workload of one of your colleagues as well as your own. Doing so may result in burnout and/or compromised patient safety. For this reason, option D, carrying on sharing her work, is not appropriate. Option F, telling her to find another profession, would be unprofessional and counter-productive as this does not solve the issue at hand. Suggesting that she seeks help from her GP (A) may be useful advice for your colleague but does not help the immediate situation. Asking another FY1 to share your workload (B) may be helpful, but it is not a long-term solution and does not deal with your colleague's problem. Asking your registrar to speak to her (C) could be an action to take in the future, but in the first instance, you should talk to your colleague yourself (E) and inform her that the current situation is not maintainable (G). Advising her to speak to her supervisor (H) is a good first step in making sure that her problem is escalated and that she receives the senior support she needs.

Recommended reading

Medical Protection Society (2012), Relating to colleagues, in *MPS Guide to Ethics: A Map for the Moral Maze*, chapter 11.

5.39 Argument

A   C   D   B   E

Disagreements are not uncommon in a busy and stressful environment such as a hospital ward. However, they should be resolved in a professional and respectful manner. In this scenario, the registrar has clearly behaved poorly, and this should not be allowed to continue. You should advise your colleague to consult with her educational supervisor (A) since they will be best placed to resolve the issue. This is preferable to encouraging the FY1 to approach the registrar herself (C) as this may result in the disagreement escalating further. Similarly, it is preferable for you not to approach the registrar yourself (D) since you are not directly involved in the disagreement and again this may escalate the problem further. It is inappropriate for you to pretend that you have not overheard (B) since you have a responsibility to act upon unacceptable behaviour by colleagues. Option E is the least acceptable response; criticising her reaction to the disagreement will only worsen the situation.

Recommended reading
General Medical Council (2013), *Good Medical Practice*, paragraphs 35–37.
Medical Protection Society (2012), Relating to colleagues, *MPS Guide to Ethics: A Map for the Moral Maze*, chapter 11.

5.40 Colleague's incompetence

C D B E A
It is the duty of a doctor to raise and act upon concerns regarding patient safety or compromise of care. Doing nothing (A) is therefore inappropriate. When there is concern over a colleague's performance, it is wise to raise these concerns with the colleague directly (C). There may be an explanation for your colleague's behaviour, such as a lack of confidence. Your registrar may be able to deal with the problem (D), although this is less direct than option C. Eliciting concerns from other members of staff (B), while giving a more detailed picture of your colleague's performance, does not solve the problem. Option E is an active approach; however, it risks damaging the professional relationship with your colleague and does not explore the cause of the situation.

Recommended reading
General Medical Council (2013), *Good Medical Practice*, paragraph 25.
Medical Protection Society (2012), Duty of care, in *MPS Guide to Ethics: A Map for the Moral Maze*, chapter 4.

5.41 Consultant kiss

C D G
The General Medical Council (GMC) has not published specific guidance on personal relationships between colleagues. While it is not recommended to pursue such relationships, it is not prohibited. It is clear, however, that a good working relationship is of paramount importance, and any personal relationships should not be allowed to jeopardise your ability to work alongside colleagues. In this scenario, the consultant has overstepped a boundary but has stopped immediately when asked. You should manage the situation in a way that allows a good professional relationship to continue. Telling the consultant that you are flattered but do not want to pursue a relationship (G) makes

your position clear while being polite, and you should continue to work the remaining time in the job (C). It would also be prudent to discuss the matter in confidence with your educational supervisor (D) so that they are already aware if any future problems were to arise relating to this consultant. At this stage, it would be inappropriate to avoid completing the time in your job, either by moving jobs (E) or taking annual leave (F), since this may result in a lack of medical cover. Similarly, you should not try to avoid the consultant (A) since this may damage your working relationship. Warning your colleagues about the consultant is unprofessional and risks his working relationship with them (H). While the consultant has overstepped a professional boundary, he has not committed a crime, so reporting him to the police (B) is completely inappropriate.

Recommended reading

General Medical Council (2013), *Good Medical Practice*, paragraph 1, 34–38.
Medical Protection Society (2012), Chapter 5: Morality and decency;
  Chapter 11: Relating to colleagues, in *MPS Guide to Ethics: A Map for the Moral Maze*.

5.42 Supporting a colleague

A C E B D

Part of your duty as a doctor is the continual improvement and development of your skills. You also have a responsibility to ensure that others are doing the same. In this scenario, your colleague is struggling to develop his skills in patient review, and you should try to support him in tackling this problem. An appropriate first response is therefore to discuss your observations with him directly (A). You could also encourage him to review more of the patients rather than asking you to do it (C). Raising your concerns with your consultant (E) is also sensible, but you should ideally have made some effort to resolve the issue with your colleague directly before involving the consultant. While patient safety is not currently compromised, it would still be inappropriate not to act when a colleague is having difficulties in an aspect of their work (B). You should not offer to give your colleague extra teaching (D) since this is not your responsibility, and their issue lies in a lack of confidence as opposed to knowledge.

Recommended reading

General Medical Council (2013), *Good Medical Practice*, paragraph 7, 8, 13, 35, 36, 43.
Medical Protection Society (2012), Chapter 10: Competence; chapter 11: Relating to colleagues, in *MPS Guide to Ethics: A Map for the Moral Maze*.

5.43 Struggling colleague

C E H

As a new FY1, starting work will be difficult, and you will make mistakes. However, if those mistakes are serious or repeated, something needs to be done about it. In this scenario, one of your colleagues seems to be struggling, and this is making the job harder for the rest of you. The best responses are those that treat your colleague respectfully and compassionately but also lead to remediation steps, such as further training or extra teaching. Option C, asking your registrar for help in this matter, is a good response; senior doctors should be made aware if one of their juniors is persistently making mistakes as they can organise appropriate training and teaching sessions to help. Option E is another appropriate response as you do not know why your colleague isn't performing well, and it could be due to a number of factors. By talking with them privately, you could both come up with a plan of how to improve their skills and work together better. Option H is the third most appropriate response: with small mistakes such as not filling in the clerking booklet fully, another FY1 is more than capable of teaching a colleague the correct way to do this. Many FY1s have different skills and strengths, and you should feel confident to both teach and learn from each other as well as from senior doctors.

Inappropriate responses include those that avoid the problem in hand, such as asking for extra locum cover to take over your failing FY1 colleague's tasks (A) and asking the nursing staff to stop giving them things to do (B). For option B, taking on more work yourself increases your responsibility and could stretch you too thin, leading to more serious errors, but it also doesn't help your colleague improve his practice in any way. Similarly, option G burdens you with extra work, which may be dangerous, and allows a colleague with sub-standard skills to progress. Getting together as a group to confront your colleague (D) is also inappropriate as it could embarrass him. Informing your colleague's educational supervisor of their difficulties (F) could argu-ably be considered appropriate. It is a good course of action because of the educational supervisor's responsibility to ensure that your colleague learns the appropriate skills of an FY1; however, to go behind your colleague's back is underhand and shows a lack of respect. Also, since FY1s do not work directly with their educational supervisors, your colleague would surely know that someone had privately informed the supervisor, and this will not aid their working relationships.

Recommended reading
Medical Protection Society (2012), Relating to colleagues, section: Commenting upon the work of others, in MPS *Guide to Ethics: A Map for the Moral Maze*, chapter 11.

5.44 Physiotherapist date

D E B A C

Having a romantic relationship with a colleague is not a problem as long as it does not affect patient care. In order to ensure that there is no impact on how you act at work, it would be preferable to postpone the date until you don't work directly together (D) rather than arranging it for next week (E).

Option E, however, is a more appropriate response than option B, turning down the date, because you should not compromise happiness in your personal life when there is no need to. If you do turn down the physiotherapist's offer, this should be with an answer and explanation (B), which allows you to continue to work together in a civil and professional manner. Avoiding dealing with the situation (A) would be both immature and potentially cause major problems with your working relationship. This could have implications for patient care. The least appropriate response would be to report the physiotherapist to their manager (C) because they have not done anything wrong by asking you out. Again, this option could lead to a lot of unhappiness and a difficult working relationship.

Recommended reading
Medical Protection Society (2012), *MPS Guide to Ethics: A Map for the Moral Maze*, chapter 5: Morality and decency, section: Relationships.

5.45 Respecting authority

A F G

This question deals with the issue of balancing a respect for authority with a genuine concern for patient care and new learning opportunities. If your colleague is neglecting his duties because he doesn't agree with the SpR's decisions, he needs to talk to the senior in question as there is the chance that patient care and safety may be compromised as a result. Both of these points need to be communicated to your colleague (options F and A). It is not unreasonable to ask seniors to explain their reasoning behind certain decisions; indeed sometimes they make mistakes, and therefore, it is good to check if you have concerns. Refusing to be proactive in response to this (C) is unprofessional, impacts the team's workload and displays a lack of respect for all your colleagues, not just those in a position of authority. Instead, you should explain to your colleague about how respect for your colleagues works (G). It is important that you give your colleague a chance to rectify his behaviour before reporting him (options D and E) as this could further jeopardise professional relationships within the team. A constructive, helpful approach would be more appropriate than simply telling him off (H). You may wish to discuss this with another FY1 (B), but this is not as appropriate as directly addressing the situation by talking to your colleague.

Recommended reading
General Medical Council (2013), Duties of a doctor, in *Good Medical Practice*.
General Medical Council (2013), *Good Medical Practice*, paragraphs 15, 16, 22, 25, 35, 36, 43, 59, 68.
Medical Protection Society (2012), Professionalism and integrity, in *MPS Guide to Ethics: A Map for the Moral Maze*, chapter 3.

5.46 Anticoagulating patients

A F G

This scenario is difficult as it puts you in an awkward position. The registrar needs to be informed that he should not be speaking to anyone in such an unprofessional manner, especially since he is incorrect in this case. Therefore the best response here is to ensure that the registrar is aware that what he said has upset you, and this is often better left until after the event to allow the person and yourself to calm down (G). You should also make sure that the registrar is aware that there is a protocol in place regarding anticoagulation and find out the reasons why they do not want the patient on low molecular weight heparin (options A and F). Getting the registrar to publicly apologise to you would be welcomed (B), but is unlikely to happen and not necessary as long as they do apologise to you at some point. Phoning the haematology registrar or your consultant (options C and H) is likely only to antagonise the registrar, so these are not good responses. If you feel that the patient should receive the medication, you should discuss your conflicting opinion with your registrar rather than blindly following their wishes (D). Displaying similarly unprofessional behavior to the registrar (E) is only going to further anger the registrar and is therefore best avoided.

Recommended reading

Medical Protection Society (2012), Professionalism and integrity, in *MPS Guide to Ethics: A Map for the Moral Maze*, chapter 3.

5.47 Punctuality

B E C A D

The best thing to do if there is a problem with one of your colleagues is to make them aware of the problem (B), otherwise it will go on to impair your working relationship with them. You should, however, make sure that this is done tactfully so that the FY1 in question doesn't feel as if you are all 'ganging up' on them. If the problem is beyond what you believe you can manage as an FY1, ensuring the consultant knows about your concerns is appropriate (E) so that they can take the matter further. This is better than going straight to the FY1's educational supervisor (C), whom you may not have had interaction with previously. Option A ranks higher than D because, although actively increasing your workload to cover for another individual is not ideal, at least in this way there is no potential risk to patient care as there is with doing nothing.

Recommended reading

Medical Protection Society (2012), Professionalism and integrity, in *MPS Guide to Ethics: A Map for the Moral Maze*, chapter 3.

5.48 Colleague not arrived for handover

C E F

Colleagues arriving for work late presents a frustrating but common ethical dilemma. You should not leave the hospital (D) because this would mean there would be inadequate cover and patients would not be safe. It would also be unsafe to stay only to give handover (H) and not to provide emergency cover before your colleague arrives. It is also inappropriate to ask another FY1 to take on additional on-call responsibility while awaiting your replacement (A). However, just because you are staying does not mean that you also need to continue working on non-urgent jobs (G) as you have finished your shift and need to rest. The most important thing is that you are available in emergencies (F). You should let your seniors know that there may be a problem (E) because they should always be aware of who is looking after their ward patients, and they are responsible for taking action if it becomes necessary to bring in extra cover. It would be an overreaction and not particularly constructive to call your colleague's supervisor (B). The simplest and most important action is to contact your colleague and find out what the situation is (C); after all they may be only a few minutes late.

Recommended reading

General Medical Council (2013), *Good Medical Practice*, paragraph 1.
Medical Protection Society (2012), Professionalism and integrity, section: Professionalism, *MPS Guide to Ethics: A Map for the Moral Maze*, chapter 3.

5.49 Consultant acting unprofessionally

A E B D C

Acting professionally includes a broad range of commitments which should be adhered to in all medical practice. One such commitment is providing impartial advice to patients. The General Medical Council (GMC) offers good advice for these scenarios: when a doctor has a financial or commercial interest in another healthcare provider, they should not be influenced by their interests when treating patients. In this scenario, it is possible that your consultant is attempting to profit from referring the patient to private healthcare. However, your consultant may have seen the patient numerous times, and there may have been other conversations that you are unaware of. Therefore, the best way to raise your concerns would be to simply ask him in private why he suggested private healthcare (A). Seeking the advice of a senior colleague could help as they may have more experience and be able to suggest an appropriate course of action (E). Challenging your consultant is an unnecessarily aggressive approach to take here and may harm your professional relationship (B), although it is preferable to other options because at least the issue is raised in private with the consultant. Doing nothing (D) may help your consultant to maintain his relationship with his patient, but if you have concerns about a fellow professional's conduct, then you should always raise these in some way. However, by raising the issue while the patient is in the room (C), you may affect your consultant's relationship with the patient without knowing all the facts that are relevant to the situation. Option C is particularly unprofessional on your part and therefore the most inappropriate answer here.

Recommended reading
General Medical Council (2013), *Good Medical Practice*, paragraphs 75 and 76.

5.50 Receiving and acting on feedback

E   C   D   A   B

On-call shifts can be very challenging for newly qualified doctors, but they can also provide numerous learning opportunities. On-call shifts are usually very busy, often with many patients requiring attention from a small team of doctors. In this scenario, the most important thing to consider is that the patient is now stable with an adequate management plan and a schedule for review. After ensuring that your patient is not in danger, you should consider how to act on the feedback you have received. So far, you have received very little feedback that you could act upon. Waiting until the end of the shift and then asking for further feedback (E) would ensure that you are not wasting the valuable time of your seniors and preventing them (and yourself) from review-ing unwell patients. Making a note of situations where there are lessons to be learnt is a valuable way of keeping your knowledge and skills up to date, and e-learning packages can be very useful to consolidate learning on a topic (C). The least appropriate response here would be to re-review the patient (B) as they have a management plan in place and a scheduled review, so this would be an inefficient use of your time and could potentially harm other patients' care. Doing nothing (A) would not waste time (making it preferable to option B), but you would not receive any feedback to allow you to learn from the situation. Immediately asking for feedback (D) would provide you with a learning oppor-tunity, but it is not appropriate to do this during a busy on-call shift.

Recommended reading
General Medical Council (2013), Duties of a doctor, in *Good Medical Practice*.
General Medical Council (2013), *Good Medical Practice*, paragraphs 9 and 13.

5.51 Derogatory comments on a social media site

A   D   E   C   B

This scenario relates to your own and your colleague's professionalism, and as part of being professional, you are expected to 'uphold the reputation of the profession, helping to maintain public confidence in it'. The most appropriate response here is option A: confronting them and making them aware that their behaviour is unprofessional. Asking a mutual friend to speak to them about it (D) may be appropriate, but it would be better for you to speak with your col-league directly if you have an issue with their comments. Writing a response on the social medical site (E) may harm your relationship with your colleague and may result in an unprofessional argument on the social media site in the public eye. Option C, informing their consultant, would be a drastic course of action and should only be taken if you have confronted your colleague to no avail or you perceive that there are more concerns regarding their professionalism. Doing nothing (B) would be the least appropriate response as this would not be upholding the reputation of the profession.

Recommended reading

Medical Protection Society (2012), Professionalism and integrity, in *MPS Guide to Ethics: A Map for the Moral Maze*, chapter 3.

5.52 Annual leave

A C B D E

You should not book a holiday without having your annual leave confirmed as it is not uncommon for annual leave requests to be denied. The ward must have the minimum level of staffing at all times to ensure patient safety, and most rotas will involve periods where you are indispensible to the team. Although you booked the holiday prior to starting work, you still have a duty to ensure adequate staffing, and in addition, you are actually only requesting the leave once you have been in the job some time. The most appropriate response would be to try and swap shifts with a colleague so that the ward is covered while you are still able take your holiday (A). The second most appropriate response, while inconvenient, is to cancel your holiday (C) since your priority in this situation is ensuring the ward is covered. Asking the rota coordinator to arrange locum cover (B) is inappropriate, since the hospital is not obliged to provide external cover for annual leave. This response is preferable, however, to simply informing the rota coordinator that you are going on holiday regardless of whether the ward is understaffed (D). Calling sick is wholly inappropriate since this is dishonest, unprofessional and potentially detrimental to patient care (E).

Recommended reading

General Medical Council (2013), *Good Medical Practice*, paragraph 38.

5.53 UTI

D E F

While going to work and caring for your patients is clearly a priority, your own health is also very important. You should be registered with a GP outside of your work or family, and you must not rely solely on your own assessment of any personal health problems. Although this may seem like a simple urinary tract infection, you should still seek advice from your GP. In this scenario, it would not be unreasonable to take sick leave in order to seek help from your GP (F). Equally, you could explain to your consultant that you need some time off to go to your GP (D). If you were able to swap a shift in order to get time off this would also be appropriate (E). Waiting until you get time off to seek assistance (G) may result in you becoming more unwell. It is strongly recommended that doctors do not prescribe for themselves, family members or friends, so options A and H are both inappropriate. In addition, FY1 doctors cannot write outpatient prescriptions (H). While your registrar can write an outpatient prescription for you (C), your needs should ideally be properly assessed by your own GP. Hospital staff should not have access to drug treatment without the correct prescription, so option B is completely inappropriate.

Recommended reading
General Medical Council (2013), *Good Practice in Prescribing and Managing Medicines and Devices*, paragraphs 17–19.

5.54 Unprofessional behaviour

D   C   B   E   A
Doctors are trusted members of society, and patients come to them in good faith to be treated professionally. If doctors are seen to laugh about patients, their conditions or their behaviour, this undermines that trust. It is important to be aware that even things said in private can easily become public, and if you would not be willing to say something publicly, should you really say it at all? The best response in this question is option D, speak privately to the individuals after the incident. This proactively deals with the situation yourself and saves embarrassment for all involved as it is likely that they didn't mean any real harm. The next best response is to speak to your colleagues there and then (C); again, it is a proactive, direct approach, but it is more confrontational. Tackling the situation in this way risks some professional friction but will deal with the problem quickly. Asking a senior for advice (B) ranks next. Your SHO should be able to help you decide how to tackle this situation and whether it needs to be taken any higher. Doing nothing when you feel like something is wrong is not a good quality in a junior doctor, so option E is an inappropriate response. Option A, however, is ranked last; joining in with inappropriate behavior to make friends or because you think it is private implicates yourself and further perpetuates the situation.

Recommended reading
General Medical Council (2013), *Good Medical Practice*, paragraphs 53–64.
Medical Protection Society (2012), Professionalism and integrity, in *MPS Guide to Ethics: A Map for the Moral Maze*, chapter 3.

5.55 Leaving on time

C   D   E
With today's shift working patterns, safe and effective handover is vital to ensure good patient care continues when you leave work. The best responses are therefore options C, D and E, which allow for a safe handover. Unfortunately, there may be some times when work impinges on your social life, although this should not be the norm. Calling your partner to explain

that you will be late (C) is an appropriate response. If you are going to hand over any of your jobs to a doctor other than the designated one, it should be to someone who is competent and who is also on call, so the evening registrar (E) would be appropriate. Handing over medical jobs to someone who is a non-medic (such as a nurse) is potentially dangerous, and there-fore, option A is inappropriate. Writing jobs down and leaving the list with nurses (H) or giving a quick handover via phone (G) are not safe handovers, so these options are also inappropriate. Calling up the registrar and com-plaining about the late FY1 (B) would achieve little in this situation and is unprofessional. The final appropriate response is option D: to maintain safe staffing and to give an effective face-to-face handover, you need to stay on the wards. If you are staying, you should continue to work through the jobs that are left so as not to leave a mountain of tasks for the evening team to complete.

Recommended reading

Junior Doctors Committee (2015), British Medical Association, *Safe Handover: Safe Patients – Guidance on Clinical Handover for Clinicians and Managers.*

Medical Protection Society (2012), Professionalism and integrity, in *MPS Guide to Ethics: A Map for the Moral Maze*, chapter 3.

5.56 Discriminating against colleagues

A   B   F

This case presents a situation in which you should encourage the nurse and sister to speak directly to the FY1 in question (F), particularly if the sister has reason to believe that this behaviour has happened before (A). This should be done before a formal complaint is made to the FY1's educational supervisor (G). You should not act as a third party when you have not heard these comments, and you should not judge your colleague on the basis of hearsay (options B, C, D, E and H).

Recommended reading

General Medical Council (2013), *Duties of a Doctor.*

General Medical Council (2013), *Good Medical Practice*, paragraphs 24, 25, 35–37, 59.

Medical Protection Society (2012), *MPS Guide to Ethics: A Map for the Moral Maze*, chapters 7 and 11.

Index

A

ABG, *see* Arterial blood gas (ABG) test
Abortion
    religious objections, 239–240, 274
    SpR, comments on, 191, 228–229
    TOP services, 42, 103–104
Accidents
    offer assistance to, 10, 63
    smart phone pictures of, 41–42, 102–103
Advanced directives, 251, 288–289
Advanced Life Support (ALS), 20, 75
Advice
    assisted suicide, 179, 214–215
    child protection, 105
    to complete death certificate, 4–5, 56–57
    consultant, 313–314, 339
    depressed colleague, 318, 345
    driving against, 29–30, 87
    to friend, 16, 70–71
    from medico-legal insurer, 251, 288–289
    police caution, 1, 52–53
    for refusing medication, 175, 209–210
    registrar, 193–194, 231
    TOP services, 103–104
    unskilled procedure, 11, 64
    for working hours monitoring, 13, 66
Aggressive patient, 43, 104
Alcohol consumption
    colleagues, 267, 307, 323, 351–352
    with friends, 167, 199
    and misdemeanours, 39–40, 100
    patients
        assessment of, 265–266, 305
        discussion with relative, 180–181, 216–217
    specialist registrar, 10, 62
Analgesia, 245, 280
Angry partner, 10–11, 63–64
Annual leave, 331–332, 362

Antibiotics
    friends, inappropriate requests from, 36, 95
    immunosuppressant drugs, prescription limits, 19, 74–75
    incident reporting, 248–249, 284
    IV antibiotics, patient's refusal to, 175, 210, 255, 293
    local clinical guidelines, 246–247,
    prescription against hospital protocol, 310–311, 336
    prophylactic antibiotics, 182, 218–219
    UTI, 332
Anticoagulation, 329, 359
Anti-emetic medication, 314–315, 340–341
Apologise
    for drinking with friends, 167, 199
    forgotten patient review, 117, 138
    for losing blood results, 3–4, 55
    for lost notes, 184, 220–221
    for lost patient list, 29, 86–87
    for ordering wrong test, 235, 268
    patient error, 131–132, 156
    poor discharge summaries, 323, 351
    X-ray reporting, 170, 203–204
Arterial blood gas (ABG) test, 126, 148
    colleague, not competent with, 315–316, 341–342
    competence, 247, 283
    inadequate equipment, 312, 337
Assisted suicide, 179, 190, 214–215, 227–228
Audit
    presentation, 118–119, 139
    professionalism, 23, 79
AWOL, 128, 150

B

Bad news, breaking, 172, 206–207
Basic life support (BLS), 24
Blind patient, 178, 213–214

Blood test
    ABG test (*see* Arterial blood gas
        (ABG) test)
    consent for, 250–251, 287
    drug level monitoring, 242, 277
    group and save, 240–241, 275
    HIV patient, 264–265, 304
    hyperkalaemia, 241–242, 276–277
Blood transfusion, 177–178, 212–213
Breaking bad news, 172, 206–207,
    244–245, 279–280
Breast examination, 37–38, 97

C
Caldicott Guardian, 15, 29, 85, 105
Campylobacter jejuni, 29
Cancer
    diagnosis, 169–170, 202–203
    difficult questions about, 172,
        205–206
    disclosure, 259–261, 299
    informing to patients, 166–167,
        198–199
    terminal diagnosis, 259, 297
Cannabis, 41, 102
Cannulation, 18, 19, 68, 73, 74, 326
Capacity, patients
    advanced directives, 288–289
    blood test, consent for, 250–251, 287
    blood transfusion, 177–178,
        212–213
    colonoscopy, 252, 289–290
    dementia, 26–27, 83, 253–254, 291
    depression, 254, 291–292
    IV antibiotics, refusal of, 175, 210,
        255, 293
    mental health illness, 300
    self-discharge, 168, 200
    treatment, refusal of, 252, 289
Cardiac arrest
    equipment, unfamiliar with, 23–24,
        79–80
    patient, assessment of, 237, 270
Cardiopulmonary resuscitation (CPR),
    134, 160, 324
Career progression, 21–22, 77
Case-based discussion (CBD), 32, 329
Catheterisation
    clinical skills, 248, 284
    inappropriate room for, 238, 271

Chaperones, 265, 304
    for breast examination, 37–38, 97
    for DRE, 263, 302
    patient's refusal of, 132–133,
        157, 303
Chest drain
    at nighttime, 237, 270–271
    removal, 17, 72
Children
    autonomy, 255, 292–293
    confidentiality, 185, 221–222
    domestic violence, 31, 89
    parents' consent, 257, 295
    protection, 191–192, 461–462,
        505–506
    safeguarding, 184, 220
    treatment, refusal of, 192,
        229–230
Chlamydial infection, 218
Clinical skills
    catheterisation, 248, 284
    medical students, 35, 94
Clostridium difficile infection, 156
Coercion, 24–25, 81, 258–259,
    295–297
Coffee house discussion, 31, 89
Colonoscopy
    knowledge limitations, 166, 198
    patient's capacity, 252, 289–290
Communication
    abortion, SpR comments on, 191,
        228–229
    alcohol consumption
        doctors, 167, 199
        patients, relative discussion,
            180–181, 216–217
    assisted suicide, 175, 190–191,
        214–215, 227–228
    blind patient, 178, 213–214
    blood transfusion, patient consent
        for, 177–178, 212–213
    breaking bad news, 172,
        206–207
    cancer
        diagnosis, 169–170, 202–203
        difficult questions about, 172,
            205–206
        informing to patients, 166–167,
            198–199
    cardiology, referral to, 170, 203

children
    confidentiality, 203, 221–222
    safeguarding, 184, 220
    treatment, refusal of, 192,
        229–230
colonoscopy, knowledge limitations,
    166, 198
complaints, patients
    against consultant, 188, 225
    inappropriate behaviour with
        relatives, 189, 226
consensual Dr–Dr relationship, 189,
    225–226
consultant names, 186, 223
contact tracing, 182, 218
contraception, young people's
    request for, 176, 211
disclosure to relatives, 174,
    208–209
drug overdose, 183, 219–220
employee disclosure, 184–185, 221
with foreign patient, 168–169,
    201–202
full-body scan, patients request for,
    168, 200–201
FY1 colleague *vs*. SpR, 187, 224
gift from patient, 194, 232
GP, patient concern, 187–188, 224
handover sheets, loss of, 185–186,
    222–223
HIV
    death certificate, 182–183, 219
    test, patient consent for, 173,
        207–208
interpreter, 195, 233
interrupting SpR, 189–190, 227
IV antibiotics, patient's refusal to,
    175, 210
knife/gunshot wounds, reporting,
    181, 217
language barriers, 175–176, 210
late colleague, 193, 230–231
medication
    new drug, patient's request for,
        171, 205
    refusal of, 175, 179, 210, 214
notes
    missing, 167, 184, 199–200,
        220–221
    writing, 165, 197

nursing staff, degradation of,
    186–187, 223
with patients family
    informing scan results, 171,
        204–205
    promise to, 194–195, 232–233
    translator, 177, 212
prophylactic antibiotics, 182,
    218–219
radiology test, request for, 165–166,
    197–198
registrars
    conflicting plans, 188,
        224–225
    responsibility, 193–194, 231
secret pregnancy, 180, 216
self-discharge, 168, 177, 200,
    211–212
smoking, patients, 173–174, 208
with suicidal patient, 169, 202
telephone conversation with relative,
    181, 217–218
uninformed consent, 174–175, 209
upset patient, 190, 227
ward round, 179–180
workplace issues
    explicit posters, response to,
        173, 207
    inappropriate clothing, 192–193,
        230
    racism, 191–192, 229
X-ray reporting, 170, 203–204
Community acquired pneumonia
    (CAP), 8, 19
Complaints
    about false statement, 117–118, 138
    about first reporting radiologist, 170,
        203–204
    lost notes, 184, 220–221
    patients, 135, 161
        against consultant, 188, 225
        gynaecology complaints, 39, 100
        inappropriate behaviour with
            relatives, 189, 226
        upset patient, 190, 227
    about specialist registrar
        contaminated sterile field,
            126, 149
        uninformed consent,
            174–175, 209

Computed tomography (CT) scan, 7, 22, 125, 236, 269, 314, 324
Confidentiality
  Caldicott Guardian, 68
  case note security, 32, 90
  child protection, 105
  disclosure after death, 27, 83–84
  doctor–patient relationship, 86, 87
  professional duty, 92
  relative discussion, 180–181
  third party, disclosure to, 33, 92
Consensual relationship, 189, 225–226
Consenting, *see* Patient consent
Conservative management, 120
Consultant names, 186, 223
Contact tracing, 182, 218
Contraception, 176, 211
Coping with pressure, *see* Pressure, coping with
Coroner statement, 135–136, 161
CPR, *see* Cardiopulmonary resuscitation (CPR)
Criminal offence, 57
Criminal records bureau (CRB), 1
CT scan, *see* Computed tomography (CT) scan

D
Death certificates, 11–12, 15, 64–65, 69–70
  HIV infection, 182–183, 219
  honesty on, 4–5, 56–57
Delirium, 254–255, 292
Demanding patient, 131, 155
Dementia
  patient's capacity, 253–254, 291
  sleeping tablets, 240, 274–275
Dentist, 266–267, 306
Depression
  colleague, 318, 345
  patient's capacity, 254, 291–292
Diabetes and driving, 33–34, 92
Diabetic ketoacidosis (DKA), 243–244, 279
Diarrhoea
  and vomiting, 48–49, 111–112
  waiter, 241, 276
Digital rectal examination (DRE), 132, 263, 302

Direct observation of practical skills (DOPS), 78, 146
Disagreement, 340
  colleague, 353, 354
  family, 253, 290
Discharge summary, 19
  patient control of, 127, 150
  quality of, 323, 351
Disclosure
  after death, 27, 83–84
  cancer diagnosis, 259–260, 298
  employee, 184–185, 221
  of mistakes, 8, 60
  to patient's relatives, 174, 208–209, 260–261, 299
  to third party, 33, 92
DKA, *see* Diabetic ketoacidosis (DKA)
DNACPR, *see* Do not attempt cardiopulmonary resuscitation (DNACPR)
Doctor–patient relationship, 1, 39, 44, 52, 99, 106
Documentation
  events, 2–3, 54
  forgot to, 6, 58
Domestic violence, 31, 89
Do not attempt cardiopulmonary resuscitation (DNACPR), 252, 324
DRE, *see* Digital rectal examination (DRE)
Dress code, 19, 112–113
Dress, inappropriate, 192–193, 230
Driver and Vehicle Licensing Agency (DVLA), 28–30, 34, 85
Driving
  and diabetes, 33–34, 92
  against medical advice, 29–30, 87
Drug chart, 19, 107
Drug errors, 146
Drug overdose, 183, 219–220
Drugs, 9, 61
Duty of Candour, 144
DVLA, *see* Driver and Vehicle Licensing Agency (DVLA)

E
Ear, nose and throat (ENT), 45, 313
ECG, *see* Electrocardiogram (ECG)

Ectopic pregnancy, 258, 296
Educational supervision, 133–134, 158
Effective communication, *see*
        Communication
E-learning certificate plagiarism,
        47–48, 110
Electrocardiogram (ECG), 239, 273,
        312–313
Employee disclosure, 184–185, 221
End of life care, 236, 264, 269, 303
E-portfolio, 133, 148, 158
Equipment
    catheterisation, inappropriate room
        for, 238, 271
    ECG machine, fault in, 239, 273
    inadequate ABG equipment, 312, 337
    unfamiliar with, 23–24, 79–80
European Working Time Directive
        (EWTD), 142, 162–163, 309
Explicit posters, 343–344

F
Facebook, 2, 53–54, 331, 361–362
Face mask, patient's refusal to,
        252, 289
Face-to-face handover, 364
False audit, 13, 66–67
False statement, 117–118, 138
Family
    disagreement, 253, 290
    informing scan results, 171, 204–205
    promise to, 194–195, 232–233
    translator, 177, 212
Feedback, 331, 361
First-aid training, 159
Flu jab, 14, 67
Follow-up tests, 242–243, 277–278
Food poisoning, 30–32, 90–91
Foreign patient, 168–169, 201–202
Foundation Programme Curriculum,
        82, 152
Francis Inquiry Report, 144
Full-body scan, patients request for,
        168, 200–201

G
General Medical Council (GMC)
    accidents, offering assistance to, 63
    community-based emergency
        situation, 69
    confidentiality guidelines, 89
    consenting, 71
    CPR, 353
    Duties of a Doctor, 61
    DVLA, 87
    emergency, clinical settings, 159–160
    equality and diversity, 43
    fabricating study data, 113
    fake thank you letters, 37
    flu vaccination, 67
    Good Medical Practice, 106
    good working relationship, 355
    guidelines, 94
    integrity and honesty, 56
    knowledge and skills, 72
    legal and professional obligation, 52
    legal/disciplinary procedures, 95–96
    patient risk, forms of, 149
    personal conduct, 59
    prescribing and referring
        practices, 103
    professional relationship, 155
    raising concerns, 35, 94
    reference number, 111
    registrar's behaviour, 128
    reporting to, 65–66
    serious infectious diseases,
        disclosures of, 86
    SHO, reporting of, 59–60
    social media, 38–39
    training courses participation, 106
Gifts
    colleagues acceptation of, 7–8,
        89–60
    from patients, 194, 232
    from patient's family, 2, 42, 53, 103
    receiving, 45–46, 107–108
Gillick competent, 296
GMC, *see* General Medical Council
        (GMC)
Good Medical Practice, 105, 106
Good Samaritan, 15, 69
Group and save blood test,
        240–241, 275
Gunshot wounds, 14–15, 181, 217
Gynae complaints, 39, 100

H
Haematology registrar, 359
Handover sheet, 185, 222–223

Health Protection Agency (HPA), 49, 86
Health Protection Authority, 32
Hearsay, acting on, 35–36, 94–95
Heparin infusion, 238, 272
HIV, *see* Human immunodeficiency
    virus (HIV)
Honesty
    death certificates, 4–5, 56–57
    mistakes, disclosure of, 8, 60
Hospital anti-microbial protocol, 311
Hospital charity, 45, 108
Hospital counselling service, 151
Hospital management, 93
Human immunodeficiency virus (HIV)
    blood test, doctor's refusal to take,
        264–265, 304
    death certificate, 182–183, 219
    test, patient consent for, 173,
        207–208
    ward round, 179–180, 215
Hungover, 46–47, 109
Hyperkalaemia, 241–242, 276–277

I
Illegal substances, 41, 61, 102
Immunosuppressant drugs, 19, 74–75
Inappropriate dress, 192–193, 230
Incident reporting, 249–250, 284
Incorrect consent, 126–127, 149
Infection control guidelines, 149
Infectious diarrhoea, 241, 276
Infectious diseases, 29, 86
Information technology (IT), 30
Informed consent, 62, 71, 97,
        194, 346
Insurance fraud, 5, 57
Intentional overdose, 169, 202
International normalised ratio (INR),
        124, 145–146
Internet printouts, 171, 205
Interpersonal relationships, 34–35,
        93–94
Interpreters, 130–131, 154, 195, 233
Intravenous (IV) antibiotics, 175, 210,
        255, 293
Intravenous drug user (IVDU) patient,
        241, 275–276

J
Jehovah's Witness, 251, 287–288

K
Knife wound, 181, 217

L
Language barriers, 175–176, 210
Legal obligation, 64, 87, 353
Local interpreter service, 130–131, 154
Lying
    blood tests, 3–4, 55
    experience, 4, 56
    hangover, 8–9, 61

M
Magnetic resonance imaging (MRI),
        168, 318, 345
Media, 34, 93
Medical admissions unit (MAU), 8, 32,
        33, 51
Medical careers, 68
Medical clerking, 159
Medical defence organisation, 135, 161
Medical defence union, 52
Medical Protection Society (MPS), 138
Medical students, 7, 59
Medication
    new drug, patient's request for,
        171, 205
    refusal of, 175, 179, 209–210, 214
Medico-legal insurer, 25, 93, 288
Medico-legal malpractice insurer, 85
Mental health, 127, 143, 262,
        300–301
Mental Health Act, 215, 255, 291, 293
Mentoring, 18, 73
Microbiology department, 313, 339
Mini-clinical evaluation exercise (mini-
        CEX), 158
Mistakes
    forgotten patient review, 117, 138
    handover task forgotten, 5–6,
        57–58
    learning from, 124–126, 147–148
    open disclosure of, 8, 60
    ordering incorrect test, 22, 78,
        235, 268
    patient error, 131–132, 156
    prescription error, 45, 107, 238,
        271–272
    SpR, contaminated sterile field,
        126, 149

struggling colleague, 327–328,
356–357
surgical error, 20–21, 75–76
wrong site surgery, 263, 301–302
X-ray reporting, 203–204
Mortality and morbidity (M&M),
39, 100
Mortuary, inappropriate comments in,
40–41, 101–102
MRI, *see* Magnetic resonance
imaging (MRI)

N
Nasogastric (NG) tube, 16, 23, 70,
78–79
National Institute for Health and Care
Excellence (NICE), 123,
125–126, 147–148
Near miss event, 16, 70
Needlestick injury, 25, 81
Negligence, 321, 348–349
DKA patient, management of,
243–244, 278–279
drug levels monitoring, 243, 278
NICE, *see* National Institute for Health
and Care Excellence (NICE)
Non-accidental injury, 239, 249–250,
273, 285–286
Notes
missing, 167, 184, 199–200,
220–221
signing sick note, 235–236, 268
writing, 165, 197
Nursing staff
colleague's appearance, commenting
on, 46, 108
harassment of, 38, 98
and patients, conflicts between, 131,
155–156
physical attributes, degradation of,
186–187, 223
prescription errors, 238, 271–272
racism, 191–192, 229
shredding, 130, 153–154
vs. SpR, 322, 349–350

O
Oesophago-gastro-duodenoscopy
(OGD), 16–17, 71, 319, 346
On-call medical registrar, 343
On-call shifts, 309, 361

Out-patient prescription, 332, 362–363
*Oxford Handbook of Clinical
Medicine*, 17, 247

P
Palliative care team, 24–25, 81
Patient consent, 25, 82
blind patient, 178, 213–214
for blood transfusion, 177–178,
212–213
delirium, 254–255, 292
dementia and, 26–27, 83
form, 126
for HIV test, 173, 207–208
for laparoscopic cholecystectomy,
9–10, 62
for medical students, 26, 82
mental health disorder, 262,
300–301
for OGDs, 16–17, 71, 319, 346
questioning consent, 256, 293–294
uninformed consent, 174–175, 209
Patient focus
ABG competence, 247, 283
advanced directives, 251, 288–289
analgesia, 245, 280
antibiotic guidelines, 246–247, 282
blood test
consent for, 250–251, 287
group and save, 240–241, 275
HIV patient, doctor's refusal to
take, 264–265, 304
hyperkalaemia, 241–242,
276–277
breaking bad news, 244–245,
279–280
cancer
disclosure, 259–261, 298, 299
terminal diagnosis, 259, 297
catheterisation
clinical skills, 248, 284
inappropriate room for, 238, 271
chest drain at nighttime, 237, 270–271
child
autonomy, 255, 292–293
parents' consent, 257, 295
protection, non-accidental injury,
239, 249–250, 273, 285–286
coercion, 257–259, 295–297
colonoscopy, capacity, 252, 289–290

consultant decisions, 244, 256, 279, 294

CT scan, request for, 236–237, 269–270

delirium, 254–255, 292

demand, 131, 155

dementia
capacity, 253–254, 291
sleeping tablets, 240, 274–275

depression and capacity, 254, 291–292

discharge summary, 127, 150

disruptive intravenous drug user patient, discharge of, 241, 275–276

drug level monitoring, team's responsible for, 242, 277

drunk colleague, 267, 307

drunken patients, assessment of, 265–266, 305

ectopic pregnancy, 258, 296

end of life care, 236, 264, 269, 303

ensuring follow-up tests, 242–243, 277–278

error, 131–132, 156

face mask, refusal of, 252, 289

family disagreement, 253, 290

faulty equipment, 239, 273

follow-up arrangements, 246, 281–282

GP treatment, 250, 286

imminent cardiac arrest, 237, 270

inappropriate images on laptop, 262, 301

incident reporting, 248–249, 284

infectious diarrhoea, 241, 276

intimate examinations and chaperones, 263–265, 302–304

keeping promises, 266–267, 305–306,

keeping up to date, 247–248, 283

mental health consent, 262, 300–301

MRSA patient, 245–246, 281

negligence
DKA patient, management of, 243–244, 278–279
drug levels monitoring, 243, 278

ordering wrong test, 235, 268

patient handover, 249, 285

prescription errors, nursing staff, 238, 271–272

questioning consent, 256, 293–294

referral, 118, 139

religious issues
abortion, objections to, 239–240, 274
Jehovah's Witness, blood products refusal, 251, 287–288

risk of falls, 252–253, 290

safeguarding, 261, 299

safety, escalating concerns for, 123, 144–145

signing sick note, 235–236, 268

staying late, 238–239, 272

STI testing, 261, 300

telephone conversation with relative, 260, 298

terminal diagnosis, 259, 297

withholding treatment, 255, 293

wrong site surgery, 263, 301–302

Patient safety, 143, 158

Phone interpreters, 130–131, 154

Phony thank you letters, 37, 96

Physiotherapist, 328, 357–358

Pleural drainage, 316, 342

Prescription errors, 45, 107, 238, 271–272

Pressure, coping with
arterial blood gas, failing to do, 126, 148
angry registrar, 136, 162
audit presentation, 118–119, 139
AWOL, 128, 150
challenging senior, 126, 149
chaperones, 132, 156–157
clerking responsibilities, 134, 159
colleague, absence of, 129, 152
community emergency, 134, 159–160
complaint, 135, 161
cope at work, 121–122, 142–143
coroner statement, 135–136, 161
demanding patient, 131, 155
discharge summary, patient control of, 127, 150
educational supervision, 133–134, 158
e-portfolio, 133, 158

EWTD breach, 136–137, 162–163
false statement, 117–118, 138
FY1 on call, 121, 142
forgotten patient review, 117, 138
incorrect consent, 126–127, 149
interpreters, 130–131, 154
jobs, list of, 119–120, 140
mean registrar, 129–130, 153
mistakes, learning from, 124–126,
146–148
not coping, 125, 147
nurse-patient breakdown, 131,
155–156
on call prioritising, 122–123,
143–144
patient error, 131–132, 156
patient referral, 113, 139
patient safety, escalating concerns
for, 123, 144–145
prioritisation, 119, 140
Bullying registrar, 128, 151
rota coordinator, 120–121,
141–142
seeking help, 120, 141
shredding nurse, 130, 153–154
stress and overwork, 122, 143
understaffing, 128–129, 151–152
unsafe on-call, 134–135, 160
unsupervised skills, 124, 146
using guidelines, 123, 145
warfarin, prescription of, 124,
145–146
workload, 141
Prioritisation, 119, 140
Private healthcare, 330, 360–361
Proactive attitude, 78
Professionalism
accidents, offering assistance to,
10, 63
advice to friend, 16, 70
aggressive patient, 43, 104
alcohol consumption
and misdemeanours, 39–40, 100
specialist registrar, 10, 62
angry partner, 10–11, 63–64
audit, 23, 79
breast examination, 37–38, 97
career progression, 21–22, 77
case note security, 32, 90
chest drain removal, 17, 72

child
domestic violence, 31, 89
protection, 43–44, 105
choosing training, 20, 75
coercion end of life, 24–25, 81
coffee house discussion, 31, 89
colleagues
appearance, inappropriate
comments on, 46, 108
embarrassing photos of, 38–39,
98–99
gifts, acceptance of, 7–8,
59–60
illegible signature, 48, 111
missing training courses,
44–45, 106
newspaper cutting of, 36,
95–96
commitments, 49–50, 113
computer files, transfer of, 30, 88
confused patient, pre-theatre,
24, 80
consenting (see Patient consent)
death certificates, 4–5, 11–12, 15,
56–57, 64–65, 69–70
diarrhoea and vomiting, 48–49,
111–112
disclosure after death, 27, 83–84
dishonest form for patient, 12, 65
doctor–patient relationship, 1, 39,
44, 52, 99, 106
documentation
events, 2–3, 54
forgot, 6, 58
dress code, 49, 112–113
driving
and diabetes, 33–34, 92
against medical advice, 29–30, 87
drugs, 9, 27–28, 61, 84
DVLA, 28–29, 85
e-learning certificate plagiarism,
47–48, 110
equipment, unfamiliar with, 23–24,
79–80
facebook, derogatory comments on,
2, 53–54
false audit, 13, 66–67
flu jab, 14, 67
food poisoning, 30–32, 88, 90–91
friends

antibiotic prescription for, 36, 49, 95, 112
with problems, 28, 84–5
test results, 3, 54–55
gifts (*see* Gifts)
Good Samaritan, 15, 69
gynae complaints, 39, 100
handover task forgotten, 5–6, 57–58
hearsay, acting on, 35–36, 94–95
hungover, 46–47, 109
illegal substances, 41, 102
inappropriate drunken stories, 12–13, 65–66
infectious diseases, disclosure of, 29, 86
insurance fraud, 5, 57
interpersonal relationships, 34–35, 93–94
keeping promises, 46, 108–109
lost patient list, 29, 86–87
lying
experience, 4, 56
hangover, 8–9, 61
results, 3–4, 55
media, 34, 93
medical students, 7, 59
mentoring, 18, 73
mistakes, open disclosure of, 8, 60
mortuary, inappropriate comments in, 40–41, 101–102
Mr/Dr, 6–7, 59
near miss event, 16, 70
needlestick injury, 25, 81
NG tube, 23, 78–79
nurse, harassment of, 38, 98
ordering incorrect test, 22, 78
out of practice, 14, 68
patients, discussion about, 32–33, 91
performing new tasks, 21, 76
phony thank you letters, 37, 96
police caution, 1, 52–53
prescribing error, 45, 107
prescribing limits, 19, 74–75
procedure confidence, 18, 73–74
racist comments, 43, 105
raising concerns, 35, 94
sexism, 37, 96–97
sexist consultant, 40, 101
shooting, 14–15, 68–69
smart phone pictures, 41–42, 102–103

surgical error, 20–21, 75–76
teaching
poor quality of, 17–18, 72
time pressures, 19, 74
third party, disclosure to, 33, 92
TOP, 42, 103–104
tourniquet, 22, 77
train late, 47, 109–110
unskilled procedure, 11, 64
working hours, monitoring, 13, 66
Prophylactic antibiotics, 182, 218–219
Punctuality, 329–330, 359

R
Racism, 43, 105, 191–192, 229
Radiologist, 165–166, 197–198, 324–325, 353
Radiology test, request for, 165–166, 197–198
Rape counselling, 34–35
Recreational drugs, 183, 219, 241, 275–276
Referral
to another specialty, 314, 340
cardiology, 170, 203
dentist, 266–267, 306
Refusal
of IV antibiotics, 175, 210, 255, 293
of medication, 175, 179, 209–210, 214
of treatment
children, 192, 229–230
face mask, 252, 289
Registrar
angry, 136, 162
bully, 128, 151
conflicting plans, 188, 224–225
illness, 316, 342–343
leaving patient list, 321, 349
mean registrar, 129, 153
nursing staff, degradation of, 186–187, 223
prescribing against protocol, 310–311, 336
responsibility, 193–194, 231–232
Relatives; *see also* Family
advanced directives, 251, 288–289
cancer disclosure, 259–261, 298, 299
disclosure to, 174, 208–209
discussion with, 180–181, 216–217

inappropriate behaviour with, 189, 226
telephone conversation with, 181,
217–218, 260
Religious issues
abortion, objections to, 42,
103–104, 239–240, 274
Jehovah's Witness, blood products
refusal, 251, 287–288
Responsibility
clerking, 134, 159
for ordering wrong test, 235, 268
registrars, 193–194, 231–232
between teams, drug level
monitoring, 242, 277
Re-training opportunities, 14, 68
Romantic relationships, 106, 357–358
Rota organiser, 334
Royal College of Obstetricians and
Gynaecologists (RCOG)
guidelines, 104

S
Safe handovers, 363–364
Secret pregnancy, 180, 216
Self-discharge, 131, 155, 168, 177,
200, 211
Senior house officer (SHO), 37–38, 97–98
ABG technique, 126, 148
advisor, 92
educational supervision, 133–134, 158
end of life care, 236, 269
gifts, acceptance of, 7–8, 59–60
honesty, 58
illegible signature, medical
notes, 48
inadequate ABG equipment, 312, 337
interpersonal relationships, 34–35,
93–94
Mr/Dr, 6–7, 59
NG tube, 79, 97
nursing staff, degradation of,
186–187, 223
patient error, 131–132, 156
post-take ward round, 134–135, 160
raising concerns, 35, 94
to supervise suturing, 124, 146
Sexism, 37, 96–97
Sexist consultant, 101, 140
Sexual harassment, 140, 326–327,
355–356

Sexually transmitted infections (STIs),
261, 300
Sexual relationships, 93
SHO, see Senior house officer (SHO)
Shooting, 14–15, 68–69
Signing sick note, 235–236, 268
Sleeping tablets, dementia, 240, 274–275
Smoking, 173–174, 208
Social media, 38–39, 53–54, 98–99,
309, 331
Specialist registrar (SpR)
abortion, comments on, 191, 228
advisor, 92
alcohol, 10, 62
competence, 342–343
DNACPR, 324
vs. FY1 colleague, 187, 224
interrupting, 189–190, 227
vs. nurse, 322, 349–350
sterile field, contamination of, 149
uninformed consent, 174–175, 209
Sterile field, 126, 149
STIs, see Sexually transmitted
infections (STIs)
Stress and overwork, 122, 143
Suicidal patient, 169, 202
Surgical error, 20, 75–76
Suturing, 21, 76

T
Teaching
attending sessions, 317, 344
colleague, missing sessions, 44–45, 106
poor quality, 17–18, 72
student, patient's consent for, 26, 82
time pressures, 19, 74
Team work
annual leave, 331–332, 362
anticoagulating patients, 329, 359
appropriate referrals, 317, 343
argument, 326, 354–355
attending teaching sessions, 317, 344
colleague
ABGs, not competent with,
315–316, 341–342
alcohol, 323–324, 351–352
bleeps, not coping with, 320,
347–348
deleting records, 310, 334–335
depressed, 318, 345

dispute, 324, 352
faking illness, 309, 334
handover, not arrived for, 330, 360
incompetence, 326, 355
patients, inappropriate comments on, 322, 350
rude, 325, 353–354
struggling, 327–328, 356–357
supporting, 327, 356
surgeon, 315, 341
tearful, 325–326, 354
competence, 313, 339
consultant
acting unprofessionally, 330, 360–361
advice, 313–314, 339
sexual harassment, 326–327, 355–356
drug level monitoring, responsible for, 242, 277
effective team player, 348
escalate care, failing to, 310, 335
extra on-calls, 309, 334
facebook, derogatory comments, 331, 361–362
feedback, receiving and acting on, 331, 361
FY1 ward round, 319–320, 347
help, beyond limits of skills, 311, 336–337
inadequate equipment, 312, 337–338
leaving on time, 333, 363–364
negligence, 321, 348–349
nurse
conflict, 322–323, 350–351
questions your competence, 314–315, 340–341
vs. SpR, 322, 349–350
OGD consent, 319, 346
physiotherapist date, 328, 357–358
poor discharge summaries, 232, 351
punctuality, 329–330, 359
radiologist, 324–325, 353
referral to another specialty, 314, 340
registrar
illness, 316, 342–343
leaving patient list, 321, 349
prescribing against protocol, 310–311, 336

respecting authority, 328–329, 358
sick patients, 311–313, 337, 338
thorough clinical examination, 318, 344–345
training, 316, 342
treatment options, 319, 346–347
unprofessional behaviour, 332–333, 363
UTI, 332, 362–363
Telephone consultations, 28, 86–85
Telephone conversation, 181, 217–218, 260, 298
Terminal diagnosis, 259, 297
Termination of pregnancy (TOP), 42, 103–104
Time-critical emergency, 336
Tourniquet, 22, 77
Translator, 177, 212

U
Understaffing, 128–129, 151–152
Uninformed consent, 174–175, 209
Unprofessional behaviour, 332–333, 363
Unsafe on-call, 134–135, 160
Unskilled procedure, 11, 64
Unsupervised skills, 124, 146
Upset patient, 190, 227
Urinary tract infection (UTI), 332, 362–363

V
Verbal handover, 272, 338

W
Ward round, 179–180, 215–216
Warfarin, 124, 145–146
Warning shots, 206
Whole body scan request, 168, 200–201
Working hours, monitoring, 13, 66
Workload, 141–142
Workplace issues
explicit posters, response to, 173, 207
inappropriate dress, 192, 230
racism, 191–192, 229
Wrong site surgery, 263, 301–302

X
X-ray reporting, 170, 203–204